Vein Diagnosis and Treatment:

A Comprehensive Approach

Vein Diagnosis and Treatment:
A Comprehensive Approach

Robert A. Weiss, MD
Assistant Professor, Department of Dermatology
The Johns Hopkins University School of Medicine,
Baltimore, Maryland; Director, Maryland Laser,
Skin and Vein Institute, Hunt Valley, Maryland
Past President, American College of Phlebology

Craig Feied, MD, FACEP, FAAEM
Director, National Center for Medical Informatics
Director of Informatics, MedStar Health / EMC Medical
Professor of Emergency Medicine, Georgetown University
President, American College of Phlebology

Margaret A. Weiss, MD
Assistant Professor, Department of Dermatology
The Johns Hopkins University School of Medicine,
Baltimore, Maryland; Director, Maryland Laser,
Skin and Vein Institute, Hunt Valley, Maryland

McGraw-Hill
Medical Publishing Division

New York   St. Louis   San Francisco   Auckland   Bogota   Caracas
Lisbon   London   Madrid   Mexico City   Milan   Montreal
New Delhi   San Juan   Singapore   Sydney   Tokyo   Toronto

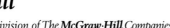

McGraw-Hill

A Division of The McGraw·Hill Companies

ISBN 0-07-069201-7

Library of Congress Cataloging-in-Publication Data

Vein diagnosis and treatment : a comprehensive approach / editors, Robert A. Weiss,
Craig F. Feied, Margaret A. Weiss
       p. ; cm.
    Includes bibliographical references and index.
    ISBN 0–07–069201–7
      1. Varicose veins. 2. Injections, Sclerosing.   I. Weiss, Robert A.   II. Feied, Craig F.
    III. Weiss, Margaret A.
       [DNLM: 1. Varicose Veins—diagnosis. 2. Sclerotherapy—methods. 3. Varicose
    Veins—therapy.   WG 620 V427 2001]
    RC695.V44   2001
    616.1'43—dc21

                                                                        00-032912

The editors were Darlene Barela Cooke, Susan R. Noujaim, and Barbara Holton.
The production supervisor was Phil Galea.
The text designer was Robert Freese.
The cover designer was Janice Bialawa.
The index was prepared by Deborah Tourtlotte.
Quebecor World Printing/Kingsport was printer and binder.

This book is printed on acid-free paper.

Dedication

This textbook is dedicated to our sons, Michael, David and Jonathan, who not only helped with some of the artwork, but who were exceptional in their ability to educate and entertain themselves during the multitude of hours we spent away from them while writing this book.   Thanks and love from Mom and Dad.

Robert & Margaret Weiss

To my wife, Julie, who makes it all worthwhile, and whose illustrations grace several chapters of this textbook.   Thanks and love from your husband.

Craig Feied

Contents

Contributors

The editors would like to acknowledge and express their gratitude to the following for their invaluable contributions to this book.

Andre Cornu-Thenard, MD
Co-Director of Phlebology Training
Cardiology and Surgery Services
St. Antoine Hospital
University Hospital Center
Paris, France

Constantino Costarangos, MD
Assistant Professor of Dermatology
The Johns Hopkins University School of Medicine
Baltimore, Maryland

Jean-Jerome Guex, MD
Secretary, International Union of Phlebology
Private Practice
Nice, France

Robert Hashemiyoon, MD
Medical Director
American Vein Institute
Vienna, Virginia
Director of Phlebology
National Center for Medical Informatics
Washington, DC

Hossein C. Nousari, MD
Assistant Professor of Dermatology
The Johns Hopkins University School of Medicine
Baltimore, Maryland

Albert-Adrien Ramelet, MD
Specialiste FMH en Dermatologie et Angiologie
Lausanne, Switzerland

Foreword

The diagnosis and treatment of venous disease is advancing each year. New developments in treating venous disease with surgical and pharmacological methods are providing patients with more efficient and cost effective care. During the last 15 years nearly one dozen medical textbooks and hundreds of peer reviewed medical articles have been published world-wide. This volume written by friends and colleagues who are all experts in Phlebology adds a great deal of practical and useful information to the field. Even though there already exists several excellent textbooks on venous disease, what differentiates this text from the rest is its practical simplicity. Useful tables and figures abound to assist the novice and improve the expert in giving care to his/her patients.

Special care has been taken to provide up-to-date information on treatment as well as classification of venous anatomy and diagnostic techniques. Although the majority of the text is written in a single style by the authors, they have chosen special colleagues to write specific chapters. One of the leaders in venous surgery, A.A. Ramelet, presents an outstanding chapter on ambulatory phlebectomy for the beginner as well as advanced surgeon. J.J. Guex provides a

practical review of sclerosing solutions presently available to the American physician with an emphasis on sclerosing solutions soon to be approved by our FDA. The chapter on venous ulcers by Andre Conu-Thenard and co-workers is simplistic, well organized and an easily understandable read.

As leaders in the field of Phlebology and former and current Presidents of the American College of Phlebology, Drs. Weiss and Feied along with their contributors are to be congratulated for spending time and effort to bring this text to fruition. Tai Tung in the 13th Century said it best in his *History of Chinese Writing:* "Were I to await perfection, my book would never be finished." The student of phlebology owes thanks to these authors for presenting their work today so that others can continue to "perfect" the art of Phlebological Medicine.

Mitchel P. Goldman, MD
Associate Clinical Professor,
Dermatology Division,
UCSD School of Medicine

Preface

We have found it very sad that venous disease has been relegated to the bottom of importance in American medicine. Time and time again we observe patients who have been told to live with their disease or even worse have been treated in far less than optimal medical and cosmetic fashion. Knowing that very little was taught about venous disease when we attended medical school in the 1970s, our motivation for this text has been to share the knowledge we have gained in treating over 14,000 patients over the last 16 years. The foundation of this knowledge began with the European phlebologists who have advanced the field to a science with detailed studies of physiology and treatment.

Until Mitchel P. Goldman published his textbook of sclerotherapy in the early 1990s there was no comprehensive American resource to help our understanding, not only of the importance of venous disease but the science and art behind the treatment. His textbook advanced the cause of phlebology and allowed great strides in physician comprehension of venous disease. His textbook still remains as the greatest resource integrating all the world's literature into a single English language volume. In contrast, our text has been written as a practical supplement to those wishing to practice phlebology in all of its many methods of treatment. Millions of adults experience the pain and the other manifestations of venous disease including edema, cellulitis and ulceration, yet because of the lack of practical knowledge in American medicine, these patients are not offered logical or comprehensive, multidisciplinary care.

We hope that this text will serve as a practical and frequently referenced guide to those physicians who wish to expand upon the very basic knowledge obtained in medical school, but we also secretly hope that this text will serve as a wake-up call to the minds assembling current medical school curriculum. Phlebology must absolutely be taught in medical school. When up to 40% of the population experiences some form of venous disease and when these patients experience pain in up to 50% of cases, physicians should be knowledgeable in diagnosis and treatment. This includes the use of compression as a treatment to reduce the signs and symptoms of venous disease and to help treat venous ulcers.

Fortunately due to educational organizations such as the American College of Phlebology (formerly the North American Society of Phlebology founded in 1986), educational symposia are readily accessible to interested physicians. For dermatologists and other interested physicians, the American Society for Dermatologic Surgery offers many opportunities to learn phlebology including a practical hands-on workshop in sclerotherapy, ambulatory phlebectomy, lasers and radio-frequency occlusion. To supplement these experiences, this textbook incorporates the results of years of patient treatment and study. We sincerely hope that reading this book will help to catapult your understanding and ability to deal with venous disease to the level of our European colleagues.

Robert A. Weiss
Margaret A. Weiss
Craig C. Feied

Linked website

More information including the companion CD-ROM demonstrating many of the procedures described in this textbook can be obtained at:

http://www.veintext.com

Other materials such as a patient education video on vein techniques are also available through this site.

Meetings and training courses are also listed at this site.

Acknowledgments

No listing of acknowledgments can ever be complete. During the writing of a textbook many different influences come together to shape the opinions expressed, and we collectively thank each and every one of the phenomenal individuals who helped us along the way.

Phlebology is a young specialty in America, and without the patient teaching of our European colleagues, the experience that allows us to create this textbook would never have occurred. We are indebted to French phlebologists in general and to Dr. Frederic Vin and Dr. Andre Cornu-Thenard in particular, whose willingness to allow us to observe their expert practice helped us immensely. Dr. Michel Schadeck taught us many aspects of Duplex diagnosis and treatment. Dr. Jean-Jerome Guex has been a source of constant friendship and valuable clinical information. The encouragement of these physicians will always be appreciated and never be forgotten.

We are also indebted to the Swiss phlebologists and in particular to dermatologic surgeon Dr. Albert-Adrien Ramelet whose ability to critically assess and solve the most complex medical and surgical problems has benefited not only us but thousands of patients. His contributions to ambulatory phlebectomy (along with those of Dr. Muller) allow phlebologists worldwide to claim this technique as their own.

The German phlebologic community also contributed to our knowledge and experience. Our observation of Dr. Ulrich Shultz-Ehrenburg in Bochum and Berlin and his workshops at the American College of Phlebology gave us a solid foundation in Doppler diagnosis. Similarly, our understanding of the science of compression and the importance of the often-neglected lateral venous system are due to the teaching efforts of Austrian dermatologic surgeon Dr. Hugo Partsch, President of the International Union of Phlebology. We have learned much through the brilliance of Dr. Gerhard Sattler and his associate Boris Sommer, and also from Dr. Alina Fratila, presently doing very exciting work in the field of intravascular laser therapeutics.

In the Netherlands, Dr. HAM Neumann has been an inspiration and a wonderful teacher not only in phlebology, but in the grace and joy of life in general. The Italian phlebologists, Drs. Allegra, Corcos, Frullini, and Georgiev have taught us much as well. Dr. Shunichi Hoshino of Japan and others in the Asian phlebologic community have also contributed greatly to our knowledge and understanding.

Our American colleagues have also been instrumental in our learning. Without the inspiration and teaching of Dr. David Duffy, none of the subsequent interactions with our European colleagues would have occurred at all. We are greatful for the guidance and encouragement of our dear friend Dr. Walter DeGroot, whose unwavering confidence helped us to advance our understanding of the venous system. Dr. John Bergan, perhaps the most eloquent and knowledgeable vascular surgeon in venous disease of this century, has been wonderfully supportive of phlebology as a specialty, and his personal guidance to us has been invaluable through the last decade. We thank Dr. Helane Fronek for always keeping things in perspective with her level-headed focus on the patient, Dr. Neil Sadick for his assistance and his superb ability to design scientific studies, and Dr. Pauline Raymond-Martimbeau for her detailed scientific work and her tireless efforts to expose American phlebologists to international viewpoints in phlebology.

Our greatest collective personal debt, however, is to Dr. Mitchel P. Goldman, whose personal friendship and guidance is the primary driving force behind this textbook. His influence has shaped our careers as it has shaped the careers of so many American phlebologists. If not for Dr. Goldman we would not be doing what we are doing, and certainly would never have produced this textbook.

We are profoundly grateful to our families and especially to our parents, who always provided encouragement and support, making it possible for us to pursue our dreams and never to be discouraged by temporary setbacks.

The Authors

Background

The Spectrum of Venous Disease

From the mild burning pain of hormonally mediated telangiectasias to the hemodynamic collapse of thromboembolism, diseases of the peripheral venous system are common today. Clinicians are faced with a spectrum of venous disease that appears in various manifestations in patients of all ages. Although venous disease in its mildest forms is merely uncomfortable, annoying, or cosmetically disfiguring, severe venous disease can produce severe systemic consequences.

The visual appearance of the lower extremities is a useful, but not always reliable, guide to the peripheral venous condition. Swelling, for example, may result from acute venous obstruction or from deep or superficial venous reflux, or it may be completely unrelated to the venous system. Hepatic insufficiency, renal failure, cardiac decompensation, infection, trauma, and environmental effects can all produce lower extremity edema that may be indistinguishable from the edema of venous obstruction or venous insufficiency.

The most common form of venous disease is venous insufficiency caused by valve incompetence in the deep or superficial veins. Deep venous insufficiency occurs when valves are damaged by deep vein thrombosis. Superficial venous insufficiency occurs when a high-pressure leakage develops between the deep and superficial systems or within the superficial system, followed by sequential failure of the venous valves in superficial veins. Venous insufficiency syndromes allow venous blood to escape its normal flow path and flow in a retrograde direction down into an already congested leg. Over time, incompetent superficial veins acquire the typical dilated and tortuous appearance of varicosities.

The presence and size of visible varicosities is not a reliable indicator of the volume or pressure of venous reflux, because a vein that is confined within fascial planes or that is buried beneath subcutaneous tissue can carry massive amounts of high-pressure reflux without being visible at all. Conversely, even a small increase in pressure can eventually produce massive dilatation of an otherwise normal superficial vein that carries very little flow.

Table 1-1
Prevalence of Varicosities by Age and Sex

Age	Female	Male
20–29	8%	1%
40–49	41%	24%
60–69	72%	43%

Data from the Tecumseh Health Study[2]

Epidemiology

The prevalence of venous disease seems to be higher in westernized and industrialized countries.[1] Incidence and prevalence also depend on the age and sex of the population. In the Tecumseh community health study,[2] for example, varicosities were observed in 72% of women aged 60–69, but in only 1% of men aged 20–29 (Table 1-1). As the baby boom generation ages, the incidence of venous disease per capita is expected to rise dramatically.[2A] Incidence in Japanese women is 45%.

Small reticular varicosities occur early in life, with only a small number of new cases developing after the childbearing years. Truncal varicosities and telangiectatic webs, on the other hand, are relatively less common in youth, and continue to appear throughout life.

Serial examinations of approximately 500 children at ages 10–12 and again four and eight years later, at ages 14–16 and 18–20, showed that symptoms are experienced (and venous tests are abnormal) before any abnormal veins are visible at the surface of the skin. Abnormal reticular veins appear first, followed several years later by incompetent perforators and truncal varicosities (Table 1-2).[3,4]

Etiology of Varicose Veins and Spider Veins

Multiple factors contribute to the development of varicose veins. Intrinsic pathological conditions combine with extrinsic environmental factors to produce a wide spectrum of

Table 1-2
Development of Varicose and Telangiectatic Leg Veins by Age

Abnormality	Age 10–12	Age 14–16	Age 18–20
Telangiectasia	0	3.7%	12.9%
Reticular	10.2%	30.3%	35.3%
Perforator	0	4.1%	5.2%
Varicose tributary	0	0.8%	5.0%
Varicose truncal vein	0	1.7%	3.3%
Saphenofemoral reflux	0	12.3%	19.8%

Data from Bochum Study I-III[10,11]

disease. Dialysis shunts and spontaneous arteriovenous malformations give ample evidence that normal veins will dilate and become tortuous in response to continued high pressure, but some people seem to have an inborn weakness of vein walls that leads to venous dilatation even in the absence of elevated venous pressures. For example, patients with varicose veins of the legs have been found to have abnormally distensible veins in the forearms and hands.[5,6]

HEREDITY

Although the specific genetic risk factors for varicosities are not known, heredity does play an important role, and seems to be particularly important in determining susceptibility to primary valvular failure. Reflux at the saphenofemoral junction is twice as likely when a parent had a similar condition.[7] Monozygotic twins are concordant with regard to varicose veins in 75% of cases. The prevalence of varicose veins in relatives of patients with varicose veins is 43% for females, but only 19% for males.[8]

ENVIRONMENTAL RISK FACTORS

Occupations that require prolonged standing can lead to chronic venous distention and secondary valvular incompetence at any level. If proximal junctional valves become incompetent, the condition rapidly progresses to become irreversible. Women seem to be more susceptible to this problem, most likely because vein walls and valves periodically become more distensible under the influence of cyclic increases in progesterone.[9]

Pregnancy is an important risk factor that causes varicosities through several mechanisms. Most important are circulating hormonal factors that increase the distensibility of vein walls and soften valve leaflets.[10] Another factor is the tremendous increase in venous capacity that develops to accommodate a greatly expanded circulating blood volume. Late in pregnancy, the enlarged uterus compresses the inferior vena cava, causing venous hypertension with secondary distension in the legs.[11] Depending on the relative contributions of these mechanisms, varicose veins of pregnancy may spontaneously regress after delivery. Treatment of varicose veins prior to pregnancy helps prevent progression during pregnancy.[12]

Age is an independent risk factor for varicosities because with advancing age the elastic lamina of the vein becomes atrophic and the smooth muscle layer begins to degenerate, leaving a weakened vein that is more susceptible to dilatation.[13,14]

Sequelae of Venous Insufficiency

Most patients with venous insufficiency have subjective symptoms of pain, soreness, burning, aching, throbbing, cramping, muscle fatigue, and restless legs. Over time, chronic venous insufficiency leads to cutaneous and soft-tissue breakdown that can be extremely debilitating.

Table 1-3
Stages of Chronic Venous Insufficiency

Edema
Hyperpigmentation
Venous stasis dermatitis
Chronic cellulitis
Cutaneous infarction (atrophie blanche)
Lipodermatosclerosis
Ulceration
Malignant degeneration

SUBJECTIVE SYMPTOMS

Subjective symptoms are typically more severe early in the progression of disease, less severe in the middle phases, and worse again with advancing age. Varicose vein symptoms do not correlate well with the size or extent of visible varices, nor with the absolute volume of reflux. Not all symptomatic patients will complain of pain; venous symptoms may be so insidious that, after treatment, patients are surprised to realize how much chronic discomfort they had accepted as "normal."[15]

Common symptoms of telangiectasia include burning, swelling, throbbing, cramping, and leg fatigue.[16] Pain associated with larger varicose veins is usually described as a dull ache that worsens after prolonged standing.[17,18] In contrast to the pain of arterial insufficiency or of venous obstruction, pain caused by venous insufficiency often is improved by walking or elevating the legs. Warmth tends to aggravate the symptoms, and cold tends to relieve them.

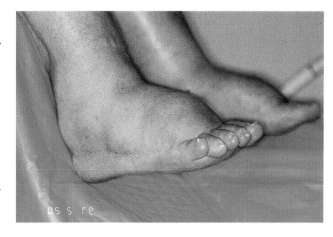

Figure 1-2. Pitting edema, the first sign of venous insufficiency with early mild stasis dermatitis.

Compression stockings may ameliorate or prevent the pain of venous insufficiency.

Pain and other symptoms may worsen with the menstrual cycle, with pregnancy, and in response to exogenous hormonal therapy, including oral contraceptives. A small number of women regularly experience pain associated with their varicose veins after sexual intercourse.[19]

OBJECTIVE SIGNS

Over time, most people with chronic venous insufficiency develop some degree of "venous stasis," chronic skin and soft-tissue changes that often begin with mild swelling and progress to include discoloration, inflammatory dermatitis, recurrent or chronic cellulitis, cutaneous infarction, ulceration, and even malignant degeneration. Chronic non-healing leg ulcers, bleeding from varicose veins, and phlebitis are serious problems that are caused by venous insufficiency, which can be relieved if the problem is corrected (*Table 1-3*). Figures 1-1 through 1-4 highlight the clinical stages of chronic venous insufficiency.

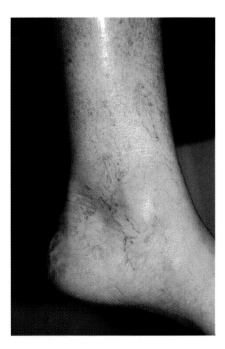

Figure 1-1. Early changes of hydrostatic pressure with violaceous telangiectasias on the medial ankle.

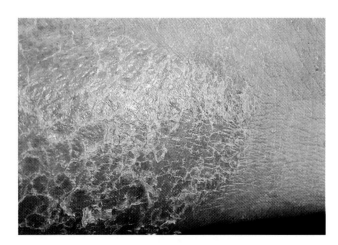

Figure 1-3. Stasis dermatitis of the medial ankle.

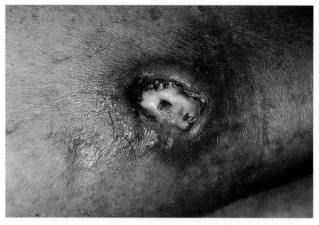

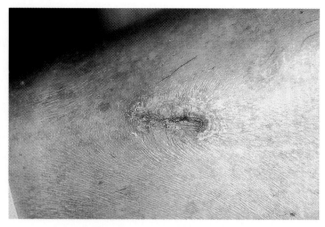

A   **B**

Figure 1-4.   **(A)** Venous ulceration. Note the erythematous border and moist ulcer surface. This is in contrast to the typical dry arterial ulcer. Without external compression these ulcers can weep continuously. **(B)** After compression therapy for 3 months there is marked improvement with reduced erythema, edema, and decreased ulcer size.

Goal of Treatment

The primary goal of treatment of a varicose vein is the improvement of venous outflow by eliminating recirculating loops of reflux, in order to increase the proportion of venous blood that returns to the central circulation. In the absence of deep-system obstruction, superficial varicosities are simply the undesirable result of high-pressure flow into a normally low-pressure system. Varicosities carrying retrograde flow are hemodynamically harmful because they cause recirculation of oxygen-poor, lactate-laden venous blood back into an already congested extremity. Ablation of these varicosities is desirable and will improve the overall circulation. When explaining this to patients, it is helpful to relate the analogy of a working fuel system (the legs are getting fuel through the arteries) with a leaky exhaust system (the leaking veins).

Summary

Venous disease is extremely common and increases with age, being present in more than half of the population by age 65. The most common type is venous insufficiency, the most visible manifestations of which are varicose veins and telangiectasias, with other cutaneous and soft-tissue abnormalities developing over time. Most patients with venous insufficiency have subjective symptoms that may range from very mild to very severe. Treatment aims to correct the underlying defect, removing or closing down points of reflux that can prevent venous blood from returning to the central circulation.

References

(1) Alexander CJ. *The epidemiology of varicose veins.* Med J Aust 1972; 1:215–218.

(2) Coon WW, Willis PW, Keller JB. *Venous thromboembolism and other venous disease in the Tecumseh community health study.* Circulation 1973; 48:839–846.

(2A) Hirai M, Naiki K, Nakayama R. *Prevalence & risk factors of varicose veins in Japanese women.* Angiology 1990; 41:228–232.

(3) Schultz-Ehrenburg U, Weindorf N, Matthes U, Hirche H. *New epidemiological findings with regard to initial stages of varicose veins (Bochum study I-III).* In: Raymond-Martimbeau P, Prescott R, Zummo M, editors. Phlebologie '92. Paris: John Libbey Eurotext, 1992: 234–236.

(4) Schultz-Ehrenburg U, Weindorf N, von Uslar D, Hirche H. *Prospektive epidemiologische studie uber die entstehunsweise der krampfadern bei kindern und jugendlichen (Bochumer Studie I und II).* Phlebol Proktol 1989; 18:10–25.

(5) Zsoter T, Cronin RFP. *Venous distensibility in patients with varicose veins.* Can Med Assoc J 1966; 94:1293–1297.

(6) Eiriksson E, Dahn I. *Plethysmographic studies of venous distensibility in patients with varicose veins.* Acta Chir Scand [suppl] 1968; 398:19–26.

(7) Reagan B, Folse R. *Lower limb venous dynamics in normal persons and children of patients with varicose veins.* Surg Gynecol Obstet 1971; 132:15–18.

(8) Gundersen J, Hauge M. *Hereditary factors in venous insufficiency.* Angiology 1969; 20:346–355.

(9) McCausland AM, Holmes F, Trotter AD. *Venous distensibility during the menstrual cycle.* Am J Obstet Gynecol 1963; 86:640–645.

(10) Barwin BN, Roddie IC. *Venous distensibility during pregnancy determined by graded venous congestion.* Am J Obstet Gynecol 1976; 125:921–923.

(11) Kerr MG, Scott D.B., Samuel E. *Studies of the inferior vena cava in late pregnancy.* Br Med J 1964; 1:532–533.

(12) van der Stricht J, van Oppens C. [*Should varices be treated before or after pregnancy?*] Phlebol 1991; 44:321–326.

(13) Bouissou H, Julian M, Pieraggi M, Louge L. *Vein morphology.* Phlebol 1988; 3(suppl 1):1–8.

(14) Widmer LK. *Peripheral venous disorders: prevalence and socio-medical importance observations in 4529 apparently healthy persons. Basle Study III.* Bern: Hans Huber, 1978.

(15) Dinn E, Henry M. *Value of lightweight elastic tights in standing occupations.* Phlebol 1989; 4:45–47.

(16) Weiss RA, Weiss MA. *Resolution of pain associated with varicose and telangiectatic leg veins after compression sclerotherapy.* J Dermatol Surg Onc 1990; 16:333–336.

(17) McPheeters HO. *The value of estrogen therapy in the treatment of varicose veins complicating pregnancy.* Lancet 1949; 69:2–4.

(18) Fegan WG, Lambe R, Henry M. *Steroid hormones and varicose veins.* Lancet 1967; 1:1070–1071.

(19) Fegan WG. *Varicose veins: Compression sclerotherapy.* London: William Heinemann, 1967.

Venous Anatomy

This text conforms to an international standard nomenclature known as the Venous Consensus Conference Classification. [1] In keeping with this nomenclature, the term "greater saphenous vein" (GSV) will be used for the vessel sometimes referred to as the "long saphenous vein." The term "lesser saphenous vein" (LSV) will be used for the vessel sometimes referred to as the "short saphenous vein." Veins that penetrate the fascia and connect the deep and superficial systems are termed perforator veins. Veins that connect to other veins within the same fascial plane are referred to as communicating veins. The principal deep vein of the thigh should be referred to as the "femoral vein," never as the "superficial femoral vein." It is not a superficial vein, and confusion on this point has led to death or disability for many patients with deep vein thrombosis (*Table 2-1*).

Anatomy Overview

The peripheral venous system functions both as a reservoir to hold extra blood and as a conduit to return blood from the periphery to the heart and lungs. Unlike arteries, which always possess three well-defined layers (a thin intima, a well-developed muscular media, and a fibrous adventitia), the smallest veins are composed of a single tissue layer. Only the largest veins possess internal elastic membranes, and at best this layer is thin and unevenly distributed, providing little buttress against high internal pressures. The correct functioning of the venous system depends upon a complex series of valves and pumps that are individually frail and prone to malfunction, yet the system as a whole performs remarkably well under extremely adverse conditions.

Table 2-1
Outline of Major Standard Nomenclature of Venous Anatomy of the Leg with Abbreviations

Superficial Venous System
 Greater saphenous vein (previous or European long saphenous)—GSV
 Lesser saphenous vein (previous or European short saphenous)—LSV
 Lateral (subdermic) venous system—LSVS
Deep Venous System
 Deep veins of the thigh
  Common femoral vein—CFV
   Femoral vein (*not Superficial femoral vein*)—FV
   Profunda ("deep") Femoral vein—DFV
  Popliteal vein—PV
 Deep veins of the calf
  Posterior tibial vein—PTV
  Anterior tibial vein—ATV
  Peroneal vein
  Gastrocnemius veins—GV
Major perforating veins and location
 Hunterian—mid-upper medial thigh
 Dodd—above medial knee
 Boyd—below medial knee
 Cockett—above ankle
 Giacomini—posterior connection between GSV and LSV

Primary collecting veins of the lower extremity are passive thin-walled reservoirs that are tremendously distensible. Most are suprafascial, surrounded by loosely bound alveolar and fatty tissue that is easily displaced. These suprafascial collecting veins can dilate to accommodate large volumes of blood with little increase in back-pressure, so that the volume of blood sequestered within the venous system at any moment can vary by a factor of two or more without interfering with the normal function of the veins. Suprafascial collecting veins belong to the superficial venous system. Outflow from collecting veins is via secondary or conduit veins that have thicker walls and are less distensible. Most of these veins are subfascial, and are surrounded by tissues that are dense and tightly bound. These subfascial veins belong to the deep venous system.

Fascial Envelope

The lower limb has both a deep and a superficial fascia to contain the high-pressure calf muscle pump and support the deep venous system. The deep fascia is a dense fibrous membrane surrounding the entire lower limb like an elastic stocking, and serving as a functional boundary between deep and superficial veins. Attached to the superficial fibers of the muscles it covers, the deep fascia is normally thin over the gastrocnemius muscles and is absent only over the perforating veins and fossa ovalis, the latter being protected by the cribriform fascia. Since the deep fascia surrounds the muscles of the limb and is relatively inextensible, contraction of the muscles causes a rise in pressure to all structures within its compartment.

The superficial fascia is composed of two layers: a superficial layer of loculated fatty tissue (Camper's fascia) and

a deep layer of collagen and elastic tissue providing stronger support (Scarpa's fascia). It is homologous with Scarpa's fascia of the anterior abdominal wall and may be considered to be single unit.[2] The superficial fascia in four-legged animals is said to provide a firmer support than that found in bipeds, which may partly explain why varicose veins affect humans but not quadrupeds.

The superficial fascia covers and supports the saphenous trunks (*Figure 2-1*), but tributaries to the saphenous veins are superficial to this fascia. Since they are not within

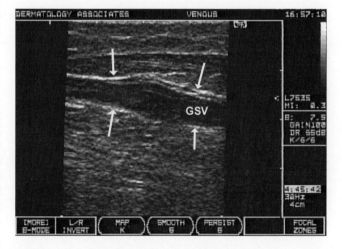

Figure 2-1. Superficial fascia covers the saphenous trunk of the greater saphenous vein (GSV) seen in this longitudinal view under duplex ultrasound. A valve is present in the central dilatation; arrows indicate the fascia.

its support, tributaries to the great saphenous vein are usually more grossly dilated than the GSV trunk itself, even in the presence of proximal high venous pressure.[3]

Although the preceding description seems simple, connections between the superficial and deep venous systems and their fascial coverings are actually very complicated. Detailed anatomic studies by Raivio[4] show an extreme variability in the connections between deep and superficial systems.

The Deep Venous System

No matter what pathway is taken, all venous blood eventually is received by the deep venous system on its way back to the right atrium of the heart. In most cases, there are five major named branches to the deep venous system of the lower extremity: three below the knee and two above the knee. The principal deep venous trunk of the leg is termed the popliteal vein (PV) from below the knee until it passes upward and anteriorly through the adductor canal in the distal thigh, becoming the femoral vein (FV) for the remainder of its course in the thigh.

DEEP VEINS OF THE CALF

In the lower leg there are three groups of deep veins: the anterior tibial vein (ATV), draining the dorsum of the foot; the posterior tibial veins (PTV) *(Figure 2-2)*, draining the sole of the foot; and the peroneal vein, draining the lateral aspect of the foot. From the ankle, the ATV passes upward anterolaterally to the interosseous membrane, the PTV pass upward posteromedially beneath the medial edge of the tibia, and the peroneal vein passes upward posteriorly through the calf. Venous sinusoids within the calf muscle coalesce to form soleal and gastrocnemius intramuscular venous plexi, which usually join the peroneal vein at mid-calf. In most patients each one of these is actually a pair of veins flanking an

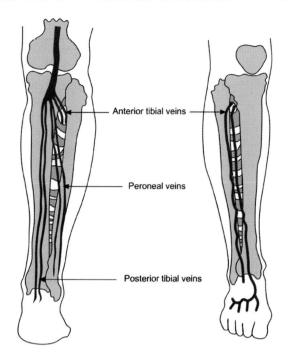

Figure 2-3. Deep veins of the calf, anterior and posterior views.

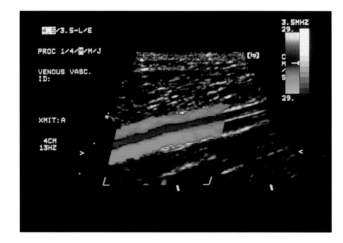

Figure 2-2. Posterior tibial veins. Duplex image of posterior tibial veins (blue) between which the posterior tibial artery lies. Abnormalities in flow can be easily discerned by this method. (Digital image from Sonos 1000, Agilent Technologies, formerly Hewlett Packard)

artery of the same name; thus there are actually six named deep veins below the knee in a typical patient *(Figure 2-3, Figure 2-4)*. Just below the knee, the anterior and posterior tibial veins join the peroneal veins at the popliteal trifurcation to become the single large popliteal vein.

DEEP VEINS OF THE THIGH

From the trifurcation, the popliteal vein courses proximally behind the knee and then passes anteromedially in the distal thigh into the adductor canal. This canal carries the femoral vein and artery from a posterior position at the knee to an anterior position just below the femoral triangle at the groin. The adductor canal is also known as the sartorial canal and (especially at its upper extent) may be referred to as the canal of Hunter.

As the PV passes above the knee, it becomes the FV, the largest and longest deep vein of the lower extremity, and sometimes incorrectly referred to as the superficial femoral vein in an attempt to distinguish it from the profunda femora, or deep femoral vein (DFV). The DFV is a short, stubby vein that usually has its origin in terminal muscle tributaries within the deep muscles of the lateral thigh, but may communicate with the PV in up to 10% of patients. In the proximal thigh the FV and the DFV join to form the common femoral vein (CFV), which passes upwards above the groin crease to become the iliac vein *(Figure 2-5)*.

Again, it cannot be overemphasized that the misleading and incorrect term superficial femoral vein should not be used, as the FV is a deep vein, not part of the superficial venous system. The incorrect term does not appear in any definitive anatomic atlas, yet has come into common use in vascular laboratory and radiology practice.[5] Because inexperienced clinicians often have the impression that throm-

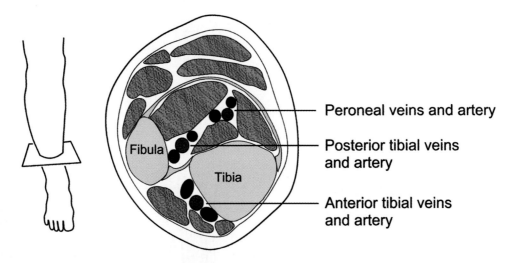

Figure 2-4.   Deep veins of the calf seen in cross-section.

bus in the "superficial femoral vein" is a superficial rather than deep vein thrombosis, they may view such thrombus as less of a threat to the patient than it actually is. Confusion arising from use of the inappropriate name thus continues to be responsible for many cases of clinical mismanagement, and even death.

Superficial Venous System

The superficial system *(Figure 2-6)* includes three major divisions: the greater saphenous, the lesser saphenous, and the lateral venous system (also known as the lateral subdermic

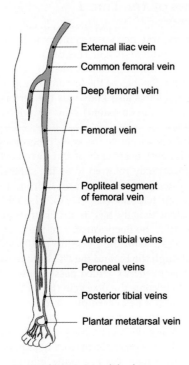

Figure 2-5.   Major deep veins of the leg.

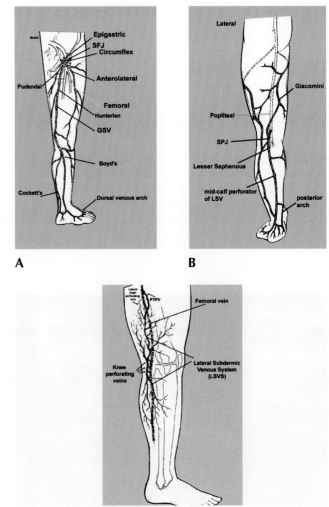

Figure 2-6.   The three major divisions of the superficial venous system: **(A)** the greater saphenous system; **(B)** the lesser saphenous system; **(C)** the lateral venous system.

venous system, the LSVS). Each of these divisions contains multiple collateral veins (accessory, anastamotic, tributary or communicating veins) and multiple points of connection that normally carry flow from the superficial to the deep system (perforating veins). Every point of connection between the superficial and the deep system is a potential point of leakage that can give rise to retrograde flow. Even tiny, unnamed veins without important connections can become dilated and tortuous when exposed to elevated venous pressures, and it is useless to pursue the identification of all but the major points of reflux. Despite the multiple variations, the vast majority of superficial vessels do belong to one of these three major divisions. The largest of these divisions is the greater saphenous system *(Figure 2-7)*.

GREATER SAPHENOUS VEIN

The greater saphenous vein (GSV) originates on the medial foot as part of the venous arch and receives tributaries from deep veins of the foot as it courses upward along the anterior aspect of the medial malleolus. Below the malleolus some of the perforating vein valves are oriented to permit flow outward (from deep to superficial), but above the malleolus all valves permit flow only inward. From the ankle, the greater saphenous vein continues along the anteromedial aspect of the calf to the knee and into the thigh, where it is found more medially. From the upper calf to the groin the GSV usually is contained within an envelope of thin fascia, and visualization of this fascial envelope is an important way to identify the greater saphenous vein on a

duplex ultrasound scan. This fascial envelope often prevents the greater saphenous vein from becoming significantly dilated, even when large volumes of reflux pass along its entire length. A normal GSV typically is 3–4 mm in diameter in the mid-thigh.

Along its course, a variable number of perforating veins may connect the GSV to the deep system at the femoral, posterior tibial, gastrocnemius, and soleal veins. Between the ankle and the knee lie Cockett's perforators, a group of perforating veins that connect the subfascial deep system with the posterior arch vein. The posterior arch vein is a tributary of the GSV that begins at the lower ankle and terminates into the GSV below the knee. Besides perforating veins, the GSV has numerous superficial tributaries as it passes through the thigh. The most important of these are the posteromedial and anterolateral thigh veins at mid-thigh, and the anterior and posterior accessory saphenous veins at the level of Hunter's canal in the upper thigh, where a fairly constant perforating vein also connects the GSV to the FV. Just below the saphenofemoral junction, the GSV receives several additional important tributary veins, including the lateral and medial femoral cutaneous branches, the external circumflex iliac vein, the superficial epigastric vein, and the internal pudendal vein *(Figure 2-7)*. These tributaries are frequently identified as the origin points of reflux, which lead to the appearance of surface varicose veins on the lower thigh or upper calf.

The termination point of the GSV into the common femoral vein is called the saphenofemoral junction (SFJ) in

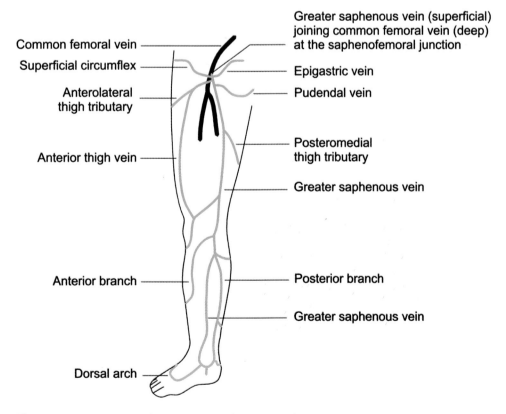

Figure 2–7. Greater saphenous vein and its major tributaries.

the English literature, but is known as the *crosse* (shepherd's crook) in the French medical literature. The terminal valve of the GSV is located within the junction itself and, in most cases, there are one or two additional "subterminal" valves within the first few centimeters of the GSV *(Figure 2-8)*. Most commonly there is a single subterminal valve that can be readily identified approximately 1 cm distal to the junctional valve.

Reflux at or near the SFJ does not always come through the terminal valve of the GSV, nor does it always involve the entire trunk of the GSV. Reflux can enter the GSV below the junction, passing through a failed subterminal valve to mimic true SFJ incompetence. Reflux can also pass directly into any of the other veins that join the GSV at that level, or may pass a few centimeters along the GSV before abandoning it for another branch vessel. It may therefore be difficult to locate the origin and primary pathway of reflux in the thigh without the use of duplex ultrasound.

Varicosities of the greater and lesser saphenous systems are referred to as axial or truncal varicosities. When these vessels carry retrograde flow, the highest reflux point is most often found at the saphenofemoral junction or the saphenopopliteal junction. These veins also possess many perforating and communicating vessels, any one of which can be the primary site of pathology. When a perforating vein is the primary site of reflux, dilatation of the vessel proceeds *both proximally and distally*. When dilatation reaches the most proximal portion of the vein, the saphenofemoral or saphenopopliteal junction is often recruited as a secondary point of reflux.

Although most large varices are tributaries of incompetent truncal vessels, failed perforating veins or connecting veins can give rise to independent varices in the greater saphenous distribution even when the saphenous system is completely normal. This can occur even when the greater saphenous vein has been surgically removed.

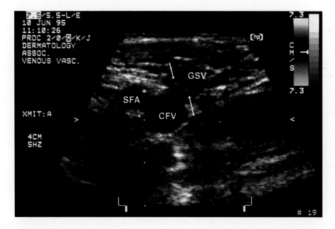

Figure 2-8. Valves at the saphenofemoral junction: CFV, common femoral vein; GSV, greater saphenous vein; SFA, superficial femoral artery (which looks like it is connected to CFV in this "Mickey Mouse" view, but it is not). Arrows indicate the terminal valve leaflets. The red circle is the deep femoral artery.

LESSER SAPHENOUS VEIN

The posterior and lateral leg below the knee is the territorial distribution of the lesser saphenous vein (LSV), which begins at the lateral aspect of the foot as a continuation of the dorsal venous arch, and passes posteriorly to the lateral malleolus. In the upper calf it ascends between two superficial fascial layers and between the gastrocnemius heads to the popliteal fossa, where under normal conditions it usually measures no more than 3 mm in diameter. Gross incompetence of the LSV usually occurs only in areas where the LSV and its tributaries are superficial to the fascia: on the lateral calf and lower third of the leg behind the lateral malleolus. As in other areas, reflux through failed perforating veins may cause tributaries to be varicose without involvement of the LSV itself.

The termination of the LSV is highly variable *(Figure 2-9)*. The most common pattern is termination in the popliteal vein at the level of, or slightly above, the popliteal fossa, but many other variations are possible. In many patients, the LSV has no upper junction at all, instead branching into multiple small deeper veins that communicate with the femoral system in the deep mid-thigh. In some patients, the LSV terminates into an oblique epifascial-communicating vein (the vein of Giacomini) that empties directly into the GSV. In other cases there may be multiple oblique veins connecting the GSV and LSV. In mid-calf a fairly constant large perforator often connects the LSV with the deep system. Multiple other perforators communicate with the deep system throughout the calf. [6]

Other superficial veins can appear within the territorial distribution of the LSV. Most important of these are the lateral and medial gastrocnemial veins, which terminate in the popliteal vein at the popliteal fossa. On ultrasound examination, these gastrocnemial veins may be confused with the LSV in a longitudinal view, but are seen as dumbbell shaped in a transverse view *(Figure 2-10)*. This dumbbell appearance is due to a small artery sandwiched between two paired and larger veins.

LATERAL SUBDERMIC VENOUS SYSTEM

Besides the greater and lesser saphenous systems, there is one other fairly constant named network of vessels that forms a distinct system: the lateral subdermic venous system (LSVS).[7,8,9] The lateral venous system is a system of small caliber veins located along the lateral aspect of the leg and extending both above and below the knee *(Figure 2-6C)*. Normal venous flow in this superficial system is, paradoxically, downward from collecting veins in the proximal thigh toward lateral thigh perforators and perforators at the knee.

The lateral venous system is an unrecognized, but important, reflux conduit in the majority of young women whose visible venous disease consists only of isolated superficial telangiectatic webs of the thigh. Varicose LSVS veins are associated with prominent telangiectasias and venulectasias along the lateral to posterior thigh, often with symptoms of burning and local sensitivity *(Figure 2-11)*. It has been postulated that varicosities of this lateral subdermic venous system often result from a defect of embryological development. Embryonic superficial veins and their

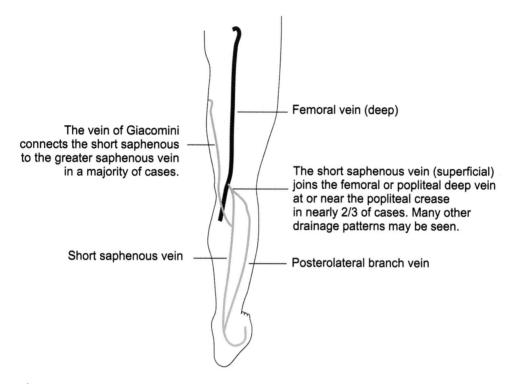

Figure 2-9. Lesser (short) saphenous vein and its major tributaries.

connections to the deep venous system at the thigh and knee fail to involute as they should.[7] They thus persist as a source of high pressure from the moment of birth. This would explain why LSVS varicosities develop at a relatively young age, often appearing in women at puberty or after pregnancy, and why (unlike other varicosities) the incidence of these lateral reticular varicosities in adults does not increase with increasing age.[10]

Although reflux at lateral and posterior perforators near the knee accounts for approximately 85% of LSVS varicosities, there are multiple other reflux pathways into this system. Patients may have reflux from superficial gluteal veins that appear proximally on the posterior thigh and often follow a zigzag path across the posterior thigh. Transfascial perforators may fail in the upper half of the lateral thigh. Reflux may begin along the medial aspect of the knee and be transmitted to the lateral leg through a peripatellar network

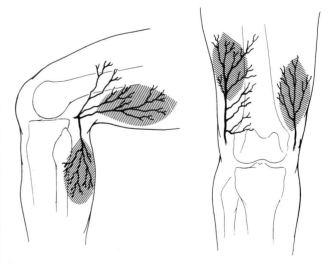

Figure 2-11.   Regions typical of burning pain from telangiectatic webs associated with the LSVS. (Reprinted by permission from *Varicose Veins and Telangiectasia: Diagnosis and Treatment,* Goldman, Weiss, and Bergan, Quality Medical Publishing, St. Louis, 1999.)

Figure 2-10.   Gastrocnemius veins seen on cross-section by duplex. SSV, lesser saphenous vein; V, vein (gastrocnemius); red circle marked A, artery.

of reticular veins. Finally, there may be reflux from the GSV via an anterolateral tributary.

Although these vessels are of very small caliber, high-resolution duplex ultrasound studies of the LSVS have allowed reconstruction of the three-dimensional structure of the typical microanatomy of these reticular veins and associated telangiectasias (*Figure 2-12*).

GASTROCNEMIAL TRIBUTARIES

Varicose veins on the posterior calf may be completely independent from the saphenous veins, instead originating from incompetent perforators connected directly to deep muscular veins of the calf, especially the gastrocnemial veins.[11-13] The gastrocnemial veins originate in venous sinuses buried deep within the gastrocnemius muscle, and normally join the peroneal vein to drain into the popliteal vein; however, the termination of the gastrocnemial veins can be highly variable. Many cases have a common termination with the LSV at the saphenopopliteal junction, some connect independently to the popliteal vein, and others terminate in the femoropopliteal vein of Giacomini.[14] When gastrocnemial veins communicate directly with the superficial venous system, it usually is by perforating veins that pass through the fascia at the level of mid-calf. These veins may communicate with the posterior arch vein or with other superficial tributaries of the GSV or LSV.

PERFORATING VEINS

Perforating veins are veins that initially lie superficially, but then pass directly or obliquely through fascial defects and between muscle bundles to carry blood from superficial

veins into the deep venous system. Most perforating veins are thin-walled, varying in diameter from less than 1 mm to 2 mm in diameter, [15] and usually containing one or several valves. Although vessels smaller than 1 mm in diameter may be valveless, their oblique orientation through muscle is usually sufficient to prevent backflow. The number of perforating veins per leg varies greatly, with individual reports ranging from 64 to more than 15,000.[2] Perforating veins are more densely concentrated in the distal leg and foot. There are roughly eight perforators in the distal leg for every one in the thigh. In a typical patient, there are perhaps 20 significant perforating veins above the knee and approximately 200 below the knee.

There are two anatomically distinct types of perforating veins. Direct perforators connect the superficial and deep veins without intermediaries, while indirect perforators connect the deep and superficial veins via muscular venous channels. The majority of perforating veins are located on either side of the sartorius and peroneal muscles and between the vastus lateralis and hamstrings, but their course beneath the deep fascia may be variable.[16] Sixty percent of perforating veins are closely accompanied by an artery.[17]

Although many names have been given to individual perforating veins, these are best considered in loose regional groupings because of the tremendous variation in the exact number and position of the perforators serving both the greater and lesser saphenous veins and their tributaries. Perforators in the upper mid-thigh often are associated with the upper extent of the adductor canal, or canal of Hunter, and therefore are often referred to as Hunterian perforators. Reflux through a Hunterian perforator is a common cause

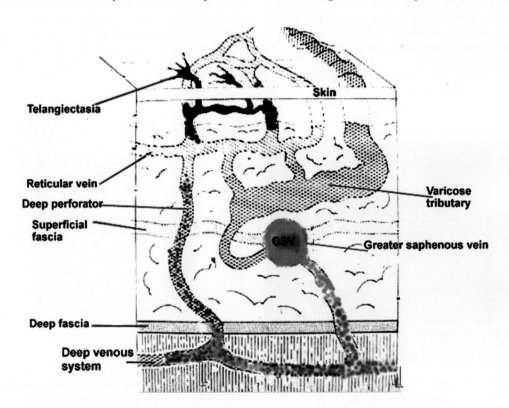

Figure 2-12. Microanatomy of the lateral subdermic venous system. (Adapted from George Somjen, M.D.)

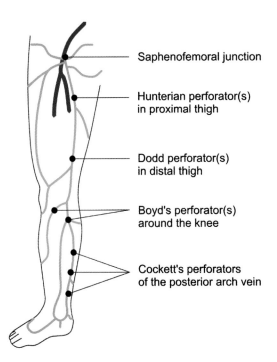

Figure 2-13.   Principal named connections between the saphenous system and the deep venous system.

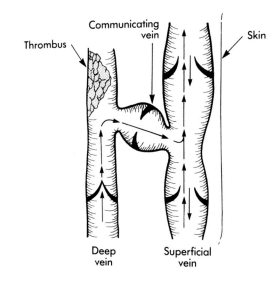

Figure 2-14.   Dilated superficial vein caused by perforator incompetence resulting from deep vein thrombosis blocking proximal flow of blood in the deep venous system. Note that with dilation of the superficial vein the valves are no longer competent. (Reprinted by permission from Goldman, M. P., *Sclerotherapy*, Mosby, St. Louis, 1995.)

for medial thigh varicose veins in patients with a competent saphenofemoral junction. Perforators in the lower medial thigh are known as Dodd's perforators, those in the medial mid-calf are called Boyd's perforators, and perforators associated with the posterior arch vein on the posteromedial ankle are known as Cockett's perforators *(Figure 2-13)*.

There are many important groups of variably present perforating veins that are unnamed. In the middle third of the lateral thigh and the midline of the posterior thigh, multiple small perforating veins may connect the GSV and its tributaries to the profunda femoris vein. A posterior tibial perforator 5–10 cm below the knee often connects the GSV to the posterior tibial veins on the medial calf. Multiple perforating veins (paraperoneal perforators) along the medial calf may connect the LSV to the deep gastrocnemius veins. Foot perforators are commonly found at sites approximately 2.5 cm below the inferior tip of the medial malleolus, 3.5 cm below and anterior to the medial malleolus, and on an arc about 3 cm anterior and below the medial malleolus. Perforating veins in the foot may be without valves or may have valves that are reversed to allow blood to flow from the deep to the superficial veins.[18]

Perforator veins often play a seminal role in the evolution of varicose veins, but are not the only source of surface varicose veins.[19] When perforator veins are incompetent, the high pressure generated by the calf muscle pump is transmitted directly to the superficial veins, causing a dilation of the superficial vessels that progresses along the vein over time *(Figure 2-14)*.[20] Incompetent perforating veins become thicker-walled and dilate to a diameter of 5 mm or more.[21] The diameter of incompetent perforators also tends to be less at the point of connection to the superficial system. This causes a "nozzle effect" of high-velocity turbulent flow

at high pressures, producing localized points of vein dilatation, colloquially referred to as "blowouts."[22]

Areas where perforators are commonly located should receive special attention in the physical examination. However, the physical exam may be unreliable because there are hundreds of palpable fascial defects that may or may not contain perforating veins. *These fascial defects often are defects within the superficial fascia (not deep fascia) and merely represent emerging surface tributaries of the saphenous system.* These tributary perforators may appear to be important origins of reflux, and can be the starting point of a varicose vein, as shown in the duplex image in *Figure 2-15*.

Duplex ultrasound frequently demonstrates areas of local venous dilatation ("blowouts") that have no evidence of an associated incompetent perforator, while many oblique incompetent perforators communicate with their superficial tributaries without giving any superficial clue to their existence. In planning treatment for a patient with venous insufficiency, the location of incompetent perforating veins is not something to be estimated or guessed at, but rather should be based on specific studies, such as duplex ultrasound or continuous-wave Doppler. The site of origin of reflux, independent of a "perforating vein" should be sought. Younger patients frequently show no sign of incompetent deep perforating veins.

Summary

The principal venous anatomy of the leg consists of only a small number of named deep and superficial vessels, yet it often confuses clinicians because of the many possible pathologic and incidental patterns that may arise, especially

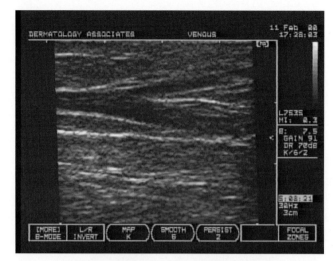

A

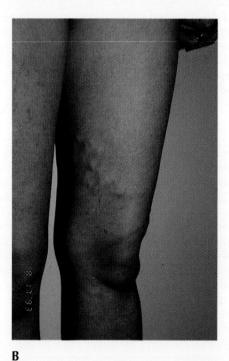

B

Figure 2-15. **(A)** One of the most common causes of axial or truncal varicose veins seen on the surface, a vein coursing to the surface becomes incompetent at its branch point off the greater saphenous vein as it "perforates" through the superficial fascia. **(B)** Surface view of this vein.

in the lower leg. Careful examination of patients, initially with hand-held Doppler, and subsequently with duplex ultrasound, is the single best way to reinforce a solid understanding of the anatomy of the venous system. Such an understanding of the venous anatomy of the leg is essential to the successful practice of phlebology.

References

(1) Beebe HG, Bergan JJ, Bergqvist D, Eklof B, Eriksson I, Goldman MP et al. *Classification and grading of chronic venous disease in the lower limbs–A consensus conference.* Vasa 1995; 24(4):313–318.
(2) Thompson H. *The surgical anatomy of the superficial and perforating veins of the lower limb.* Ann R Coll Surg Engl 1979; 61:198–210.
(3) Miller SS. *Investigation and management of varicose veins.* Ann R Coll Surg Engl 1974; 55:245–245.
(4) Raivio EVL. *Untersuchungen die venen der unteren extremitaten mit besonderer bevuckgichtigunu der gegenseihgen verbindungen zwischen den oberflachlichen und tiefen venen.* Ann Med Exp Fenn 1948; 26(suppl):1–21.
(5) Bundens WP, Bergan JJ, Halasz NA, Murray J, Drehobl M. *The superficial femoral vein, a potentially lethal misnomer [see comments].* JAMA 1995; 274(16):1296–1298.
(6) Somjen GM, Royle JP, Fell G, Roberts AK, Hoare MC, Tong Y. *Venous reflux patterns in the popliteal fossa.* J Cardiovasc Surg (Torino) 1992; 33(1):85–91.
(7) Albanese AR, Albanese AM, Albanese EF. *Lateral subdermic varicose vein system of the legs: its surgical treatment by the chiseling tube method.* Vasc Surg 1969; 3:81–89.
(8) Weiss RA, Weiss MA. *Doppler ultrasound findings in reticular veins of the thigh subdermic lateral venous system and implications for sclerotherapy.* J Dermatol Surg Onc 1993; 19(10):947–951.
(9) Somjen GM, Ziegenbein R, Johnston AH, Royle JP. *Anatomical examination of leg telangiectases with duplex scanning [see comments].* J Dermatol Surg Onc 1993; 19(10):940–945.
(10) Hirai M, Naiki K, Nakayama R. *Prevalence and risk factors of varicose veins in Japanese women.* Angiology 1990; 41:228–232.
(11) Vandendriessche M. *Association between gastrocnemial vein insufficiency and varicose veins.* Phlebol 1989; 4:171–184.
(12) Thiery L. *La vena fossa poplitea.* Phlebologie(Brussels) 1983; 2:649–651.
(13) May R, Nissl R. *Die Phlebographie der Unteren Extremitat.* Stuttgart: Thieme, 1959.
(14) Georgiev M. *The femoropopliteal vein—ultrasound anatomy diagnosis and office surgery.* Dermatol Surg 1996; 22(1):57–62.
(15) Bjordal RI. *Circulation patterns in incompetent perforating veins of the calf in venous dysfunction.* In: May B, Partsch H, Staubesant J, editors. Perforating Veins. Munich: Urban and Schwarzenberg, 1981: 71–88.
(16) Stolic E. *Terminology, division, and systematic anatomy of the communicating veins of the lower limb.* In: May R, Partsch H, Straubesand J, editors. Perforating veins. Munich: Urban & Schwarzenber, 1981: 21–33.
(17) Limborgh J. *L'anatomie du systeme veineux de l'extremite inferieure en relatio avec la pathologie variqueuse.* Folia Angiologica 1961; 8:3–8.
(18) Askar O, Kassem KA, Aly SA. *The venographic pattern of the foot.* J Cardiovasc Surg 1975; 16:64–70.
(19) Sherman RS. *Varicose veins: further findings based on anatomic and surgical dissections.* Ann Surg 1949; 130:219–224.
(20) Arnoldi CC. *Venous pressure in patients with valvular incompetence of the veins of the lower limb.* Acta Chir Scand 1966; 132:628–640.
(21) Linton R. *Communicating veins of the lower leg and the operative technique for their ligation.* Ann Surg 1938; 107:582–591.
(22) Wuppermann T, Mellmann J, von Schweder WJ. *Morphometric characteristics of incompetent perforating veins in primary varicosis of the lower leg.* Vasa 1978; 7:66–70.

CHAPTER 3

Histology

Vein Walls
  Intima
  Media
  Adventitia
  Innervation
Venous Valves
Venules
Telangiectasias and Venulectases
Summary

It is useful to understand the histology of normal and pathologic veins and venous valves because the structure of the vein determines its normal mode of function and its common modes of failure. It is also important to understand the zones that must be injured in order to permit sclerosis and closure of veins.

Vein Walls

Collection of venous blood begins with the end-capillary venule, which is about 20 μm in diameter and consists of an endothelium surrounded by a thin layer of collagenous fibers. As it carries blood proximally, the venule increases in diameter and gains smooth muscle cells within the fibrous sheath. At a diameter of 200 μm, the muscular layer becomes more well-defined, and by the time the vessel is large enough to be clinically visible, three distinct layers can be recognized. This is the case for venules of the leg that comprise telangiectatic webs. As veins become larger, they include elastic fibers and demonstrate a more organized structure with three tunicas: intima, media, and adventitia (Figure 3-1).

In its relaxed state, the normal vein contains an intrinsic rest volume, and is slightly oval or elliptical in cross-section, with the short axis perpendicular to the skin. When the volume of blood increases, the vein accommodates this by becoming circular in cross-section, increasing its volume without significantly increasing the intravascular pressure (Figure 3-2). This contributes to the large intrinsic capacitance of the venous system.[1] When further volume must be accommodated, the vessel stretches and the pressure rises according to the tension developed in the muscular, elastic, and fibrous tissues of the vein wall. Prolonged exposure to high pressures causes the vein to increase its intrinsic rest volume by permanently increasing its length and diameter, becoming dilated and tortuous and often following a spiral path. Varicose saphenous veins have been shown to have significantly larger wall areas and higher amounts of collagen. Collagen content and wall area are larger proximally

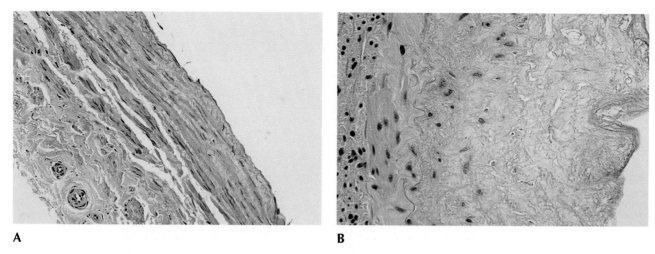

A   B

Figure 3-1.   Cross section of adult normal vein. **(A)** Note three distinct layers of intima (facing right), media and adventitia (hematoxylin and eosin stain, 200x). **(B)** Same vein after in vivo exposure to 3% sodium tetradecyl sulfate for 10 minutes. Note marked destruction of media with necrosis of smooth muscle cells.

compared to distally in both control and varicose veins, with a higher content of smooth muscle and elastin in varicose veins[2] *(Table 3-1).* Varicosis is therefore thought to be a dynamic response to venous hypertension.

INTIMA

The intima includes a layer of endothelial cells and a fenestrated basement membrane covered by an incomplete elastic lamina. Endothelial cells have multiple microvilli on their intravascular surfaces, and while easily damaged, have a remarkable regenerative ability. For successful sclerosis this layer must be completely destroyed *(Figure 3-3).*

MEDIA

Three layers of smooth muscle bundles make up the media: an inner layer of longitudinally arranged muscle fibers with loose connective tissue and small elastic fibrils separating the bundles, a middle layer of circumferentially arranged muscle bundles separated by layers of elastic fibrils, and an outer layer of thick fibrous tissues with longitudinal muscle bundles running through it. The smooth muscle content is higher in veins that are exposed to higher pressures, in distal (rather than proximal) veins, and in superficial (rather than deep) veins.[2] The greatest amount of circular muscle occurs near the insertion of the valve leaflets, making this region the last to dilate when a vein becomes varicose.[3] Patients who lack this relative increase in muscular fibers encircling the valves are prone to develop primary valvular insufficiency. For sclerosis to occur, these layers of smooth muscle must be significantly damaged *(Figure 3-1B, Table 3-2).*

ADVENTITIA

The adventitia is a thick layer of interlacing fibers of collagen in longitudinal, circular, and spiral orientations. The adventitia of large vessels may also contain an extensive

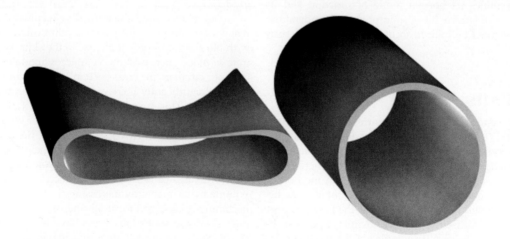

Figure 3-2.   Transformation of shape from oval to circular to accommodate increased volume without raising pressure.

Table 3-1
Histologic Variations of Varicose Veins

Increase in diameter
Larger wall areas
Higher amounts of collagen
Increased smooth muscle
Increased elastin

Table 3-2
Changes in Histology for Sclerosis of Veins

Intima: must be destroyed, connections between endothelial cells broken
Media: smooth muscles must be damaged and replaced by collagen
Adventitia: destruction of vasa vasorum, sclerotic changes

network of elastic fibers that extends along the vein from valve to valve.[4] The outer part of the collagen layer merges with perivenous connective tissue and contains vasa vasorum and adrenergic nerve fibers. These nerve fibers transmit pain when a sclerosing solution makes its way to this layer. The vasa vasorum supply blood to the tissues of the vessel wall, arising as branches of perivenous arterioles and draining into venules in the perivenous connective tissue. At 10 days following venous thrombosis, sclerotic changes are noted in the adventitia.[5]

INNERVATION

Muscular veins lack direct innervation, but cutaneous veins respond to both alpha- and beta-adrenergic stimulation.[6] Venous muscular constriction can occur in response to a wide variety of stimuli, including temperature change, position, activity, sensation, emotion, acid–base status, respiratory phasicity, and many circulating substances such as common medications.[7]

Venous Valves

Venous valves are thin sheets of collagen and smooth muscle covered by endothelium. At the base of the valve cusp, an increased number of muscle fibers extends both circumferentially and longitudinally. Elastic fibers are evenly dis-

tributed along the entire length of the cusp, while collagen fibers are thicker at the base and thinner toward the free edge of the cusp. The valve itself is avascular, its circulatory needs served by the venous blood carried within the vein. In young patients, valves are extremely flexible, but in older patients the valves become less flexible due to increased amounts of collagen and thicker muscular layers. Commissural reflux may occur through inflexible valve leaflets that oppose correctly.

Venules

The term "venule" describes a series of vessels ranging from the tiniest post-capillary venule (15–20μm in diameter) consisting only of endothelial cells and a basement membrane to the largest venules with a structure identical to that of larger veins, having three distinct and well-organized tissue layers. Even tiny venules contain valves, most often located where a venule passes from the dermis into the deeper adipose tissues or where it joins a larger venule at a branch point. The valves are always pointed in the direction of the larger vessel, as would be expected in a collecting vein.[8]

Telangiectasias and Venulectases

Telangiectasias are dilated blood channels in the dermis that histologically resemble much smaller capillary venules in consisting of a single endothelial cell lining with only a rudimentary media and adventitia (Figure 3-4).[9] Most telangiectasias of the lower extremities begin as tiny vessels that have become dilated in response to increased pressure (often due to reflux in underlying larger veins).[10] The ectasia response is more common than a proliferation of the number of blood vessels, as proposed in telangiectatic matting. Larger veins that appear in a "starburst" or "sunburst" pattern have histologic characteristics suggesting that they arise from normal small cutaneous veins that have enlarged and become dysplastic. The results of light and electron microscopy of 18 punch biopsies of sunburst telangiectases indicate that these are widened cutaneous veins located within the superficial vessel network, as well as within descending branches, often with an asymmetrically thickened wall. Only a few elastic fibers have been detected, as opposed to numerous oxytalan fibers.[11] Electron microscopy reveals an interfibrillar collagenous dysplasia, lattice collagen, and some matrix vesicles. The center of sunburst vessels is found at depths ranging from 175–382 μm below the stratum granulosum.

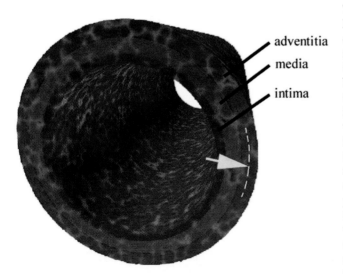

adventitia
media
intima

Figure 3-3. Schematic of histologic layers of vein showing to which depth destruction must occur (*yellow arrow*) for sclerosis to be successful.

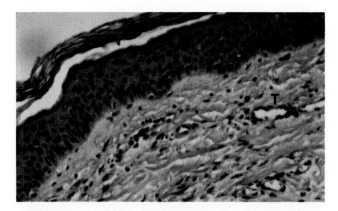

Figure 3-4. Telangiectasia (T) cross section showing single endothelial cell lining taken from biopsy of leg (hematoxylin and eosin stain, 20x).

The source of high pressure that causes these veins to enlarge is most often reflux in one of the major superficial venous systems, but high pressure from small arteriovenous malformations may be responsible for some of these starburst clusters. Pressure from arterioles, in an unknown way, may also stimulate a process of angiogenesis that may account for new vessels that occur following elimination of the original telangiectasias. Protuberant telangiectasias that are violaceous and between 1–2 mm diameter are often referred to as venulectases.

Summary

Normal veins are structures whose thin walls permit them to dilate easily, providing an important capacitance reservoir for the overall circulation. Prolonged high pressure causes predictable changes of dilatation, wall thickening, and tortuosity. Successful destruction involves elimination of the intima and media with some damage extending to the adventitia.

References

(1) Van Cleef JF, Hugentobler JP, Desvaux P, Griton PH, Cloarec M. *Etude endoscopique des reflux valvulaires sapheniens.* Journal des Maladies Vasculaires 1992; 17:113–116.

(2) Travers JP, Brookes CE, Evans J, Baker DM, Kent C, Makin GS, et al. *Assessment of wall structure and composition of varicose veins with reference to collagen, elastin and smooth muscle content.* European Journal of Vascular & Endovascular Surgery 1996; 11(2):230–237.

(3) Gaitini D, Torem S, Pery M, Kaftori JK. *Image-directed Doppler ultrasound in the diagnosis of lower-limb venous insufficiency.* Journal of Clinical Ultrasound 1994; 22(5):291–297.

(4) Griton P, Vanet P, Cloarec M. [*Anatomic and functional features of venous valves*]. J Mal Vasc 1997; 22(2):97–100.

(5) Baeshko AA, Berlov GA, Rogov I, Kriuchok AG, Markautsan PV, Sysov AV, et al. [*Morphologic changes in the thrombus and venous wall in experimental phleobothrombosis and thrombophlebitis*]. Morfologiia 1998; 114(5):59–64.

(6) Rudner XL, Berkowitz DE, Booth JV, Funk BL, Cozart KL, D'Amico EB, et al. *Subtype specific regulation of human vascular alpha(1)-adrenergic receptors by vessel bed and age. Circulation* 1999; 100(23):2336–2343.

(7) Daniel EE, Low AM, Lu-Chao H, Gaspar V, Kwan CY. *Characterization of alpha-adrenoceptors in canine mesenteric vein.* J Cardiovasc Pharmacol 1997; 30(5):591–598.

(8) Braverman IM, Keh-Yen A. *Ultrastructure of the human dermal microcirculation. IV. Valve- containing collecting veins at the dermal-subcutaneous junction.* J Invest Dermatol 1983; 81(5):438–442.

(9) Braverman IM. *Ultrastructure and organization of the cutaneous microvasculature in normal and pathologic states.* J Invest Dermatol 1989; 93(2 Suppl):2S–9S.

(10) Braverman IM. *The cutaneous microcirculation: ultrastructure and microanatomical organization.* Microcirculation 1997; 4(3):329–340.

(11) Wokalek H, Vanscheidt W, Martay K, Leder O. *Morphology and localization of sunburst varicosities: an electron microscopic and morphometric study.* J Dermatol Surg Onc 1989; 15:149–154.

Venous Physiology and Pathophysiology

In order to treat venous problems properly, it is essential to understand the normal pattern of venous blood flow and the effects of venous valves. For practical purposes, the venous system of the leg can be considered to have two major parts: a deep component and a superficial component. The superficial veins serve as a primary collecting system, and are connected through perforating veins to the deep veins, which normally carry about 90% of the blood from the leg back to the central circulation.

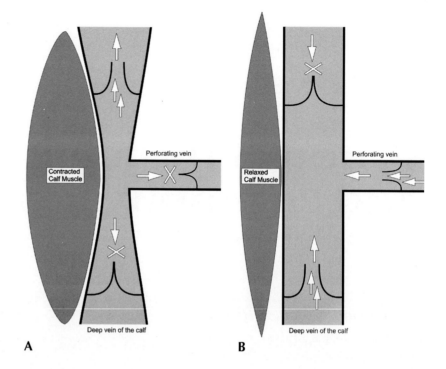

Figure 4-1. **(A)** The calf muscle pump with muscle contracted, 2 atmospheres of pressure force the vein segment to empty. **(B)** The calf muscle pump with muscle relaxed; zero or negative pressure permits the vein segment to refill.

A   B

Normal Venous Physiology

As arterial blood flows into the leg, distal superficial veins and venous reservoirs constantly fill, must be regularly emptied into the deep veins, and then the blood somehow returned to the right side of the heart. Venous return from the leg must flow uphill against gravity, against fluctuating thoraco-abdominal pressures, and sometimes in the face of additional backpressures such as the elevated right atrial pressure of congestive heart failure. This process depends on the patency of the flow circuit and on the correct functioning of a complex series of valves and pumps.

CALF MUSCLE PUMP

When muscles of the calf and leg contract, they compress deep veins within the muscles, forcing the blood in those veins to flow upward past venous valves. When the muscles relax, the deep veins expand and draw in more blood from superficial collecting veins (*Figure 4-1*). This system is known as the calf muscle pump, often referred to as a peripheral heart. Veins and muscles of both the calf and the foot play an important role in the normal function of this system, which can achieve pumping pressures of several hundred torr before valve failure will occur.[1] Particularly important venous capacitance reservoirs are found within the soleus muscle and the deep muscles of the foot.

VENOUS VALVES

Normal deep and superficial veins contain one-way valves that permit flow from the superficial system into the deep system and from distal to proximal. The calf muscle pump cannot function without competent valves both above and below. Venous valves are bicuspid, and are located every few centimeters in all normal veins below the level of the

common femoral vein.[2] Recent studies of venous valves indicate that there may be several different types of valves, including some that offer some resistance but do not shut completely.[3] Normal venous valves can withstand pressures of up to 3 atmospheres, but congenitally weak valves and valves that have softened due to hormonal influences may malfunction to permit retrograde flow at lower pressures.

AMBULATORY VENOUS PRESSURE

Immediately after ambulation, the normal pressure within the veins of the lower extremity is extremely low because a normally functioning muscle pump has emptied both the superficial and deep venous systems. Normal inflow to the lower extremity veins is purely via arterial inflow, thus the normal venous system will be refilled only after 3–5 minutes of standing. After prolonged standing, the entire venous system is filled, the valves float open, and venous pressure rises to a maximum that is exactly equal to the height of the standing column of venous blood from head to foot (*Figure 4-2*). This condition triggers an urge to move the legs, activating the muscle pumps and re-emptying the legs. Any condition that increases venous inflow or impedes venous outflow will cause an elevated venous pressure during or immediately after ambulation.

Venous Pathophysiology

Impaired venous outflow and abnormal (retrograde) venous inflow are the two principal causes of venous circulatory pathology. Venous pathology can be related to the deep system, the superficial system, or can be of mixed etiology. It can result from primary muscle-pump failure, venous ob-

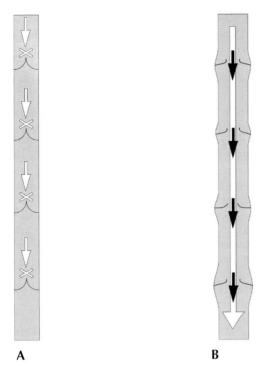

A   B

Figure 4-2. **(A)** Immediately upon standing, veins are empty and valves are closed. Hydrostatic pressure is limited to the height between valves. **(B)** After prolonged standing, veins are full and valves have opened. Hydrostatic pressure rises to the full height of the column of blood.

struction (thrombotic or nonthrombotic), or venous valvular incompetence, which may be deep, superficial and segmental, or whole-leg. Nearly any abnormality of venous circulation will ultimately result in the development of varicose veins *(Table 4-1)*.

Table 4-1
Physiologic Causes of Venous Insufficiency

Failure of calf muscle pump leading to high ambulatory venous pressure
    Muscle wasting
    Neuromuscular disease
    Prolonged standing
Failure of valves
    Venous distension
    Valve deformation
Deep obstruction
Deep incompetence
    Primary agenesis
    Prior valve damage
    Direct trauma
    Dilation with secondary valve failure
Perforator incompetence
Superficial incompetence
    Gravitational hydrostatic pressure

VALVE FAILURE

Valve failure permitting venous reflux is the most common cause of symptomatic venous pathology. Many different mechanisms can lead to valve malfunction and reflux. Reflux is common after thrombosis or other inflammatory processes have damaged valve leaflets. Chronic turbulent blood flow may also lead to reflux by causing atrophic changes of the valves. Congenital conditions may result in malformed valve leaflets. When a vein becomes distended due to overfilling, the base of the valve (the valve sinus) may expand so far that normal valve leaflets can no longer form a tight seal. Even when the valves themselves function normally, leakage around the base (commisural reflux) may be induced by any process that deforms the base. Superficial vein walls are inherently weak because (with the exception of the greater saphenous vein in the thigh) they are supported only by subcutaneous tissue and skin rather than by fascia and muscle. With prolonged standing, hydrostatic pressure can cause even "normal" veins to become distended to the point where they permit reflux.[4] External compression may therefore play an important role in the protection of a "normal" leg by supporting the veins and minimizing distention.

PRIMARY MUSCLE PUMP FAILURE

The calf muscle pump can fail to operate because of muscle wasting, neuromuscular disease, local edema, deep fasciotomies, or local vein-valve failure within the muscle fascia sheath. When there is complete failure of the calf muscle pump, venous blood is never effectively pumped out of the distal extremity at all.[1] The immediate post-ambulatory venous pressure will be nearly as high as the pressure after prolonged standing; and the volume of venous blood that suffuses the extremity will be increased. A smaller fraction of the extremity's venous blood will return to the central circulation each minute, and because arterial blood must flow into congested tissues with elevated hydrostatic pressure, the volume of arterial inflow will actually be reduced. This situation often leads to ulceration of the lower extremity.[5]

DEEP OBSTRUCTION

Partial obstruction of the deep veins may have little effect upon venous outflow, but severe obstruction of the deep veins produces secondary muscle pump failure. In this case the muscle pump produces an appropriately high outflow pressure with each contraction, but the volume of venous blood pumped out of the calf is reduced because of the reduced diameter of the outflow tract.

DEEP INCOMPETENCE

If outflow tracts are open and the muscle pump itself is functional, but the valves of the deep veins permit reflux (because of primary agenesis, prior valve damage, direct trauma, or dilation with secondary valve failure), then venous blood will be pumped out of the calf in normal volumes; however, extremity refill will include both normal arterial inflow and pathologic deep venous retrograde flow. Total failure of all deep vein valves allows venous blood to flow backwards rapidly from the vena cava down into the legs upon standing, and can produce orthostatic hypotension.

In patients with deep venous valve incompetence, the venous pressure immediately after ambulation may be slightly elevated or even normal, but the veins will refill and dilate very quickly. After only a few seconds of standing, the venous pressure will be nearly as high as the normal pressure after prolonged standing. The volume of venous blood that suffuses the extremity will be increased. A smaller fraction of the extremity's venous blood will return to the central circulation each minute, and because arterial blood must flow into congested tissues with elevated hydrostatic pressure, the volume of arterial inflow will be reduced, as in primary pump failure.

PERFORATOR INCOMPETENCE

Under ordinary circumstances the bulk of venous blood moves strictly from the superficial system to the deep system. Failure of the valves of communicating perforator veins can permit a significant volume of blood to flow backwards from deep to superficial veins, producing local congestion and venous hypertension. More importantly, perforator incompetence allows the extremely high pressures generated within deep veins by the calf muscle pump to be communicated to the superficial veins, which are not strong enough to tolerate the pressure. This high pressure (even if intermittent and highly localized) can produce excessive venous dilation and secondary failure of superficial vein valves. This is one of the major mechanisms for the develop-

ment of superficial venous incompetence and varicose veins. Perforator incompetence plays an important role near the ankle, where higher venous pressures result in typical physical signs of venous insufficiency.

SUPERFICIAL INCOMPETENCE

Superficial venous incompetence is the most common form of venous disease. In contrast to catastrophic deep-system incompetence, severe reflux limited to the superficial system alone rarely produces a severe hemodynamic response. Instead, when a series of superficial vein valves fail, hydrostatic pressure causes localized pooling of venous blood and localized sequelae.

Retrograde flow through the superficial venous system occurs when venous valves no longer perform their usual function, which can happen for a variety of reasons. Direct injury or superficial phlebitis may cause primary valve failure. Congenitally weak vein walls may dilate under normal pressures to cause secondary valve failure, or congenitally abnormal valves may themselves be incompetent at normal superficial venous pressures. Normal veins and normal valves may become excessively distensible under the influence of hormones (as in pregnancy). In most cases, however, superficial venous reflux is simply the inevitable end result of the introduction of high pressures into otherwise normal superficial veins that were intended to function as a low-pressure system. High pressure causes normal superficial veins to dilate so widely that the thin flaps of venous valves simply no longer meet in the middle *(Figure 4-3)*.

High pressure can enter the superficial veins by failure

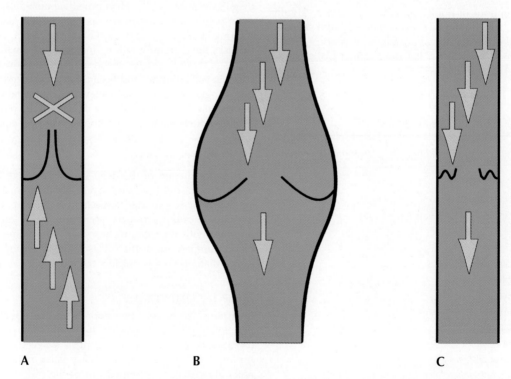

Figure 4-3.   **(A)** Normal valve allows forward flow, but prevents backwards flow. **(B)** Dilated vessel prevents normal valve leaflets from meeting, thus failing to prevent retrograde flow. **(C)** Damaged valve has scarred leaflets that cannot seal properly, permitting retrograde flow.

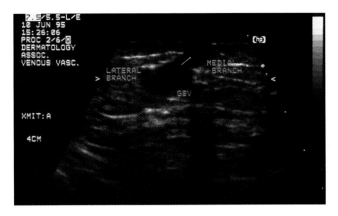

Figure 4-4. A branch point off the greater saphenous vein, a site at which reflux often begins, is seen on Duplex ultrasound in the transverse view. Note the perforation through the superficial fascia (*arrow*).

of key valves at any point of communication between the deep and superficial systems or in branching points. Branching points such as tributaries of the greater saphenous vein are inherently more distensible, partially due to lack of superficial fascial protection (*Figure 4-4*). Junctional high-pressure disease results from failure of the primary valve at the junction between the greater saphenous vein and the common femoral vein (the saphenofemoral junction, or SFJ), or at the junction between the lesser saphenous vein and the popliteal vein (the saphenopopliteal junction, or SPJ). Perforator high-pressure disease results from failure of the valves of any perforating vein. The most

common sites of primary perforator valve failure are at the canal of Hunter in the mid-proximal thigh and in the proximal calf.

Junctional reflux produces a fairly constant hydrostatic elevation of venous pressure, but when calf perforators fail, a high-pressure jet of blood is squirted out from the deep system towards the surface of the skin with every muscle contraction. This can result in a visible and palpable localized dilatation ("blow-out") at the site where an incompetent perforator joins a superficial vessel (*Figure 4-5*). This may even occur in the posterior thigh and be linked to the lateral venous system.[6] A blow-out situation also occurs when a saphenous vein tributary perforates through the superficial fascia (*Figure 4-4*). While not true perforating veins, these tributaries may produce local recirculation in the same way that incompetent true perforating veins do. Incompetent tributaries that course through the superficial fascia may balloon anywhere between the superficial fascial plane and the skin surface.

VARICOSE VEINS

Varicose veins are nothing more than superficial veins that have expanded in response to increased pressure and turbulence. No matter where the initial valve failure occurs, a leakage of high pressure into the superficial veins causes a predictable progression of disease, with sequential failure of valve after valve as the superficial veins become progressively more dilated in response to the increased blood pressure. When the initial point of reflux is proximal, vein dilation proceeds from proximal to distal and patients perceive that a large varicose vein is "growing down the leg." When the initial point of reflux is distal, patients first notice large

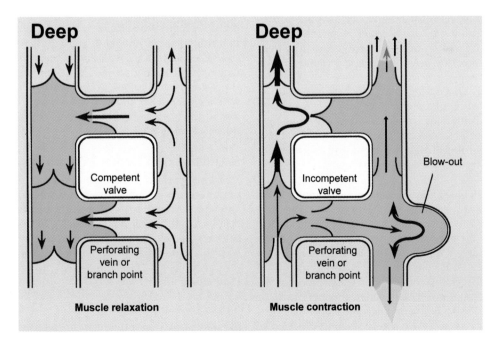

Figure 4-5. Schematic of blow-out at perforator site. High pressure during muscle contraction forces blood to the surface via incompetent valves in superficial, deep perforating, or branch veins, leading to a superficial varicosity.

clusters of veins in the lower leg, with large varicose veins eventually "growing up the leg" toward the groin.

Primary varicosities sometimes develop from a localized weakness of the wall itself, but are more often caused by failure of a single valve structure in a critical location, allowing high pressure to pass from the stronger deep system into fragile, easily distended, unsupported superficial veins. Whether the valve failure results from vein wall elasticity or a primary valvular defect is unimportant since the end result is identical. Secondary varicosities occur when thrombophlebitis causes deep system and perforator valve damage, allowing high pressure to pass into unsupported superficial veins.

Venous Insufficiency

MECHANISMS

The normal pressure in the venous system of the lower leg during ambulation is near zero, and the early standing pressure in the normal leg is, at most, the hydrostatic pressure of a column of blood as high as the nearest competent valve. Failed valves permit this hydrostatic pressure to increase. Failure of the calf muscle pump increases it more. High venous pressure is directly responsible for many aspects of venous insufficiency syndrome, including edema, protein deposition, fibrin cuffing, and red cell extravasation.

Venous hypertension accounts for many of the sequelae of peripheral venous disease, but not for all. For example, not all patients with venous hypertension will develop ulceration, and some patients with venous ulceration do not have marked venous hypertension. Poor clearance of lactate, CO_2, and other products of cellular respiration also contribute to the development of the syndrome. A defect in clearance of extraneous substances can be quantified: If albumin labeled with a radioactive tracer is injected into the foot tissues, the clearance rate is markedly slowed by deep venous obstruction or by deep or superficial venous incompetence.[7]

Although this effect is referred to as venous stasis, reduced clearance of cellular metabolites is not always due to true venous stasis. In many cases venous blood moves at a normal speed, but a local recirculation of venous blood prolongs the average transit time for blood to pass from the heart and lungs through the legs and back to the central circulation (*Figure 4-6*).

The concept of blood aliquot transit time is similar to the cardiac output measure used for the heart. A tracer substance is injected into the femoral artery and recorded as it is cleared through the femoral vein. In the normal patient, a bolus of tracer makes a rapid transit of the leg and is cleared as a slightly spread-out bolus. In a patient with venous reflux and venous recirculation the first appearance of the tracer is very slightly slowed, but the remainder of the tracer is cleared very slowly. For venous insufficiency, one measures a low level of tracer over a very prolonged period of time.[8] A prolonged time for an aliquot of radiolabeled blood to pass from the femoral artery through the leg and back to the central circulation correlates extremely well with the development of leg ulcers.

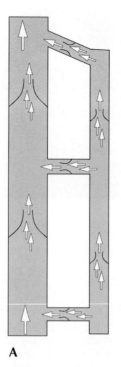
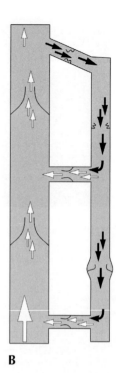

A   B

Figure 4-6. **(A)** With normal valves between the deep and superficial systems, there is no recirculation, thus there is a normal clearance time. **(B)** With injured or dilated valves connecting the deep and superficial systems, local recirculation occurs, leading to a prolonged clearance time.

Superficial varicosities always produce venous recirculation, and can result in prolonged clearance that may be very localized or may affect the whole leg. As a practical matter, progressive visible "stasis dermatitis" and ulceration will not occur if the peak retrograde flows in the greater and lesser saphenous veins and in the popliteal vein add up to less than 10 cc per second. If the sum of these reflux flows is greater than 15 cc per second, the incidence of ulceration will be very high.[9] In some cases a local or regional reflux that is purely superficial and is more than 7 cc/sec may produce local ulceration.[10,11]

SEQUELAE OF VENOUS INSUFFICIENCY

Venous hypertension and reduced venous clearance are important causes of morbidity and disability in patients with varicose venous disease. Chronic pain, swelling, recurrent cellulitis, and chronic nonhealing leg ulcers (ulcer cruris) are common sequelae, but superficial venous disease can also lead to death either from hemorrhage or from superficial thrombophlebitis that progresses to cause pulmonary thromboembolism (*Table 4-2*).

Subjective symptoms

Symptoms may be present in up to 98% of patients with "clinically relevant" alterations of venous circulation,[12] but even small telangiectasias are often symptomatic: 53% of patients presenting with telangiectasias less than 1 mm in diameter complain of symptoms that resolve with treat-

Table 4-2
Sequelae of Venous Insufficiency

Chronic pain
Swelling (edema)
Recurrent cellulitis
Nonhealing leg ulcers (ulcer cruris)
Hemorrhage
Superficial phlebitis
Deep vein thrombosis
Pulmonary embolism

Table 4-4
Stages of Progressive Tissue Damage
Due to Venous Insufficiency

Edema
Hyperpigmentation
Venous dermatitis
Chronic cellulitis
Cutaneous infarction (atrophie blanche)
Ulceration
Malignant degeneration

ment.[13] Many common symptoms of small reticular and varicose veins are caused when high pressure reaches distal branch veins with no major runoff connections (Table 4-3).

Episodic pain and other symptoms associated with superficial venous disease may be temporally related to physiologic and pharmacologic hormonal changes. Half of all pregnant women with varicose veins complain of pain related to the varicosities, and 17% are unable to remain standing upright more than 1 to 2 hours at a time because of the severity of the pain.[14]

Objective signs

Up to 50% of people with varicose veins have secondary cutaneous abnormalities.[15,16] The most common physical signs of venous disease are related to progressive syndromes of chronic venous stasis and chronic venous hypertension. Table 4-4 lists the stages of progressive tissue damage commonly seen in lower extremity venous stasis.

Leg ulcers

Chronic nonhealing leg ulceration can be so debilitating as to produce complete functional disability. Venous insuffi-

ciency is the underlying cause in most patients, and superficial system reflux is involved in more than half of those with venous ulcers. Approximately 1 million persons in the United States have ulceration due to superficial venous disease, and about one out of ten are functionally disabled.[17]

Variceal hemorrhage

Bleeding from lower extremity varicosities can be fatal, especially in elderly or debilitated patients. There were 23 such fatalities reported in England and Wales in 1971.[18] Treatment of these bleeding varicosities is a medical emergency (Figure 4-7).

Superficial thrombophlebitis

The lifetime incidence of superficial thrombophlebitis in patients with untreated varicose veins has been estimated at 20–50%. This is not a benign condition, as unrecognized deep vein thrombosis is present in up to 45% of patients with what appears to be a purely superficial phlebitis. The risk of deep vein thrombosis has been reported to be 3 times higher in patients with superficial varicosities.[19]

Table 4-3
Symptoms of Pain from Telangiectatic Webs

Fatigue
Heaviness
Focal burning or aching
Focal pruritus
Sharp intermittent stabbing pain (focal)
Diffuse burning
Night cramping
Restless legs

Adapted from ref. 13

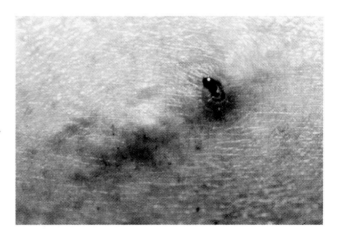

Figure 4-7. Bleeding varicosity. This small ruptured vessel led to several hours of unnoticed nocturnal hemorrhage. The previously healthy patient presented to the emergency department with a hematocrit of 19.

Summary

The normal physiologic functioning of the peripheral venous system depends upon a complex interaction among fragile and delicate structures. Abnormalities of any component of the system can lead to venous insufficiency syndromes in which venous clearance from the lower extremities is impaired. Varicose veins and telangiectasias are dilated refluxing veins that usually appear early in the progression towards end-stage venous circulatory disorders. Refluxing veins play a central role in the progression of venous insufficiency syndrome, and treatment of these refluxing veins can arrest or reverse the progression of disease.

References

(1) Araki CT, Back TL, Padberg FT, Thompson PN, Jamil Z, Lee BC, et al. *The significance of calf muscle pump function in venous ulceration.* J Vasc Surg 1994; 20:872–77.

(2) Boisseau MR. [*Venous valves in the legs: hemodynamic and biological problems and relationship to physiopathology*]. J Mal Vasc 1997; 22(2):122–127.

(3) Griton P, Vanet P, Cloarec M. [*Anatomic and functional features of venous valves*]. J Mal Vasc 1997; 22(2):97–100.

(4) Schadeck M. [*Reflux in healthy valves of the great saphenous vein*]. Phlebol 1991; 44:603–613.

(5) Labropoulos N, Giannoukas AD, Nicolaides AN, Veller M, Leon M, Volteas N. *The role of venous reflux and calf muscle pump function in nonthrombotic chronic venous insufficiency. Correlation with severity of signs and symptoms.* Arch Surg 1996; 131(4):403–406.

(6) Labropoulos N, Delis K, Mansour MA, Kang SS, Buckman J, Nicolaides AN, et al. *Prevalence and clinical significance of posterolateral thigh perforator vein incompetence.* J Vasc Surg 1997; 26(5):743–748.

(7) Gajraj H, Browse NL. *Fibrinolytic activity of the arms and legs of patients with lower limb venous disease.* Br J Surg 1991; 78:853–856.

(8) Konstantinova GD, Shkuro AG, Frolov VK, Karalkin AV, Virganskii AO. [*Evacuation function of a musculovenous "pump" of the leg in varicose veins of the lower extremities*]. Vestn Khir Im I I Grek 1981; 127(7):58–62.

(9) Nicolaides A. *Quantification of venous reflux by means of duplex scanning.* J Vasc Surg 1990; 10:670–677.

(10) Christopoulos D, Nicolaides AN. *Noninvasive diagnosis and quantitation of popliteal reflux in the swollen and ulcerated leg.* J Cardiovasc Surg (Torino) 1988; 29:535–539.

(11) Christopoulos DC, Belcaro G, Nicolaides AN. *The hemodynamic effect of venous hypertension in the microcirculation of the lower limb.* J Cardiovasc Surg (Torino) 1995; 36(4):403–406.

(12) Fischer H. *Socio-epidemiological study on distribution of venous disorders among a residential population.* International Angiography 1984; 3:89–94.

(13) Weiss RA, Weiss MA. *Resolution of pain associated with varicose and telangiectatic leg veins after compression sclerotherapy.* J Dermatol Surg Onc 1990; 16:333–336.

(14) McCausland AM. *Varicose veins in pregnancy.* West J Surg 1939; 47:81.

(15) Almgren B, Eriksson I. *Valvular incompetence in superficial, deep and perforator veins of limbs with varicose veins.* Acta Chir Scand 1990; 156:69–74.

(16) Hobbs JT. *The problem of the post-thrombotic syndrome.* Postgrad Med 1973; J (Aug Suppl):48.

(17) Coon WW, Willis PW, Keller JB. *Venous thromboembolism and other venous disease in the Tecumseh community health study.* Circulation 1973; 48:839–846.

(18) Evans GA, Evans DM, Seal RM, Craven JL. *Spontaneous fatal haemorrhage caused by varicose veins.* Lancet 1973; 2:1359–1361.

(19) Nicolaides AN, Kakkar VV, Field ES, Fish P. *Venous stasis and deep-vein thrombosis.* Br J Surg 1972; 59(9):713–717.

CHAPTER 5

Common Patterns of Abnormal Veins: A Visual Guide

The Regional Anatomy of Varices
>   Medial Thigh
>   Posterior Thigh
>   Lateral Thigh
>   Anterior Thigh
>   Posterior Calf
>   Lateral Calf
>   Medial Calf
>   Anterior Calf (Pre-tibial)
>   Popliteal Fossa
>   Ankle

Summary

The Regional Anatomy of Varices

For a regional consideration of the anatomy that gives rise to varices, the leg is divided into eight quadrants: lateral, medial, anterior, and posterior, then above or below the knee. This chapter seeks to provide both the novice and experienced phlebologist with a visual guide to the common (and less common) pattern of abnormal veins that one is likely to encounter in everyday practice. A regional approach leads to some unavoidable repetition in discussion and presentation, as many veins extend through different regions or have tributaries that cross many boundaries. Clinical photographs accompanied by simplified diagrams and tables can facilitate rapid identification of the root causes of an unfamiliar pattern of reflux, but there is no substitute for a complete understanding of normal venous anatomy.

MEDIAL THIGH (TABLE 5-1)

Pudendal. Most proximally, visualization of blue reticular to 3–4 mm varicose veins can be seen extending from external genitalia. These indicate reflux through the pudendal tributary of the greater saphenous vein (GSV). These veins, when varicose, may cause pain during sexual intercourse, when they become engorged. In early stages of pudendal reflux, the saphenofemoral junction (SFJ) is not involved and treatment is easily performed (Figure 5-1).

31

Table 5-1
Quadrant 1—Medial Thigh

Pudendal vein
Incompetent saphenofemoral junction
Hidden reflux at saphenofemoral junction (only palpable on standing)
Superficial axial branch veins (medial tributaries) of GSV
Hunterian perforator connection—mid-thigh
Distal saccular saphenous vein dilation (just above knee)
Resistant telangiectatic matting (just above knee)

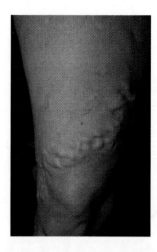

Figure 5-2.   Large varicosity beginning on the upper thigh extending downwards across it (beginning from a main branch varicosity of the GSV).

Bulging GSV at inguinal fold from SFJ reflux. Although rare, long-standing reflux at the saphenofemoral junction in a thin individual may allow visualization of a flesh-colored spongy bulge, which is the incompetent SFJ.

Hidden GSV reflux. Because of its depth in the proximal thigh, the greater saphenous vein is usually not visible in this region, even when it carries high-grade reflux from a widely incompetent saphenofemoral junction. The subterminal valve may also be incompetent in younger patients. Continuous-wave Doppler or duplex ultrasound examination in this region is essential if a proper diagnosis and treatment plan are to be made. It may be palpable only with the patient standing.

Superficial tributaries of the GSV. Visible veins on the medial portion of the thigh are often superficial tributaries of the GSV that accept reflux from the GSV below and proximally. *(Figure 5-2)* Visualization by duplex ultrasound shows the clear origin point at a superficial fascial gap at the point of termination of the tributary. Novices incorrectly assume that the varicose vein at the medial thigh surface either represents the GSV or the originating point of reflux.

Hunterian perforator. Varicose veins that become palpable or visible in the mid-medial thigh may be due to terminal or subterminal saphenofemoral incompetence, or may result from reflux through a thigh perforator, such as a Hunterian perforator. These dilated veins may be portions of the greater saphenous vein, but may also be accessory saphenous veins that pursue a parallel course *(Figure 5-3)*. Reflux below the medial thigh can be the result of a failed Dodd's perforator.

Distal segment saccular GSV dilatation. On the most distal portion of the medial thigh, just above the knee, the greater saphenous vein becomes more superficial, courses posteriorly, and may be apparent as an enlarged bulbous segment. Superficial phlebitis in this area can produce a painful palpable mass of surprising size. The most common cause is reflux from higher in the thigh *(Figure 5-4)*.

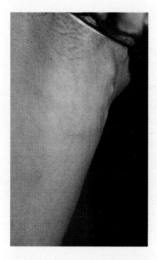

Figure 5-1.   Pudendal vein varicosities on the uppermost medial thigh extending upwards to the genitalia. Rapid response to sclerotherapy or phlebectomy is typical.

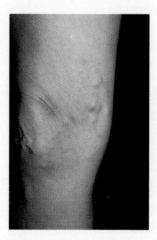

Figure 5-3.   Large varicosity on lower medial thigh from Hunterian perforator insufficiency; duplex exams showing origin of perforator incompetence in Hunterian canal are shown in Chapters 2 and 10.

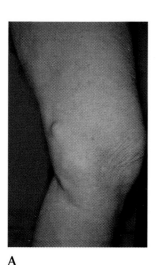 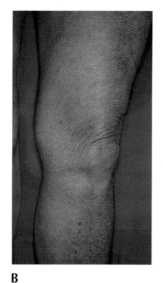

A   B

Figure 5-4. **(A)** Saccular GSV dilatation above the knee. This vein is usually a branch of the GSV, however, rarely, as in this case, is the GSV itself in a superficial location. **(B)** Excellent results are seen 2 months after saphenofemoral ligation followed by ambulatory phlebectomy.

Resistant telangiectasias. The medial thigh just above the knee can also be the site of telangiectasias that are persistent and difficult to treat. Sometimes saphenous system reflux is responsible for these vessels, and sometimes they are fed by reticular veins that originate from the lateral subdermic venous system (LSVS) via peripatellar veins. New telangiectasias in this area are common when drainage pathways below are ligated, removed, or sclerosed while there remains a source of high-pressure reflux from above *(Figure 5-5)*. Sometimes no source of reflux can be found for telangiectasias in this area. When duplex ultrasound fails to identify any source of reflux, it is possible that the telangiectasias

Table 5-2
Quadrant 2—Posterior Thigh

Superficial gluteal
S-shaped reticular vein of posterior thigh
Posterior thigh perforators (PTPV) emptying into LSVS
S-shaped reticular vein of posterior thigh
Giacomini vein
Incompetent saphenopopliteal junction
Greater saphenous vein (rarely)

may have resulted from local injury and resulting angioneogenesis. Hypothetically, oxygen deprivation from sleeping in the lateral position with knees pressed together may further stimulate angioneogenesis.

POSTERIOR THIGH (*TABLE 5-2*)

Superficial gluteal. The most prevalent pattern of veins on the posterior thigh is a central zig zagging reticular vein whose origin is in the gluteal region. Often running just below the dermis and appearing immediately below the gluteal fold, it is thought to be a superficial branch of the inferior gluteal vein. This reticular vein often terminates into a branch of the LSVS in the posterolateral portion of the popliteal fossa *(Figure 5-6)*. Multiple telangiectasias often arise from these reticular veins.

Posterior thigh perforating veins emptying into LSVS. Posterior lateral thigh perforatoring veins (PTPV), have been shown to dive 3–8 cm in the posterior thigh to join tributaries of both femoral veins. Some of these PTPV veins give rise to superficial tributaries that extend to the lower lateral and posterior thigh, whereas some give rise to tributaries alongside the lesser saphenous vein and the anterior arch of the greater saphenous vein.[1] On the posterior lateral portion of the distal posterior thigh lie the multiple reticular

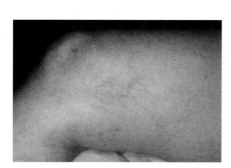

Figure 5-5. Resistant telangiectasias on the medial thigh above the knee: the most troublesome region for persistent failure or recurrence after sclerotherapy. These may occur even after GSV reflux is totally eliminated.

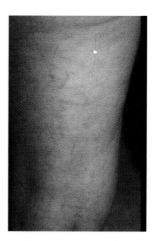

Figure 5-6. Reticular varicosity originating from superficial gluteal venous network with a possible contribution from posterior thigh perforating veins.

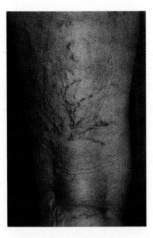

Figure 5-7.   Posterior thigh perforators leading to large reticular varicosities and telangiectasias. This lower posterior thigh pattern responds extremely well to sclerotherapy.

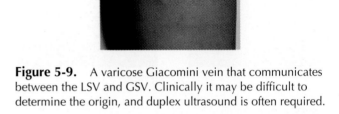

Figure 5-9.   A varicose Giacomini vein that communicates between the LSV and GSV. Clinically it may be difficult to determine the origin, and duplex ultrasound is often required.

veins of the LSVS, which can communicate with the PTPV. These interconnect with the smaller reticular varicosities that populate the popliteal fossa. The exact position of these is quite variable. When coursing within 2 cm of the popliteal fossa, reflux originating from the lesser saphenous vein–popliteal vein junction must be excluded by Doppler examination before proceeding with treatment *(Figure 5-7)*.

S-shaped reticular vein of posterior thigh. This reticular vein courses along the posterior thigh, resulting from reflux from PTPV or gluteal branches. It may also be considered a posterior component of the lateral subdermic venous system *(Figure 5-8)*.

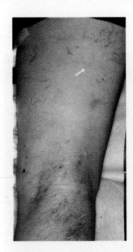

Figure 5-8.   S-shaped reticular vein on posterior thigh connecting with LSVS. This pattern is the most common on the posterior thigh and often accounts for pain during prolonged sitting. *Arrow* indicates possible connection with posterior thigh perforating veins.

Giacomini vein. The medial port of the posterior thigh is often the location of a communicating vein connecting the lesser saphenous vein with the greater saphenous vein. In some patients the LSV terminates into an oblique epifascial communicating vein (the vein of Giacomini) that empties directly into the greater saphenous vein. Its location and length are quite variable, and it may be easily confused with an extension of the lesser saphenous vein on to the mid-posterior thigh or with a more posteriorly located greater saphenous vein *(Figure 5-9)*.

Incompetent saphenopopliteal junction. Rarely this enlargement at the terminal portion of the LSV may be visible or palpable with the patient standing, usually 2–3 cm above the popliteal fold.

Greater saphenous vein. Very rarely, when large amounts of reflux are present or when the GSV is very superficial, the GSV itself may be visible on the posterior medial aspect of the thigh just above the knee. More typically, a larger vein in this location is a branch varicosity of the GSV. The varicosity seen in *Figure 5-4* coursed posteriorly after its bulge above the knee.

LATERAL THIGH (*TABLE 5-3*)

Lateral subdermic venous system (Albanese). This is the classic lateral thigh pattern of cosmetic reticular veins with associated telangiectatic webs. Reflux through reticular veins may occur retrograde due to movement of the knee as these veins normally drain distally, by gravity rather than having the usual venous pattern of proximal drainage. Many cases, however, originate from gluteal or posterior thigh-perforating veins and follow the classic pattern of reflux in a retrograde fashion down the lateral and posterior thigh. As varicosities and telangiectasias on the lateral thigh most often arise due to reflux through the lateral subdermic venous system, successful treatment of these seemingly iso-

Table 5-3
Quadrant 3—Lateral Thigh

Lateral subdermic venous system (Albanese)—most common cosmetic pattern
Anterolateral tributary of the GSV
Branch varicosity of lesser saphenous vein

---

lated telangiectatic webs depends on ablation of the underlying source of reflux.

Knowledge of the lateral and posterior thigh anatomic patterns is crucial to successful treatment. The pattern may become more complex with age (*Figure 5-10*). The pattern most commonly seen in young women is this "bridge" of telangiectasias associated with central reticular varicosities (*Figure 5-11*), which typically responds well to sclerotherapy of the entire network. Early on these may be due entirely to reflux originating at the lateral or posterior knee, but in half the individuals reflux originates from an incompetent lateral mid-thigh or posterior thigh perforator vein (PTPV) with normal venous flow at the knee. When reflux originates from the upper thigh, the so-called "feeding" reticular veins below the telangiectatic webs may be more prominent as the reflux drains inferiorly into the perforating veins of the lateral knee. It is important to eliminate reflux both above and below the telangiectatic webs.

Anterolateral tributary of the GSV. (ALT) One of the major tributaries at the terminal of the greater saphenous vein in the groin, this larger varicosity typically traverses the entire anterior thigh and ultimately intersects and interacts with the lateral venous system. Early on this may not be seen traversing the anterior thigh or it may appear as small superficial reticular veins. When varicose, the ALT causes a more significant dilatation and varicosis of LSVS reticular veins (*Figure 5-12*).

Branch varicosity of the lesser saphenous vein. In some cases, a dilated LSVS vein slightly above the knee may arise from a relatively small communicating tributary of the lesser saphenous vein and will be most prominent posteriorly, but it is typically seen predominantly at and below the popliteal fossa (*Figure 5-13*).

ANTERIOR THIGH (*TABLE 5-4*)

Incompetent saphenofemoral junction. Although mentioned as being primarily in the medial quadrant, occasionally the SFJ may appear in the central upper anterior thigh.

Inguinal reticular veins. The most proximal portion of the anterior thigh frequently reveals small reticular veins that drain ultimately into the GSV or into the pudendal vein. Occasionally these small reticular veins receive flow from superficial lower abdominal veins. They are most often accompanied by reflux of the pudendal branch in the genital region. They may be anterior and/or medial (*Figure 5-14*).

Anterolateral tributary. The largest vein on the anterior thigh is often the anterolateral tributary of the GSV that allows direct communication between the GSV and the LSVS. Nearer the inguinal region, very small varicosities (3–4 mm) may indicate reflux through a pudendal branch of the GSV, but more often are due to reflux through an anterolateral branch (*Figure 5-15*). Any terminal branch vein of the greater saphenous that normally appears in the medial thigh may also be seen on the anterior thigh when it courses more laterally.

Small anterior branches of the LSVS. Some anterior thigh varicosities and telangiectasias are fed from reticular veins that ultimately connect with the LSVS (*Figure 5-16*).

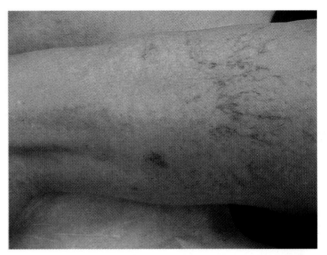

A

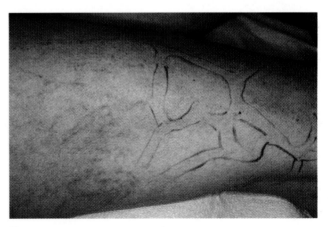

B

Figure 5-10. LSVS variations in severity: the most common region for appearance of cosmetic veins without associated saphenous reflux. **(A)** Some LSVS have a simple single reticular vein connection to the lateral knee. **(B)** More complex communications and networks develop over time, involving multiple lateral and posterior thigh perforating veins, and making treatment much more difficult and time consuming.

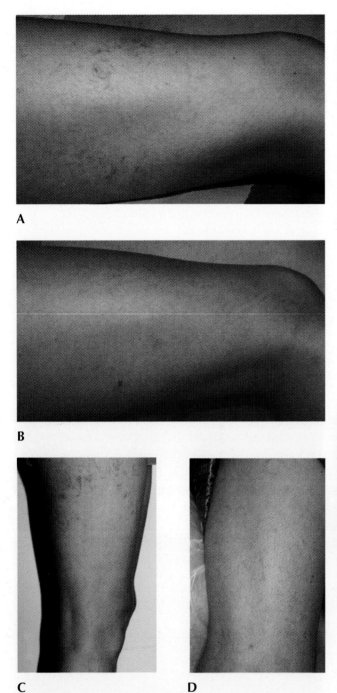

A

B

C D

Figure 5-11. Excellent results may be achieved in younger patients after one or two treatments. Recognizing this relatively straightforward pattern is of utmost importance for treatment of the cosmetic patient. **(A)** Before sclerotherapy of reticular veins and telangiectasias. **(B)** Three weeks after one treatment. **(C)** Before sclerotherapy of both telangiectasias and associated reticular veins. **(D)** After two sessions, three-year follow-up with continuing excellent results.

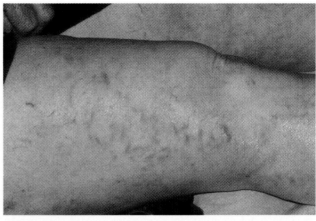

Figure 5-12. Anterolateral tributary (lateral view) of the GSV traversing the anterior thigh communicating with the LSVS. These reticular veins will become quite large in diameter over time, often up to 5 mm or more.

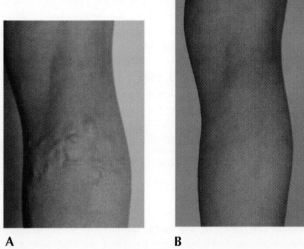

A B

Figure 5-13. A branch varicosity originating as a branch point directly from the LSV without saphenopopliteal reflux, thus sclerotherapy is successful. **(A)** Before sclerotherapy. **(B)** Six months after two treatments.

Table 5-4
Quadrant 4—Anterior Thigh

Anterolateral tributary of GSV
Inguinal fold reticulars
Incompetent saphenofemoral junction
Superficial axial branch veins (lateral tributaries) of GSV
Small anterior branches of the LSVS
Patellar

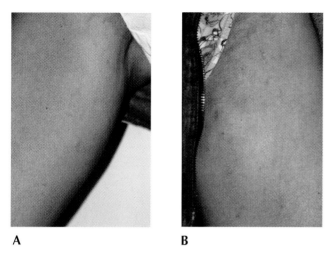

A   **B**

Figure 5-14.   Inguinal reticular veins communicating with the pudendal vein. **(A)** Early presentation is usually more medial. **(B)** A more advanced case extends onto the anterior thigh. Some contribution from abdominal wall veins may occasionally be seen.

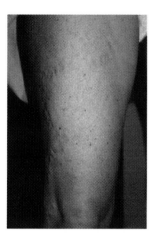

Figure 5-15.   Anterolateral tributary. The anterior view shown here, but this vein extends onto the lateral thigh.

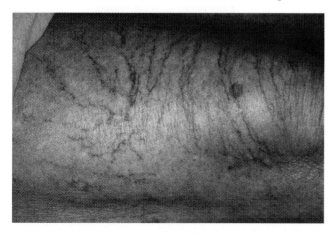

Figure 5-16.   Small anterior branches of the LSVS seen as a spray of telangiectasias. The key to efficient reduction is through elimination of reflux in the LSVS.

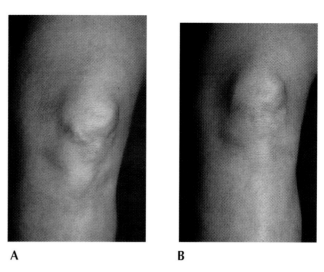

A   **B**

Figure 5-17.   **(A)** Patellar reticular vein communicating with the LSVS. **(B)** One week after a two-puncture ambulatory phlebectomy. Remarkable results, and far better than the probable hyperpigmentation post-sclerotherapy.

Patellar. A small varicose vein extending superior to the patella often represents a communication between a GSV tributary and the peripatellar reticular veins that communicate with the LSVS *(Figure 5-17).*

POSTERIOR CALF *(TABLE 5-5)*

Lesser saphenous vein. The dominant vein of the posterior calf is the lesser saphenous vein. Even when varicose, it is rarely visible from the surface at the level of the popliteal fossa to the mid-calf. Thus, diagnosis of reflux of the saphenopopliteal junction is difficult to make by visual inspection alone. An enlarged LSV can often be palpated in a standing patient, but reflux is most reliably detected by Doppler or duplex examination. Confusion may arise when a superficial reticular vein (usually associated with the LSVS) overlies this region, since the LSV may not be positioned at the exact center of the popliteal fossa. Duplex ultrasound may be the only reliable method of properly diagnosing an abnormality of the origin of the LSV. Recent evidence indicates many small unnamed arteries are associated with the proximal portion of the LSV so that any treatment of reflux in this segment must be undertaken with extreme caution *(Figure 5-18).*[2] This is the region where duplex-guided sclerotherapy is the most hazardous.

Table 5-5
Quadrant 5—Posterior Calf

Lesser saphenous vein
Mid-calf perforator of LSV
LSV major tributaries
LSVS
Greater saphenous vein

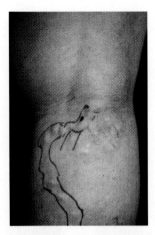

Figure 5-18. A bulge that is seen in the popliteal fossa suggests reflux of the LSV. LSV reflux must always be ruled out before treating this pattern, as occurred in this case.

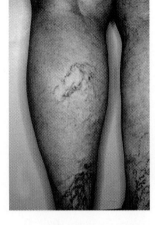

Figure 5-20. Large reticular vein of LSVS progressing over 35 years, now mimicking LSV reflux but terminating in telangiectatic webs. LSVS dilatation, similar to other varicosities, is progressive over decades.

Mid-calf perforator. This aptly named perforator is a large perforating vein connecting the lesser saphenous vein with the surface. It is a superficial perforating vein, perforating only through the superficial fascia. The mid-calf perforator is the most prominent and is most commonly seen as the origin of a varicose vein on the calf. It occurs frequently in the absence of reflux at the SPJ. Our many duplex exams have confirmed the origin of reflux at the point at which this vein travels through the superficial fascia. This is one of the many situations in which there is primary superficial vein reflux with an associated competent saphenous trunk.[3] Small varicosities on the central posterior calf frequently communicate via small perforating veins connected to the lesser saphenous vein. These smaller veins may be seen in the superior or mid portion of the posterior calf (Figure 5-19).

LSVS. The lateral posterior calf is very frequently the site of posterior extensions of the LSVS with associated telangiectasias (Figure 5-20). These groups of telangiectasias must be distinguished from telangiectasias arising from reflux on the lesser saphenous vein. Visual inspection allows the examiner to trace the reticular vein origin to the LSVS.

LSV major tributaries. Larger varicosities near the region of, and just lateral to, the Achilles tendon may indicate reflux from the LSV. However, near the ankle it is possible for crossover from reflux from the GSV to also be manifest (Figure 5-21).

Greater saphenous vein. When large amounts of reflux are present or when the GSV is very superficial, the GSV itself

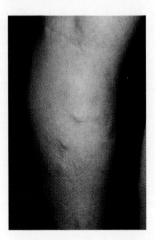

Figure 5-19. Mid-calf perforator gives rise to this large centrally located varicosity of the LSV on the calf. This is the most common perforator on the calf, but has no "official" name.

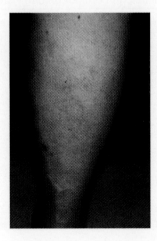

Figure 5-21. Vein of posterior ankle that arises from incompetent LSV. LSV varicosities terminate at the lateral ankle.

Table 5-6
Quadrant 6—Lateral Calf

Lateral subdermic venous system
Branch varicosities of the lesser saphenous vein (rare)

Table 5-7
Quadrant 7—Medial Calf

Most common site for initial varicosities
Boyd's perforators
Thigh GSV branch reflux

may be visible on the posterior medial aspect of the thigh just below (or above) the knee. More typically, a larger vein in this location is a branch varicosity of the GSV.

LATERAL CALF *(TABLE 5-6)*

LSVS. This region is primarily populated by reticular varicose veins of the LSVS with multiple associated telangiectatic webs. An extension from a greater saphenous vein tributary to the LSVS can cause a greatly dilated vein on the lateral portion of the calf, but this is unusual. Occasionally, a tributary of the GSV just above or below the knee traverses along the anterior calf so that it is also visualized in the lateral calf. A tributary of an incompetent LSV may traverse posteriorly to reach the lateral calf *(Figure 5-22)*.

Branch varicosities of the lesser saphenous vein. In association with reflux of the LSV, larger varicosities may be seen coursing posteriorly. When the LSVS is enlarged through reflux from the anterior lateral tributary of the GSV, larger varicosities may also be seen on the lateral calf. Visual inspection of the thigh should permit accurate diagnosis of the source. Duplex ultrasound may be necessary to rule out SPJ reflux.

MEDIAL CALF *(TABLE 5-7)*

Branch varicosity of the GSV. Although this is the most common site for varicosities to first appear, it is very common to see the origin of reflux begin in the lower medial thigh approximately 1.5 cm below the skin surface (see medial thigh). Again, reliable diagnosis of reflux origin requires Doppler examination at a minimum, but duplex ultrasound is best for identifying vessels 1 cm or more below the surface.

Additionally, reflux at the SFJ may initially reveal itself as surface varicosities in this region *(Figure 5-23)*.

Boyd's perforators. Varices along the medial calf most often arise as greater saphenous tributaries, but perforator-fed varices are also common in this area. This site is where larger varicosities first appear clinically. Many of these have been labeled incompetent Boyd's perforators, when in fact they are incompetent superficial branches or tributaries of the GSV. They occur from reflux originating where the GSV tributary exits through superficial fascia *(Figure 5-24)*.

ANTERIOR CALF (PRE-TIBIAL) *(TABLE 5-8)*

Superficial anterior tibial reticular vein. A frequent occurrence is a small reticular vein that traverses the anterior tibial plateau and which demonstrates reflux. It typically drains into the greater saphenous vein medially. Our observation has been that this vein occurs in the absence of any reflux in the GSV. Occasionally reticular veins from the LSVS can be associated superiorly with this vein. Clinically it may cause a throbbing sensation when incompetence progresses *(Figure 5-25)*.

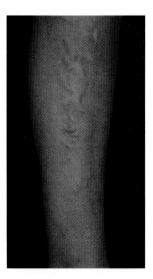

Figure 5-23.   Large varicosity that is a main branch off the GSV. This is the primary region for new varicosities or recurrent varicosities when GSV or SFJ reflux is not addressed, and is called Boyd's perforator region. Most early varicosities in this region actually originate from branches off the GSV, not from perforating veins connected to the deep system.

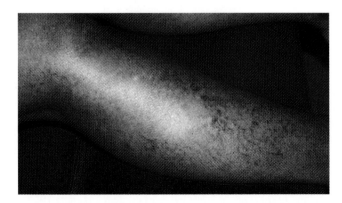

Figure 5-22.   Lateral subdermic venous system extends onto the lateral calf, another very common cosmetic pattern.

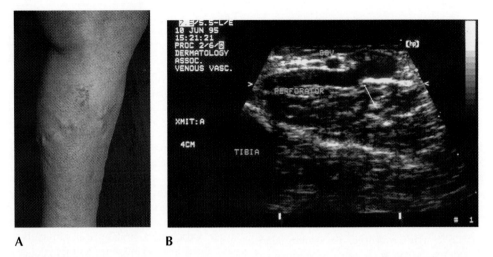

A   B

Figure 5-24. **(A)** Another example of this common pattern, here an incompetent Boyd's perforator (not a branch varicosity of the GSV), leads to a large varicosity on the medial calf. **(B)** Duplex exam shows the large perforating vein extending from below, but not directly connected to, the GSV in this plane. *Arrow* indicates "perforation" through the superficial fascia that is palpable from the surface as a filling defect. Most commonly a direct connection with a branch of the GSV is seen with no perforating vein.

GSV. When incompetent throughout its full length, the GSV itself may be visualized just above the ankle anteriorly.

GSV tributaries. Just above the ankle, multiple incompetent tributaries of the GSV may be visualized as large veins, particularly in more advanced cases of venous insufficiency. These are the typical ropelike varicosities on the anterior and medial calf *(Figure 5-26)*.

POPLITEAL FOSSA *(TABLE 5-9)*

LSVS. The popliteal fossa contains many superficial reticular veins with reflux originating from the PTPV, as described above *(Figures 5-8 and 5-27)*.

Giacomini's vein. It may connect the greater and lesser saphenous veins in this region.

Lesser saphenous vein. As described in the posterior calf quadrant above. It should be mentioned that gastrocnemius vein reflux may terminate in this region. Loud reflux may be heard by Doppler, but its anatomic origin can be distinguished only by duplex. Gastrocnemius reflux terminating in the popliteal fossa veins may be impossible and dangerous to treat, often resulting in treatment failures for associated LSV reflux.

Table 5-8
Quadrant 8—Anterior Calf (Pre-tibial)

    Superficial anterior tibial vein
    GSV tributaries
    GSV

ANKLE *(TABLE 5-10)*

GSV advanced disease. Large varices at the medial ankle indicate a minimum of superficial venous system disease, most likely GSV reflux, but may indicate concomitant deep venous system insufficiency. Because of the distal location, venous pressures can be very high, leading to hyperpigmentation.

Cockett's perforators. When venous disease progresses from superficial venous disease to that involving Cockett's perforators, communications with the posterior arch vein,

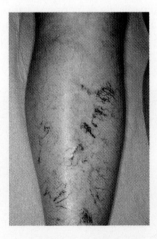

Figure 5-25. The superficial anterior tibial reticular vein is a small reticular varicosity that courses along the pretibial plateau. In this patient it has led to multiple telangiectasias. This reticular vein may be painful, and may or may not be connected with the LSVS.

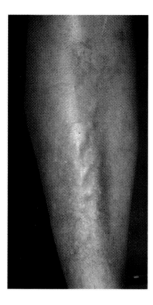

Figure 5-26. The pre-tibial region is also a very common site for larger branch varicosities of the GSV. Many of these large varicosities have multiple branch points and originate from reflux in the GSV that originates in the thigh.

Table 5-9
Popliteal Fossa

Lateral subdermic venous system from posterior thigh perforating veins
Giacomini's vein
Lesser saphenous vein
Gastrocnemius vein reflux

Table 5-10
Ankle

GSV advanced disease
Cockett's perforators
LSV advanced disease
Corona phlebectasia
Anterior dorsal vein

and posterior tibial veins, many enlarged veins are seen on the surface, particularly posterior to the medial malleolus. This appearance may also be the result of deep venous insufficiency *(Figure 5-28)*.

LSV advanced disease. When a large vein is seen posterior to the lateral malleolus it is wise to check for reflux at the termination of the LSV in the popliteal fossa. When the LSV has enlarged at the ankle location, advanced disease is typically suspected.

Corona phlebectasia. Multiple small blue reticular varicosities that "crown" the proximal ankle indicate increased venous pressure. Moderate to severe venous insufficiency involving the GSV is the most common origin. Other veins, including the LSV, may be involved, but this is much less common. When present, these telangiectatic veins typically indicate high venous pressure from above and are frequently associated with major reflux of the GSV *(Figure 5-29)*.

Anterior dorsal vein. Often observed traversing the anterior ankle is an extension of GSV, LSV, or prominent LSVS reflux channeled through a single large rubbery varicosity that terminates in the dorsal venous arch. This vein is a leading indication for ambulatory phlebectomy *(Figure 5-30)*.

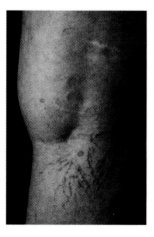

Figure 5-27. Reticular veins of the LSVS terminating in telangiectasias in the popliteal fossa. This straightforward pattern quickly responds to treatment. It is a region often shown for dramatic response to just one treatment. These may originate from reflux in the PTPV.

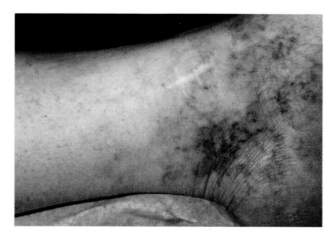

Figure 5-28. Varicose vein arising from reflux in Cockett's perforators. This is usually advanced disease with a high risk of venous ulceration. A scar from previous vein stripping is visible, but reflux has persisted or recurred through connections with the posterior arch and/or posterior tibial veins.

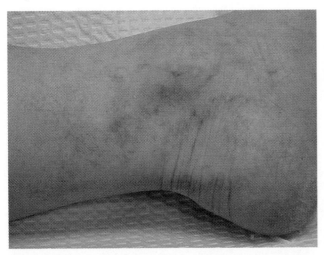

A

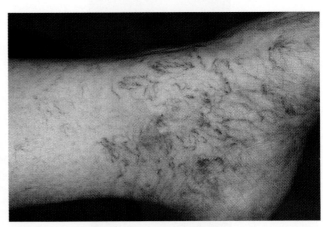

B

Figure 5-29.   Corona phlebectasia: multiple telangiectasias of the ankle are frequently a reliable sign of reflux in the GSV. **(A)** Early presentation. **(B)** More advanced presentation. The wise clinician hunts for GSV reflux as the etiology of this pattern instead of rushing to treatment.

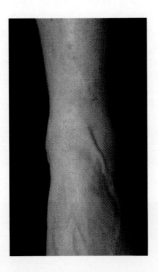

Figure 5-30.   Anterior dorsal vein of the ankle. Although reflux may originate from a number of sources (even local perforating veins), this thick-walled rubbery vein responds best to ambulatory phlebectomy, even though sclerotherapy has been utilized. These veins may be painful and have associated fibrotic nerves that may be unavoidably avulsed during a phlebectomy.

Summary

With practice, it is possible to quickly recognize a large number of common patterns of abnormal varicose veins and telangiectasias. Recognition is important, but alone not sufficient to guide treatment: pathways of reflux can be extremely complex and variable, involving many veins that are not visible on the surface of the skin. Common pattern recognition and a good understanding of the anatomy and physiology will direct an appropriate examination and diagnostic evaluation, permitting a correct diagnosis and treatment plan.

References

(1) Labropoulos N, Delis K, Mansour MA, Kang SS, Buckman J, Nicolaides AN, et al. *Prevalence and clinical significance of posterolateral thigh perforator vein incompetence.* J Vasc Surg 1997; 26(5):743–748.

(2) Bergan JJ, Weiss RA, Goldman MP. *Extensive tissue necrosis following high-concentration sclerotherapy for varicose veins.* Dermatol Surg. 2000; 26(6):535–541.

(3) Labropoulos N, Kang SS, Mansour MA, Giannoukas AD, Buckman J, Baker WH. *Primary superficial vein reflux with competent saphenous trunk.* Eur J Vasc Endovasc Surg 1999; 18(3):201–206.

PART II

Diagnosis

CHAPTER 6

History and Physical Exam

Introduction: Organization of the Clinical Exam

The physician must first explore the patient's presenting complaint and its history, along with his or her general and vascular history. Functional disorders and aesthetic complaints are addressed. The physical examination (including Doppler auscultation) is initially performed with the patient standing, and then in the supine and prone positions. A preliminary assessment is thus performed that includes diagnosis of the primary varicose veins and their regions of involvement. Further evaluation is required to quantify functional and aesthetic impairment, to assess the risks of possible complications, and to establish a plan for management that will be medically appropriate and acceptable to the patient.

History

As in all good medical practice, evaluation of the patient with varicosities begins with a complete history. The clinical history should include general medical and surgical information, as well as information about vascular disease. Besides the presenting complaint, it is important to document the onset of the problem and the clinical course of the disease. Any predisposing or aggravating factors and any situations that improve the symptoms are also recorded. The patient should be explicitly asked about each of the common symptoms that are seen with venous insufficiency, including leg heaviness, exercise intolerance, pain or tenderness along the course of a vein, pruritus, "restless" legs, night cramps, edema, and paresthesias. The history form that patients complete prior to the physical examination is shown in Chapter 27, Appendix B, Figure 3.

PRESENTING COMPLAINT

Patients may consult the phlebologist because of symptoms or aesthetic concerns, for advice on the medical implications of varicose veins, or simply seeking to know methods of treatment. Some visits are prompted by complications such as the rupture of a varicose vein with bleeding or the recent development of dermatitis, thrombophlebitis, cellulitis, or ulceration. Treatment that does not properly address the patient's primary concerns will not result in a satisfactory overall outcome. Patients also need to have a thorough understanding of the nature of gravitational influence on the formation of new veins.

GENERAL HISTORY

- Sex, age, weight, height.
- Medical history, including hypertension, diabetes, allergy history, tobacco consumption, rheumatological history, and general disease.
- Surgical history, including any fractures or surgical operations.
- Gynecological and obstetric history, including the number of pregnancies and miscarriages; plan for future pregnancies;[1] duration, dosage, and effect on venous complaints of hormone replacement therapy or oral contraception; and any variation of symptoms with the menstrual cycle.

HISTORY OF VASCULAR DISEASE

- History of venous insufficiency, including the date of onset of visible abnormal vessels and of onset of any symptoms.
- Presence or absence of predisposing factors such as heredity, trauma to the legs, occupational prolonged standing, or sports participation.
- History of edema, including the date of onset, predisposing factors, site, intensity, hardness, and modification after a night's rest.
- History of any prior evaluation of or treatment for venous disease, including medications, injections, surgery, or compression.
- History of superficial or deep thrombophlebitis, including the date of onset, site, predisposing factors, and sequelae.
- History of any other vascular disease, including peripheral arterial disease, coronary artery disease, lymphedema, or lymphangitis.
- Family history of vascular disease of any type.

ACTIVE SYMPTOMS

Symptoms present at the time of the visit are documented and described in terms of their site, their time of onset, character, and any factors that aggravate them or improve them. Symptoms of venous disease are most often, but not exclusively located on the medial surface of the leg. Symptoms often are increased by heat, prolonged standing, or during the premenstrual period in women, and are typically relieved by cold, ambulation, rest with leg elevation, or wearing of gradient elastic stockings.[2]

Characteristics of venous pain include a dull ache, burning, or pruritis. This pain may be localized to a protruding varicose or reticular vein. It is rarely described as a sharp stabbing pain or pain radiating down the back of the thigh. Surprisingly, nighttime muscle cramping can be caused by venous insufficiency. Restless legs may rarely be caused by venous insufficiency.

Physical Examination

INTRODUCTION

Physical examination of the lower extremities, while extremely important, is not always the most reliable guide because clinical findings common in venous disease are also common to many other entities. Findings of special importance to the phlebologist on physical examination are listed in Table 6-1. Some of these physical findings may help guide the choice of treatment modality and its degree of difficulty. For example, if a patient is a runner with muscular, well-toned legs, the veins will have a thick adventitia, and may pose a greater therapeutic challenge. Ambulatory phlebectomy of such thick-walled veins is more time-consuming and tedious; this type of vein is often more resistant to sclerosing solutions.

Swelling may result from acute venous obstruction (such as is seen in deep vein thrombosis), from deep or superficial venous reflux, or from other non-venous causes. Hepatic insufficiency, renal failure, cardiac decompensation, infection, trauma, and environmental effects can all produce lower-extremity pitting edema that may be indistinguishable from the edema of venous obstruction or venous insufficiency. Edema due to lymphatic system mal-

Table 6-1
Physical Examination Findings Associated with Venous Reflux

Asymmetry of limbs
    Size, length, ankle diameter
Scars
    Previous venous surgery
    Previous venous ulcers
Cutaneous signs of chronic venous insufficiency
Superficial vascular malformations such as port wine stains
Muscular tone and development
    Hypertrophy of veins and thickening of vein walls

function may be due to primary obstruction of lymphatic outflow, may be secondary to overproduction of lymph due to severe venous hypertension ("venolymphatic syndrome").

Despite the increasing popularity of technical laboratory investigations, clinical evaluation of the patient with venous disease remains the basis on which the diagnostic and therapeutic approach is built. The presenting complaint and the patient's goals for treatment must be defined and clearly understood. Knowledge of the patient's medical, social, work, and family environment is important. A general assessment of the patient's venous disease, including its severity and consequences, is critical to judging the risks of complications, both vascular (superficial venous thrombosis, prehemorrhagic bulla, ulceration) and trophic (eczema, cellulitis, leg ulcer).

Rather than being considered a special diagnostic modality, the use of Doppler for auscultation is an integral part of the clinical examination of patients with venous disease.[3] Doppler is so important to the physical examination that it may be considered the stethoscope of the phlebologist. Handheld Doppler helps to confirm the clinical findings of the physical examination, and is particularly valuable because it can reveal clinically undetectable subsurface reflux. Doppler helps define the topography of varicose disease and the hemodynamic status of the deep venous system. Repeated examinations over time help document the results of treatment or the natural course of the disease.

EQUIPMENT

The clinical examination requires a medical file, an examination platform, excellent lighting, a phlebological examination table, a continuous-wave Doppler apparatus, and a small amount of miscellaneous equipment.

Examination platform

Having the patient stand on a platform consisting of two or three steps will greatly increase the physical comfort for the physician and allow for a more complete examination. Thus, the patient can be examined in a standing position without requiring the physician to contort his or her body in a nonergonomic manner. Platforms may include a railing to increase safety and to reduce any patient anxiety (*Figure 6-1*).

Lighting

Lighting should be even and consistent. The simplest approach is to have a 75W lamp on each side of the patient. Uniform overhead fluorescent lighting is satisfactory. Hot spots from strong halogen lamps will bleach out reticular veins and should be avoided. Magnifying lamps or magnifying glasses are sometimes helpful when small lesions are to be examined in more detail. A new useful device to examine smaller telangiectasias is the cross-polarized lamp known as the Syris v600, Syris Scientific LLC, Gray, ME. The visual enhancement of fine telangiectasia and hard-to-see reticular veins is seen in Figure 6-2 (see also Figure 27-6). Transillumination may be helpful to map out reticular veins within 1–2 mm of the skin surface, as discussed further in Chapter 27.

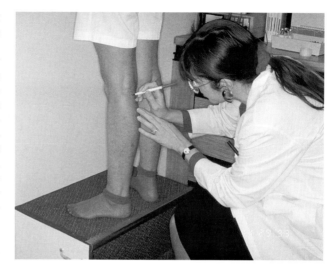

Figure 6-1. Examination platform: Having the patient on either steps or a stool makes examination easier for the physician.

Examination table

The examination table can be simple and inexpensive, but should allow examination of the patient either in a half-seated or a totally supine position. A hydraulic examination table will facilitate the examination by permitting the patient to be raised to a level convenient for the examiner and to be tilted into Trendelenburg and reverse Trendelenburg positions as needed. A hydraulic table will also be useful for subsequent treatments.

Doppler apparatus

The continuous-wave Doppler examination is the simplest, least expensive, and most rapid method by which to enhance the physical examination of patients with chronic venous insufficiency, provided it is performed by an experienced operator with a good knowledge of pathophysiology and all venous anatomical variants. The Doppler equipment and examination are described in detail in Chapter 8, with manufacturers and distributors listed in Chapter 27.

Minor equipment

Elastic tourniquets can be useful for Trendelenburg maneuvers. Either a 35-mm camera with a macro lens or a digital camera is essential to provide documentation of the current state of disease. (Cameras are further discussed in Chapter 27.) A tape measure must be available for leg diameter measurements, and a set of calipers will assist in measuring the diameter of the largest varicose veins.

PHYSICAL EXAMINATION (STANDING)

Complete physical examination of the lower extremities allows recording of the cutaneous complications of venous insufficiency and subsequently directs non-invasive diagnostic examination prior to treatment. This examination is initially performed with the patient standing, and then por-

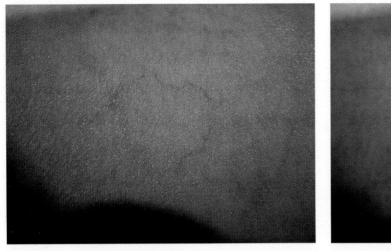
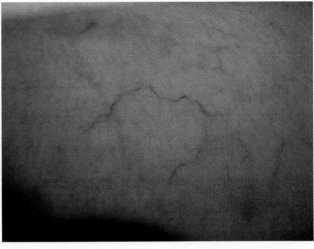

A

B

Figure 6-2. Enhancement of view of telangiectasia. **(A)** View with normal fluorescent lighting. **(B)** View with Syris v600 polarizing vision device.

tions are repeated with the patient supine or prone. The upright position corresponds to the position of maximal venous dilatation, while in the supine position the effect of hydrostatic pressure disappears and varicose veins collapse. As mentioned, the physical examination begins with inspection, palpation, and percussion, followed by Doppler auscultation. It is not uncommon for patients to feel lightheaded or even to faint while undergoing this examination. A cool room, particularly for patients with a previous history of vasovagal reactions, will help to minimize this. Patients should be warned to alert the physician immediately if they are feeling faint.

Inspection

Inspection is performed in an organized way from distal to proximal and from anterior to posterior, with the patient positioned on the highest step of the exam platform. Lighting should be even, without any zones of shadow. The examination is bilateral with comparison of findings on each leg. The examiner should always begin with the same limb in order to avoid being detoured by the most obvious lesions while skipping the subtle ones. In addition to the legs, the perineal region, pubic region, and abdominal wall must also be examined. The presence of a chaperone is highly recommended when examining a patient of the opposite sex.

Inspection should detect morphological abnormalities such as an abnormally large toe, flat feet, frozen ankle, swollen leg, hourglass leg, knee joint alignment abnormalities, or lengthening or trophic changes of one lower limb compared to the other. Further inspection should identify any cutaneous disorders, such as ulceration; telangiectasias of the leg, foot or ankle; acrocyanosis; eczema; brown spots; ochre dermatitis; flat angiomata; prominent varicose veins (small, large, rectilinear or tortuous); scars from a prior surgical operation; or evidence of previous sclerosant injections. Particular attention must be made to identify any ve-

nous dilatations within the perineal, suprapubic, or abdominal regions.

Normal veins are typically visibly distended at the foot and ankle, and occasionally in the popliteal fossa. For other regions of the leg visible distension usually implies disease. Translucent skin may allow normal veins to be visible as a light blue subdermal reticular pattern, but dilated veins above the ankle usually are evidence of venous pathology.

One of the primary goals of inspection is to determine the predominant "zone of influence" of involvement. The examiner must consider whether the veins arise from regions of the greater saphenous vein (GSV), lesser saphenous vein (LSV), or lateral venous system. Many patients will have a combination, but this is the foundation of a rational approach to treatment *(Figure 6-3)*. A comprehensive discus-

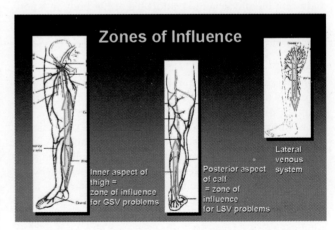

Figure 6-3. Zones of influence of varicose veins. **Left:** GSV region of influence (medial leg). **Center:** LSV region of influence (posterior lower leg). **Right:** Lateral venous system region of influence (lateral leg).

sion of the patterns of presentation of venous disease found on visual inspection is presented in Chapter 5.

Darkened, discolored, stained skin is often a sign of chronic venous stasis, particularly if it is localized along the medial ankle and the medial aspect of the lower leg. As these areas require drainage from a competent and patent full length of the GSV and all of the perforating veins attached to it, they are particularly susceptible to suffering from GSV malfunction. Nonhealing ulcers in this area are also most likely due to underlying venous stasis. Skin changes or ulcerations that are localized only to the lateral aspect of the ankle are much more likely to be related to prior trauma or to arterial insufficiency than to pure venous insufficiency.

Abnormalities of the posterior lower leg may be related to problems in the LSV. The typical appearance of involvement of only the lateral venous system is a common presentation. Since telangiectasia on the lower lateral and posterior leg may result from a more proximal refluxing lateral system at the knee or thigh, it is critical to fully examine the entire leg as part of the initial assessment.

Obvious varicosities or telangiectasias may be easily observed. The sudden appearance of "new" vessels, whether large or small, is often a clue to acute venous obstruction (such as deep vein thrombosis) for which the newly dilated vessels serve as a bypass pathway. The new appearance of varices and telangiectasias is often noted during pregnancy. Venous outflow obstruction from uterine compression of the pelvic outflow tracts was once thought to be the cause, but it has been shown that this is an uncommon mechanism for the development of varicose veins of pregnancy. It is now believed that nearly all of the effect is due to hormonal changes that render the vein wall and the valves themselves more pliable. Although the appearance of hormonally mediated varicosities of pregnancy is a common occurrence, the sudden appearance of new dilated varicosities during pregnancy still warrants a full evaluation for the possibility of acute deep vein thrombosis, which may occur during pregnancy.

Light palpation

Light palpation is often performed as a part of the process of inspection. The entire surface of the skin is lightly palpated with the fingertips because dilated veins may be palpable even where they are not readily seen. Palpation helps to locate both normal and abnormal veins, but it sometimes is possible to distinguish the soft collapsibility of a normal vein from the "distended inner tube" sensation when palpating a varicosity. This is only useful with the patient standing.

Starting with the right leg and asking the patient to turn every so often, the physician palpates the entire anteromedial surface of the lower limb (the territory of the greater saphenous vein) *(Figure 6-4)*, the lateral surface (collateral varicose veins of large trunks and nonsaphenous varicose veins), and finally the posterior surface (territory of the lesser saphenous vein) of both lower limbs. The location, size, shape, and course of all varicosities are documented, and the diameter of the largest vessel is measured as accurately as possible.

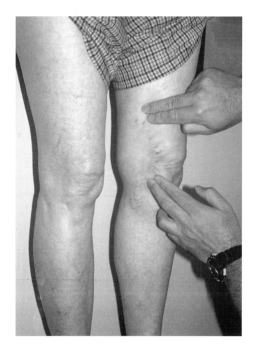

Figure 6-4. Palpation being performed of the anteromedial leg with large varicosities present.

After a few minutes of standing, the arch of the greater saphenous vein may be palpated in some thin patients, particularly when reflux is present at the junction. It is best appreciated two fingerbreadths below the inguinal ligament and just medial to the femoral artery. In patients with saphenofemoral incompetence, a forced coughing maneuver may produce a palpable thrill or sudden expansion at this level. The lesser saphenous vein is often more difficult to examine manually, but it may be palpable in the popliteal fossa in some slender patients after a period of standing or when involved with reflux. Other normal superficial veins above the feet should not be palpable, even after prolonged standing.

Deep palpation

Once inspection and light palpation have identified the locations of the principal superficial veins and varices, deeper palpation in those areas may reveal much more about these veins.

Palpation of an area of leg pain or tenderness may reveal a firm, thickened thrombosed vein. These palpable thrombosed vessels are virtually always superficial veins. However, one cannot assume the benign nature of a pure superficial thrombosis, since combined deep and superficial venous thrombosis commonly occur. A completely thrombosed popliteal vein may itself sometimes be palpated in the popliteal fossa, and the same is true of the common femoral vein at the groin. Palpation for deep thrombosis is not reliable since the vast majority of cases of deep vein thrombosis do not produce any palpable abnormality.

Varices of recent onset may easily be distinguished from chronic varices by palpation: newly dilated vessels sit on the surface of the muscle or bone, while chronic varices will have eroded into the underlying muscle or bone, often creating deep "boggy" or "spongy" pockets in the calf muscle, and deep palpable notches, especially over the anterior tibia.

If there are dilated varicosities in the lower leg, palpation often reveals numerous deep fascial defects in the calf along the course of the abnormal vein. These fascial defects often are sites through which incompetent perforating veins connect the superficial and deep venous systems. Unfortunately, not every palpable fascial defect contains an incompetent perforator, and not every incompetent perforator produces a palpable fascial defect. Fascial defects palpable from the surface primarily represent superficial tributaries emerging through openings in the superficial fascia (*Figure 6-5*). Traditionally, physicians have been taught that palpation of these fascial defects locates deep perforators, but in the author's experience of thousands of duplex examinations, these defects are saphenous vein branch points through superficial fascia. The deep perforators are physically located much more deeply, typically too deep to palpate.

The presence of significant obesity or of edema may make the underlying varicose veins difficult to palpate. Sometimes varices may be more readily palpable after edema has been reduced by a few minutes of compression with a blood pressure cuff. A muscular hernia can simulate a varicose vein on palpation, but the two can be distinguished because muscular herniae usually are situated in the anterolateral compartment of the leg. Hernias, not veins, will collapse on standing and during forced flexion of the foot on the leg.

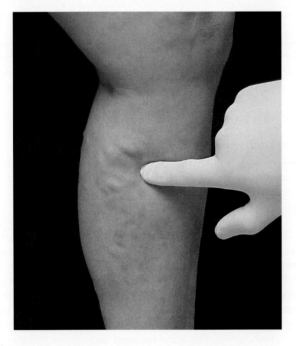

Figure 6-5. Palpation of a fascial defect at the site of a branch point through the *superficial* fascia. This is the most common fascial defect palpable in early stages of venous disease. These fascial defects typically do not arise from deep perforating veins.

Percussion

Venous percussion (sometimes referred to as Perthe's test, which must be distinguished from Perthe's maneuver to detect venous outflow obstruction) is a classic percussive physical examination finding that is useful to determine whether two venous segments are directly interconnected. Percussion can be used to trace out the course of veins already detected on palpation, to discover varicose veins that could not be palpated, and to assess the relationships between the various varicose vein networks.

The patient stands, and a vein segment suspected of containing incompetent valves is tapped at one position while an examining hand feels for a "pulse wave" at another position. The propagation of a palpable pulse wave demonstrates a patent superficial venous segment with incompetent valves connecting the two positions. The examination must be carried out with caution, because prolonged standing will cause even a normal vein to become distended, and if valves have floated open, a pulse wave may be propagated even in the absence of pathology. The technique is most valuable when a large bulging venous cluster in the lower leg has no obvious connection with a varicosity in the upper thigh, yet palpable pulse wave propagation between the two demonstrates the existence of an unseen connection.

Percussion can also be used to elucidate the course of any major vein. With the patient standing, the physician taps the lowest portion of the vein gently with the middle finger of the right hand (in the same way as to detect dullness over the lungs). The opposite hand searches above for a percussion wave, and the two hands (one over the other) then repeatedly ascend along the course of the vein to the proximal part of the limb. This entire procedure is repeated as often as necessary, vein by vein, until a clear anatomical picture has been brought into focus.

Veins and their connections gradually become better defined through inspection, palpation, and percussion to form a "venous map" that will later guide treatment. The courses of all the dilated veins that are identified may be marked along the leg with a pen, and later transcribed into the medical record as a map of all known areas of superficial reflux. An image of this penned map may be taken as well. This preliminary evaluation will be confirmed, more precisely defined, and completed through Doppler auscultation.

Doppler auscultation

The physical examination as described thus far can locate areas of venous dilatation, but it cannot distinguish between dilated veins of normal function or true varicosities that carry venous blood in a retrograde direction. Doppler examination is the easiest method used to distinguish incompetent refluxing varicose veins from large veins that carry antegrade flow. A complete description of the Doppler examination appears in Chapter 8.

When used as part of the physical examination, the upper hand holds the Doppler transducer along the axis of a vein to be examined, with the probe at an angle of 45° to the skin (*Figure 6-6*). If there are obviously dilated veins that have the appearance of varicosities, gentle tapping on the underlying vessel produces a strong Doppler signal and confirms the correct positioning of the transducer. The

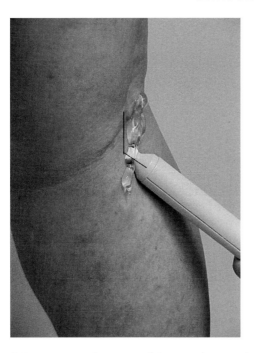

Figure 6-6. Correct placement of the Doppler transducer relative to the vein for maximal detection of flow sounds.

---

lower (or distal) hand then performs "augmentation" by compressing and releasing the underlying veins and muscles below the level of the probe. Compression causes forward flow in the direction of the valves, and release causes backward flow through incompetent valves. No signal occurs if the valves are competent and the blood cannot flow backwards.[3] These distal compression–decompression maneuvers are repeated while gradually ascending the limb to a level where the reflux can no longer be appreciated.

When telangiectasias are noted on the lateral surface of the thigh, the Doppler may be able to demonstrate reflux in feeding reticular veins that originate around the knee.[4] If there are no visible or palpable dilated varices, the presence or absence of retrograde flow is documented at the top, middle, and bottom of the long and short saphenous veins on each leg.

The Doppler examination adds a great deal of information to the physical examination, but it is not an actual imaging study. When there is any uncertainty or ambiguity about the physical examination or Doppler findings, duplex ultrasound should be performed.

PHYSICAL EXAMINATION (SUPINE)

After the standing examination, the patient is placed in a supine position on the examining table in order to carry out an exam without venous filling. When a patient is in the supine or prone position, the superficial vessels are empty, thus neither percussion nor Doppler auscultation provide any useful diagnostic information.[5,6] The deep venous system remains full when the patient is supine, and Doppler examination of the deep veins is best carried out with the patient in this position.

Inspection and light palpation

Each limb is again inspected, starting with the toes and moving proximally to the plantar arch, dorsum and surfaces of the feet, ankle, leg, knee, thigh, groin, and lesser pelvis. This inspection should detect interdigital mycosis, plantar callus, microulcers on the edges of an area of "atrophie blanche," and other small problems that may have been missed on the standing examination. If signs of pigmentation with stasis dermatitis, ulceration, or any other trophic disorder are noted, the lesions should be measured and photographed. At this time distal and proximal arterial pulses are palpated. An ankle-brachial index is obtained if there is any suspicion of arterial insufficiency.

Deep palpation

Deep palpation with the patient supine is useful to assess the texture of the deep subcutaneous planes and to detect the presence of edema, cellulitis, arteriovenous fistulas, and abnormal lymph nodes.

The examiner should firmly pinch and release the dorsum of each toe to detect edema. A normal toe can be pinched without leaving a skinfold upon release, but edema due to venous congestion causes the skin to remain tented in a skinfold after pinching. If there is lymphatic edema, the toe usually cannot be pinched, as the examiner's fingers slip over the toe.

Edema above the level of the toes is detected by applying gentle and prolonged pressure with the thumb, which will sink as far as the underlying hard plane (the medial surface of the tibia, for example). The amount and extent of edema are documented by measuring the leg with a tape measure at the narrowest part of the ankle, at the widest part of the leg, and at a point 10 cm above the superior margin of the patella.

Cellulitis may be recognized in the lower third of the leg, generally on the medial surface. At times it may be clinically very difficult to distinguish between chronic cellulites and lipodermatosclerosis. Cellulitis typically has clearly defined limits with a firm consistency. Varicose veins traversing the cellulitis may appear as large "canyons."

Doppler auscultation

Continuous-wave Doppler examination of the deep venous system is performed as described in Chapter 8. Evidence of obstruction or reflux are sought in the common iliofemoral trunk above the saphenofemoral junction and in the popliteal segment of the femoral vein.

COMPLEMENTARY CLINICAL MANEUVERS

Several traditional maneuvers are useful to help demonstrate classic venous pathophysiology, but none are reliable enough to displace the Doppler examination, which gives the same information and is far more reliable.[7,8]

Perthes' maneuver

Perthes' maneuver is intended to distinguish antegrade flow from retrograde flow in superficial varices.[9] Antegrade flow in a variceal system is an indication of deep venous obstruction. When the deep veins are not patent, superficial varices are an important pathway for venous return, and must not be sclerosed or surgically removed. To perform Perthes' maneuver, a tourniquet is placed over the proximal part of the varicose leg and the patient is made to ambulate. Increasing varicose congestion is a sign of deep system obstruction. The patient then lies down with the tourniquet in place, and the leg is elevated (Linton test). If varices distal to the tourniquet fail to drain after a few seconds, obstruction is suspected. These maneuvers are not consistently reliable, and are of primarily historical interest.

Trendelenburg's test
Another classical physical examination maneuver, the Trendelenburg test, may often distinguish distal venous congestion caused by superficial venous reflux from a problem caused by incompetence of the valves within the deep venous system.[10] To perform the Trendelenburg test, the leg is elevated until the congested superficial veins have all collapsed. A tourniquet (or the examiner's hand) is used to occlude a vein at a point of suspected reflux from the deep system into the superficial varicosity. Most often the greater saphenous vein is manually occluded just below the saphenofemoral junction at the groin, but any large vein may be investigated in a similar manner. The patient is made to stand, with the occlusion still in place. If the distal varicosity remains more or less empty, or fills very slowly, then the occluding hand or tourniquet is suddenly removed. Sudden dilation of the varicosity means that the principal entry point of high pressure into the superficial system has been correctly identified. Rapid filling of the varicosity despite manual occlusion of the suspected high point of reflux means that another reflux pathway is involved. If the filling is unusually rapid, it usually means that deep vein valves are incompetent between the groin and the level at which the reflux "escapes" the deep system (through an incompetent perforating vein) into the superficial system.

FURTHER CLINICAL ASSESSMENT
Examination of the arterial system, particularly of the lower limbs, consists of detection of peripheral pulses, palpation and auscultation of the arteries, and use of the Doppler to measure the systolic blood pressure at the ankle and the elbow to determine an ankle-brachial index. Clinical assessment may also include the osteoarticular system; particularly the ankles, knees, and hips, as well as a sensory and deep tendon reflex evaluation of the neurological system.

CHARTING
Varicose vein mapping
The anatomical and hemodynamic data that has been acquired through physical examination and Doppler investigation must be unambiguously recorded on a chart diagram. It is important to adopt some uniform system for documenting complex findings in the clinical chart that is consistent from one patient to the next in the phlebology practice. Color-coding can be helpful, but one must keep in mind that these colors will not be reproduced on photocopied records. Distribution of varicosities, sites of reflux

heard by Doppler, and location of surgical scars are important to record.

Preliminary assessment
A preliminary assessment is an important guide to determine subsequent management, and must address a number of interrelated issues:

- The severity of the functional and esthetic impairment
- The diagnosis of essential varicose veins
- The patency and valve competency of the deep venous system
- The absence of deep system angiodysplasia
- The topography of all varicose lesions
- The topography of the greater and lesser saphenous veins
- The degree of tissue sequelae
- The possible need for additional investigations to confirm, refute, or complete the diagnosis, or to guide the choice of treatment

Classification and quantification
A consensus document defines two alternative classification schemes for patients with venous disease: patients may be classified either by the type of chronic venous insufficiency or by the severity of the varicose disease.[11] This classification system of venous disorders is based upon clinical, etiological, anatomical, and pathophysiological data (CEAP classification, see Chapter 26). Each category is assigned a number according to a scale. The total value assigns a clinical stage of chronic venous disease (CVD). An alternative system is a varicose disease scoring system based on the maximum clinical diameter (MCD) as determined by palpation and measurement by calipers or tape measure after digital detection of the vessel margins. A Clinical Identification Grid is established by taking into account the MCD determined in each of the greater saphenous, lesser saphenous, and non-saphenous territories of each limb. This grid can be used to follow the course of the varicose disease in a quantitative fashion and to conduct studies on patients with a comparable varicose state.

Summary
The clinical examination of a patient suffering from superficial or deep venous insufficiency is complex because there are many pitfalls related to the high frequency of anatomical variants. The initial evaluation will thus include an appropriate clinical interview, including a description of the main presenting complaint and its history, the history of venous and other diseases, and any prior treatments together with their results. The results of complete inspection, detailed palpation, careful percussion, and Doppler auscultation are carefully recorded. It is helpful to use a standard drawing of the lower limbs to map the precise location of varicose dilatations and the information provided by Doppler auscultation (see Chapter 27 Appendix B, Figures 4 and 6). Other

Table 6-2
Goals of the Initial Examination

Determine the zones of involvement: GSV, LSV, lateral venous system

Assess for reflux in the inguinal region and popliteal fossa

Map superficial varicosities

Observe and record associated physical findings of venous disease

Doppler examination to determine if further testing is required to finalize treatment plan

Determine contraindications to treatment (see Chapters 12, 15, and 18)

physical findings, such as the margins of a leg ulcer, can also be indicated on the same drawing.

A summary of the examination, the proposed diagnosis, and documentation of decisions concerning any complementary investigations and treatment will also be included. In the majority of cases, this assessment allows a precise positive venous mapping, facilitating evaluation of the current and long-term risks of venous insufficiency *(Table 6-2)*. The medical record documents the presenting complaint, history, symptoms and signs, as well as a detailed set of anatomical and venodynamic diagrams. Integration of all this data allows the formulation of an appropriate management program for each patient.

References

(1) Sparey C, Haddad N, Sissons G, Rosser S, De Cossart L. *The effect of pregnancy on the lower-limb venous system of women with varicose veins.* Eur J Vasc Endovasc Surg 1999; 18(4):294–299.

(2) Weiss RA, Duffy D. *Clinical Benefits of Lightweight Compression: Reduction of Venous- Related Symptoms by Ready-to-Wear Lightweight Gradient Compression Hosiery.* Dermatol Surg 1999; 25(9):701–704.

(3) Weiss RA. *Evaluation of the venous system by Doppler ultrasound and photoplethysmography or light reflection rheography before sclerotherapy.* Semin Dermatol 1993; 12:78–87.

(4) Weiss RA, Weiss MA. *Doppler ultrasound findings in reticular veins of the thigh subdermic lateral venous system and implications for sclerotherapy.* J Dermatol Surg Onc 1993; 19(10):947–951.

(5) Weiss RA, Weiss MA. *Continuous wave venous Doppler examination for pretreatment diagnosis of varicose and telangiectatic veins.* Dermatol Surg 1995; 21:58–62.

(6) Schultz-Ehrenburg U, Hubner H-J. *Reflux diagnosis with Doppler ultrasound (monograph).* Stuttgart: Schattauer, 1989.

(7) Raju S, Fredericks R. Evaluation of methods for detecting venous reflux. Perspectives in venous insufficiency. Arch Surg 1990 Nov; 125(11):1463–7.

(8) McMullin GM, Smith PDC, Scurr JH. *A study of tourniquets in the investigation of venous insufficiency.* Phlebol 1991; 6:133–139.

(9) Perthes G. *Uber die operation der unterschenkelvaricen nach trendelenburg.* Deutsche Med Wehrschr 1895; 21:253–261.

(10) Sherman RS. *Varicose veins: anatomy re-evaluation of Trendelenburg tests and operating procedure.* Surg Clin North Am 1964; 44:1369–1377.

(11) Kistner RL, Eklof B, Masuda EM. *Diagnosis of chronic venous disease of the lower extremities: the "CEAP" classification* [see comments]. Mayo Clin Proc 1996; 71(4):338–345.

CHAPTER 7

Common Clinical Presentations

There are many illustrative cases in each of the chapters on treatment, but several clinical situations are common enough to warrant special presentation. In addition, there are some more unusual presentations that are commonly misdiagnosed. These are important for the clinician to recognize, and are presented here.

Case No. I: Axial Varicosities in a Young Male

A 29-year-old computer-networking consultant who travels extensively presents with varicose veins present since the age of 20 years and painful for the last 2 years. He noticed the initial onset while playing tennis. Both parents have a history of varicose veins. The presenting veins are situated along the anterior surface of the left thigh and the medial surface of the left lower limb.

EXAM

On the left leg, a varicose vein is visible and palpable extending from the upper anterior thigh (not to the groin), down to the knee. Another large varicose vein is seen originating at the medial calf length (mean diameter: 12 mm). Percussion allows a fluid wave to be felt on the thigh portion when the calf portion is tapped repeatedly *(Figure 7-1A,B)*.

DOPPLER

No incompetence is noted at the left saphenofemoral junction, even with the Valsalva maneuver. Marked incompetence is heard along the entire visible vein, in the region of the greater saphenous vein (GSV) at the level of the knee and in the lower segment of the varicosity in the calf. There is no reflux in the left lesser saphenous vein.

FUNCTIONAL TESTS

D-PPG shows refill time of 19 seconds.

DUPLEX EXAMINATION

A duplex ultrasound exam is ordered with an RVT knowledgeable in the superficial venous system, but the patient's insurance plan only pays for a duplex exam at a specific radiology group. The exam report reads, "No evidence of deep venous thrombosis. Reflux seen in some superficial veins."

TREATMENT

Based on the fact that the patient does not desire surgery nor is reflux detected at the SFJ by the general radiologist's duplex ultrasound technician, the patient is treated with 3% STS (sodium tetradecyl sulfate) injections of 1 cc at three sites total. At one month, significant reduction of the diameter of the varicosities is noted. A second treatment is performed with 1% STS at 6 sites. Follow-up one month later shows complete resolution.

LONG-TERM FOLLOW-UP

The patient returns in two years with a slight recurrence in the calf *(Figure 7-1C)*. Duplex examination reveals reflux at the SFJ and along the GSV. Treatment consists of ligation at the SFJ followed by stripping of the thigh portion of the GSV. The calf varicosity is injected with 1% STS one month after surgery. The patient remains free of disease at 5 years.

COMMENTARY

Reflux in the anterolateral tributary of the GSV extending down the leg resulted in reflux in a branch varicosity of the calf. Recurrence at two years was due either to new development of reflux in the GSV related to genetic susceptibility, or to the possible failure to initially diagnose SFJ incompetence because of an inadequate duplex examination.

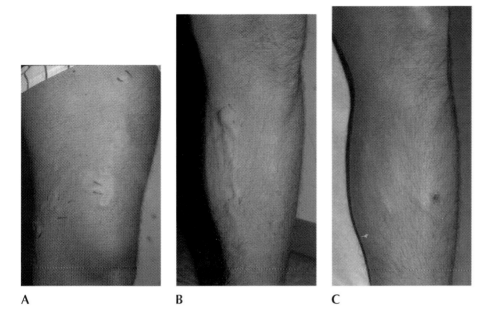

Figure 7-1. **(A)** Thigh varicosities before treatment. **(B)** Calf varicosities before treatment. **(C)** Recurrence of calf varicosities (although smaller) two years after initial sclerotherapy.

A   B   C

Case No. II: Axial Varicosities in a Middle-Aged Woman

A 45-year-old woman who works as a cashier presents with a large varicose vein on the medial surface of the right leg. This lesion is very bothersome aesthetically, and is "hot at the end of the day" with associated aching of the leg. There is a history of superficial venous thrombosis during the second pregnancy 10 years earlier, during which this vein was noted to develop. Family history is positive for varicose veins in the mother and sister.

EXAM

Inspection and palpation reveal a large spongy varicose vein that originates in the groin, splits on the anterior thigh and terminates near the ankle. A few small telangiectasias are seen near the ankle. The clinical diameter of the dilatation is 12 mm standing, but 8 mm at 30 degrees reverse

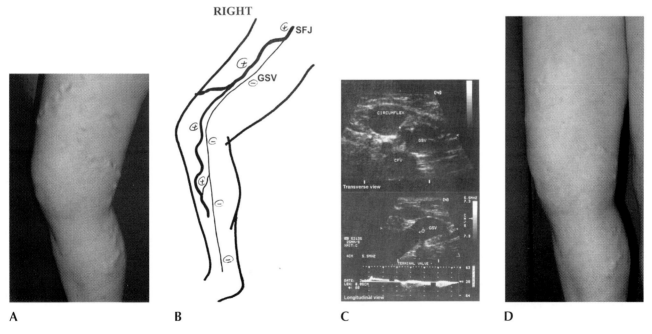

A   B   C   D

Figure 7-2. **(A)** Varicosities before treatment. **(B)** Map of duplex findings indicates sites of reflux. **(C)** Duplex image of the incompetent SFJ in the inguinal region. Upper transverse view highlights enlarged circumflex branch. Lower longitudinal view shows enlarged GSV and terminal valves during Valsalva maneuver. **(D)** Improvement after ligation of the SFJ alone. Acoustic signal graph shows reverse flow.

Trendelenburg. Percussion suggests a continuous varicose vein from the thigh to the mid-calf *(Figure 7-2A)*.

DOPPLER

Doppler auscultation (slowly ascending with the transducer from the dilatation to the groin) reveals incompetence of the upper greater saphenous vein, particularly at its junction: cough and the Valsalva maneuver reveal severe reflux. No reflux can be heard in the thigh portion of the greater saphenous vein.

FUNCTIONAL TESTS

Not performed; patient referred directly for duplex ultrasound.

DUPLEX EXAMINATION

Duplex examination reveals reflux originating at the SFJ but diverted through the circumflex tributary and extending down the leg as a branch varicosity. The vast majority of the GSV is normal. *Figure 7-2B* shows the mapping of duplex findings; the duplex image is seen in transverse and longitudinal views in *Figure 7-2C*.

TREATMENT

The patient undergoes ligation alone at the SFJ, without stripping of the GSV, since the vast majority of the GSV is normal with a diameter of 4 mm. The patient experiences marked reduction in varicosities after ligation at the SFJ without an additional treatment *(Figure 7-2D)*. Within one month, the remaining shrunken branch varicosity is treated with 1% STS with complete resolution after two treatments one month apart.

COMMENTARY

A branch varicosity originating with an incompetent SFJ but with a normal thigh GSV could be treated by a number of methods, including ambulatory phlebectomy after ligation at the junction. Due to the normal thigh portion of the GSV, this patient did not require GSV stripping or RF endovenous occlusion of the GSV. Only when the thigh portion of the saphenous vein is incompetent and larger than 7 mm when standing are surgical stripping or the equivalent typically required. Ligation with accompanying sclerotherapy (duplex or non-duplex guided) or ambulatory phlebectomy may suffice in these cases.

Case No. III: New Onset of a Varicose Vein in a Teenager

A 17-year-old female develops a varicose vein during puberty. Family history is non-contributory. The patient presents for treatment due to the appearance, as there are no symptoms.

EXAM

Inspection reveals a blue varicose vein on the medial calf in Boyd's region *(Figure 7-3A)*. Palpation and percussion do not reveal a varicose greater saphenous vein or lesser saphenous vein.

DOPPLER

Doppler auscultation demonstrates reflux in the visible varicose vein with some reflux detectable in the thigh. Both saphenous veins are competent at and below the junctions.

FUNCTIONAL TESTS

Not performed.

DUPLEX EXAMINATION

Due to the reflux detectable in the thigh on Doppler examination, a duplex examination is performed, showing a medial branch varicosity originating off the GSV in the thigh extending directly to the visible varicose vein. *Figure 7-3B* shows the mapping of duplex findings; the duplex image of the incompetent branch off of the GSV is seen in *Figure 7-3C*.

TREATMENT

Duplex-guided sclerotherapy in the thigh is performed; 1% STS is used at origin of the branch point *(Figure 7-3D)*, followed by 0.2% STS injection in the visible portion of the vein. Visible disappearance and contraction are noted immediately *(Figure 7-3E)*. Complete resolution occurred after one treatment.

COMMENTARY

Even a patient as young as 17 can develop a single branch varicosity in the thigh leading to a "reticular" varicose vein on the medial aspect of the calf. In this early stage, it can be efficiently and effectively treated by duplex-guided sclerotherapy with just one treatment.

Case No. IV: Lateral Venous System

A 46 year-old woman complains of the appearance of the veins on her thigh. These had developed during pregnancy and gradually worsened over the following 15 years. She has no significant symptoms.

EXAM

Clinical examination reveals a prominent blue reticular vein network with associated telangiectasias of the lateral thigh that faded from sight below the knee. No other abnormal veins *(Figure 7-4A)*.

DOPPLER

Doppler auscultation reveals mild reflux along the lower course of the reticular vein, loudest near the lateral knee.

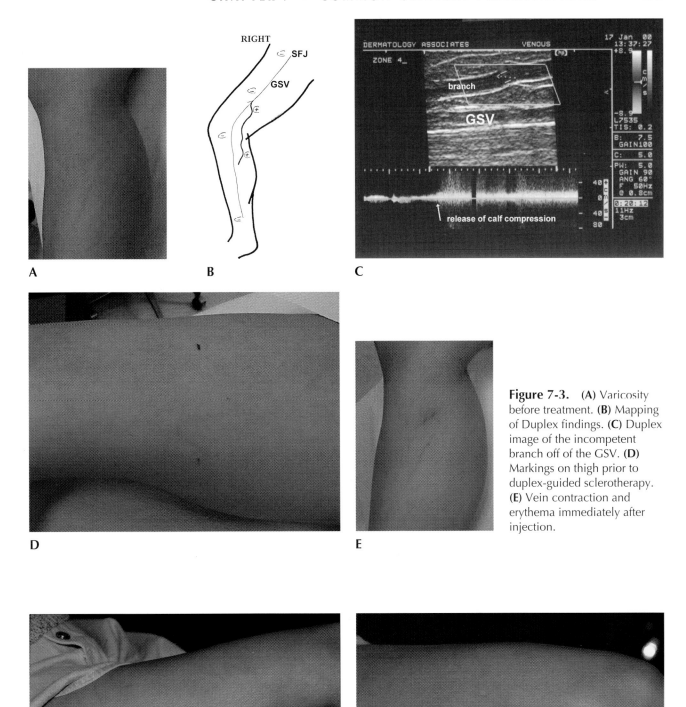

Figure 7-3. (A) Varicosity before treatment. (B) Mapping of Duplex findings. (C) Duplex image of the incompetent branch off of the GSV. (D) Markings on thigh prior to duplex-guided sclerotherapy. (E) Vein contraction and erythema immediately after injection.

Figure 7-4. (A) Lateral venous system before sclerotherapy. (B) Lateral venous system after sclerotherapy.

FUNCTIONAL TESTS
Not performed.

DUPLEX EXAMINATION
Not performed.

ASSESSMENT
Incompetent lateral venous system manifesting in prominent reticular veins and some associated telangiectasias.

TREATMENT
A series of two treatments are performed. The first uses 1% STS, 0.3–0.5 cc into each of several sites 4–6 cm apart along the reticular veins with a total of 4 cc, and 0.1% STS 0.5 cc into each group of telangiectasias with a total of 3 cc. Compression hosiery (18–20 mm Hg at the ankle) are worn for two weeks after each treatment.

At the second treatment, the reticular veins have greatly shrunk. A few hyperpigmented nodular areas are drained of blood (see Chapter 24). A total of 3 cc of 0.5% STS are injected into the remaining reticulars, and 1.5 cc total of 0.1% STS into the telangiectasias. After two months, the leg has cleared nicely *(Figure 7-4B)*.

COMMENTARY
This patient is an example of the commonly seen pattern of an abnormal lateral venous system without other venous abnormalities, which usually responds extremely well to compression sclerotherapy.

Case No. V: Doppler-Guided Sclerotherapy of Non-truncal Varicosity and Telangiectasia

A 26-year-old woman presents for cosmetic varicosity and telangiectasias on the medial aspect of the right lower leg. Occasional burning is noted in the region of telangiectasias.

EXAM
A blue reticular varicose vein protrudes slightly, beginning just above the medial aspect of the knee and terminating in the mid-calf in a cluster of telangiectasias *(Figure 7-5A)*.

DOPPLER
Doppler auscultation shows slight reflux at the proximal end of the visible varicosity at the medial aspect of the knee, with negative augmentation on Valsalva maneuver.

FUNCTIONAL TESTS
Not performed.

DUPLEX EXAMINATION
Not performed. (Note: This patient's treatments were performed in 1990 and early 1991. At that time, the author had not yet acquired a duplex ultrasound machine, and so relied on Doppler to initiate treatment.)

ASSESSMENT
Non-truncal varicosity with associated telangiectasias and venulectasias, with reflux of a branch of the GSV. Normal SFJ.

TREATMENT
Injections are performed on two occasions, one month apart, using a total of 2 cc of 1% polidocanol (POL) into the varicosity and 1.5 cc total of 0.5% POL into the telangiectasias at each session. Compression hosiery (18–20 mm Hg at the ankle) are worn for two weeks after each treatment.

After doing very well initially, the patient returns six months later complaining of the emergence of new, deeper violet vessels just below the knee *(Figure 7–5B)*. The original blue varicosity is gone. No reticular vein can be easily seen. There is faint audible reflux at the site of the matting that can be traced above the knee to the lower thigh, but attempts to cannulate that site are unsuccessful. Therefore, only the matting vessels are injected with 0.2% STS.

One month later, she has significantly improved *(Figure 7-5C)*.

Four months later, she returns with a worsened pattern: a reemergence of the matting below the knee with new areas of matting above the knee *(Figure 7-5D)*. At this time, the Doppler exam is repeated, with marking of the leg at the site of loudest reflux. Valsalva maneuver is negative, and exam of the saphenofemoral junction with Doppler is negative. This time, the author is able to aspirate venous blood at the marked site (about 1 cm below the skin surface on the medial aspect of the thigh about 4 cm above the knee), and 1 cc of 1% STS is injected. The telangiectasia are again injected with 1 cc of 0.2% STS.

At three months since the last treatment, the patient's leg has cleared very well *(Figure 7-E)*. She has been seen at intervals for other conditions, and the vessels have stayed clear for nearly nine years. Had this patient not cleared, she would have been referred to a vascular lab in the hope of finding the location of the reflux by duplex.

COMMENTARY
This patient illustrates the difficulty that can arise when one relies only on Doppler findings in treating varicose branches of axial veins. Initial Doppler examination, whether due to physician inexperience or to variation in the clinical presentation of the vein on that day, did not detect the highest point of reflux. This led to only short-term success, followed by early recurrence and matting. Only after the highest point of reflux was diagnosed and treated was long-term success achieved. When a patient presents today with these clinical findings on the medial lower leg, the author always follows the positive Doppler exam with a duplex study of the affected leg, in order to be sure that the highest source of reflux is accurately treated from the very beginning.

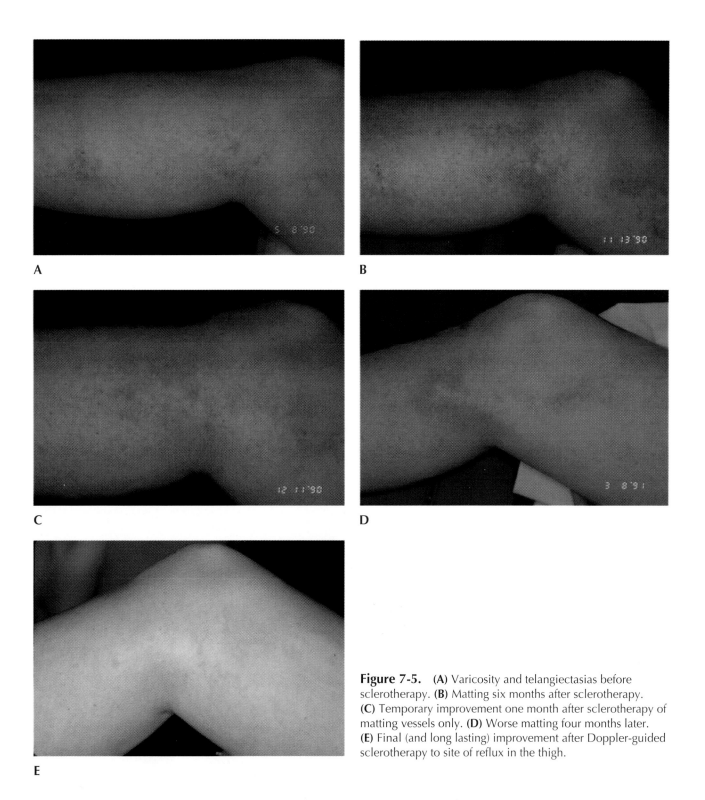

Figure 7-5. **(A)** Varicosity and telangiectasias before sclerotherapy. **(B)** Matting six months after sclerotherapy. **(C)** Temporary improvement one month after sclerotherapy of matting vessels only. **(D)** Worse matting four months later. **(E)** Final (and long lasting) improvement after Doppler-guided sclerotherapy to site of reflux in the thigh.

Case No. VI: Varicose and Spider Veins during Pregnancy

A 32-year-old woman, seven months into her first pregnancy, presents with widely disseminated varicose veins and associated "roadmap" legs that have appeared explosively over the preceding two months. Family history is positive for large varicose veins. The patient is very anxious, not only because of the cosmetic appearance, but because of worsening pain over the preceding two weeks. She is willing to undergo any treatment to relieve the symptoms and to reduce the "horrible" appearance of her legs.

EXAM

Physical examination reveals numerous tortuous varicose veins (maximum clinical diameter: 7 mm) extending over the entire medial and lateral surface of the both thighs down to the ankles. While standing, large rubbery veins are palpable extending into the inguinal fold on the anteromedial thigh. Large reticular vein networks are extensive. Addi-

tionally there are myriads of violaceous telangiectatic webs that make visible identification of the larger varicose veins difficult (*Figure 7-6A and Figure 7-6C*).

DOPPLER

Reflux is detected over almost every visible vein, including the telangiectatic webs.

FUNCTIONAL TESTS

D-PPG reveals a refill time of 12 seconds on the right leg and 15 seconds on the left leg.

DUPLEX EXAMINATION

Duplex ultrasound shows no evidence of DVT. Superficial system not examined.

TREATMENT

Compression hose of 30–40 mm Hg significantly relieve the pain. The patient is told that since this is the first pregnancy, spontaneous resolution is highly likely, but that she should return for re-evaluation 4–6 months postpartum. The pa-

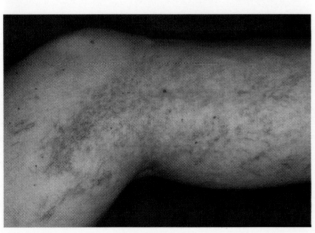

A

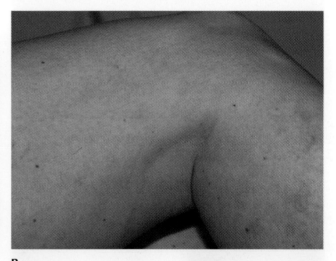

B

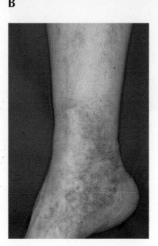

C

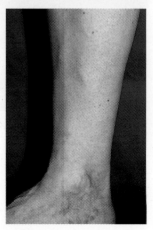

D

Figure 7-6. **(A)** Pregnant woman's thigh. **(B)** Postpartum spontaneous improvement. **(C)** Pregnant woman's ankle. **(D)** Postpartum spontaneous improvement.

tient returns in 6 months. Her leg is examined and shows marked spontaneous resolution of all except some small reticular veins (*Figure 7–6B and Figure 7-6D*). No reflux is detected by Doppler along any of the saphenous veins. She is told to wear graduated compression support hose at the earliest knowledge of her next planned pregnancy. Should any residual varicose veins occur following subsequent pregnancies, they will be addressed at that time.

COMMENTARY

Multiple saphenous varicose veins with associated venous hypertension changes seen on the skin surface that develop during pregnancy can clear spontaneously postpartum, even when severe, as in this case. With a positive family history, a woman should use compression as an important preventive component of the treatment of varicose veins, especially during a first pregnancy. Such compression can relieve symptoms in nearly all cases, and allow treatment to be deferred until enough time has passed for natural postpartum improvement to occur.

Case No. VII: Spider Angioma at the Ankle

A 66-year-old woman is seen with a red to violaceous spider telangiectasia of the lateral surface of the right ankle. She states that she has no symptoms, and that this is a purely cosmetic concern. Family history is negative for varicose veins. No edema is present.

EXAM

Physical examination does not reveal any varicose veins, edema, or trophic disorders. A spider telangiectasia is an isolated finding on the ankle (*Figure 7-7A*).

DOPPLER

Doppler auscultation demonstrates no incompetence of any saphenous veins.

FUNCTIONAL TESTS

Not performed.

DUPLEX EXAMINATION

Not performed.

TREATMENT

Since no associated venous system abnormalities are found, laser treatment of the vessels is performed with 14-millisecond pulses of 1064 nm laser with a 6 mm spot size. Resolution is achieved with one treatment (*Figure 7-7B*).

COMMENTARY

This isolated ectatic telangiectasia is related to sun or aging, with collagen degeneration of the vessel wall. It may also be a small A–V malformation. This is a primary indication for laser treatment, as sclerotherapy for a vessel with a possible arterial connection would require greater caution and entails greater risks. Additionally, note that patients aged 65 and over generally respond with a more vigorous destructive reaction to sclerosing solutions, so that sclerosant concentrations should be halved.

Case No. VIII: Unusual Case of Minocycline-induced Hyperpigmentation after Sclerotherapy of the Lateral Venous System

A 39-year-old woman complains of the appearance of the veins on her thigh. These have developed gradually over the preceding 20 years without symptoms. The patient also has a history of cystic acne requiring multiple courses of various antibiotics for control. At the time sclerotherapy starts, she has been on minocycline 100 mg twice daily for the preceding 18 months.

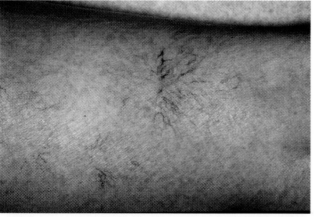

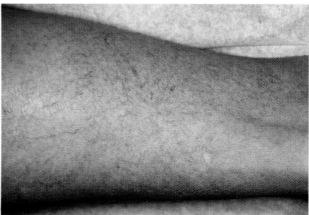

A

B

Figure 7-7. **(A)** Spider telangiectasia of ankle before treatment. **(B)** Improvement after one treatment with the 1064 nm laser.

EXAM

Physical examination does not reveal any varicose veins. There are some telangiectasias scattered on the upper lateral thigh associated with a prominent blue reticular vein that courses distally onto the lateral aspect of the calf *(Figure 7-8A)*.

DOPPLER

Doppler auscultation demonstrates incompetence of the reticular vein, loudest at the lateral knee.

FUNCTIONAL TESTS

Not performed.

DUPLEX EXAMINATION

Not performed.

ASSESSMENT

Typical abnormal lateral venous system.

TREATMENT

Two sessions are performed a month apart using 0.1% STD injected into the telangiectasias (0.2 cc at each site) and 0.5% STD (0.5% at several sites, 4–6 cm apart, 3 cc total) along the reticular vein. Compression hosiery (18–20 mm Hg at the ankle) are worn for two weeks after each treatment. The veins fade over two months, leaving in their place a blue-gray linear area where the reticular vein had been *(Figure 7-8B)*.

No nodules are present, and no blood can be drained. She is switched to doxycycline to control her acne. Very gradually, the pigmentation begins to fade. No further sclerotherapy is necessary, as no residual veins are present. At one year, the pigmentation has completely cleared *(Figure 7-8C)*.

COMMENTARY

Minocycline has been associated with unusual depositions of blue-gray pigmentation in the skin. Two of the authors have seen this in approximately four patients over 16 years of experience with more than 14,000 patients. In each case, cessation of the minocycline resulted in very slow, but satisfactory, fading of the pigmentation.

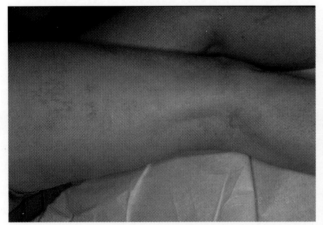

A

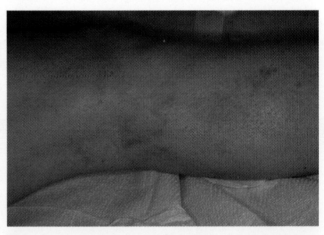

B

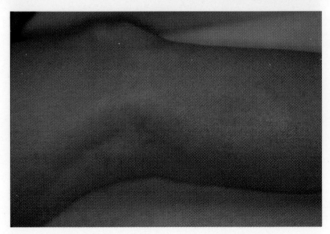

C

Figure 7-8.   **(A)** Lateral venous system before sclerotherapy. **(B)** Blue-gray linear post-sclerotherapy pigmentation due to minocycline. **(C)** Clearing one year after cessation of minocycline.

Case No. IX: Initial Presentation with "Matting"-Type Telangiectasias on the Medial Thigh

A 41-year-old woman complains of the appearance of the veins on her medial thigh. These have developed gradually over the preceding 15 years without symptoms.

EXAM

Physical examination does not reveal any varicose veins. There is an arclike grouping of tiny telangiectasias on the upper medial thigh with an abrupt cut-off, and no visible associated reticular vein *(Figure 7-9)*. Transillumination fails to reveal any reticular vein.

DOPPLER

Doppler auscultation is negative.

FUNCTIONAL TESTS

Not performed.

DUPLEX EXAMINATION

Negative for any vessels feeding into this group of telangiectasias.

ASSESSMENT

Prominent group of tiny telangiectasias with pattern that suggests a reticular vein should be present, but none can be found.

TREATMENT

Using the polarizing lighted headpiece for better visualization, the telangiectasias were injected with 0.1% STS, 0.5 cc

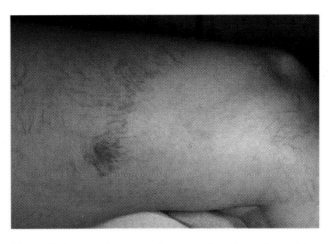

Figure 7-9. Matting-type telangiectasia without detectable reticular vein on medial thigh prior to any type of treatment.

total. Two sessions were necessary for adequate improvement. The patient wore 18–20 mm compression hosiery for one week after each session. Two years later, recurrent vessels were treated successfully with sclerotherapy.

COMMENTARY

In this situation, after attempts to find a reflux source are unsuccessful, one can begin treatment. Given the very small diameter of the telangiectasias and the patient's fair skin, one has more flexibility in treatment choices. Sclerotherapy, laser, and intense pulsed light can all be considered. Even though no reticular vein could be detected, the authors would still recommend one-week compression hosiery after any type of treatment. Use of the polarizing lighted headpiece improved visualization and facilitated successful sclerotherapy. The need for retreatment of re-emerging telangiectasias as years pass is common, especially on the medial lower thigh.

CHAPTER 8

Continuous-Wave Doppler

When to Perform a Doppler Examination

When there is a need to supplement the physical examination, continuous-wave Doppler (CWD) is the test modality most often available to the clinician. Most leading phlebologists regard the CWD examination as an essential part of every physical examination of the venous system, and consider the handheld Doppler to be the "stethoscope" of the phlebologist. There are some practitioners, however, who perform a Doppler examination only when there is clinical evidence to suggest that the patient has more than just end-branch spider vein abnormalities.

Continuous-wave Doppler can provide essential information in many clinical presentations: when a patient complains of pain related to varicosities, when the physical examination reveals varicosities larger than 3 mm in diameter, when varicosities of any size extend into the groin or the popliteal fossa, and when a feeding vessel is sought for a focal area of grouped venulectases (1–2 mm).[1] Guidelines for the use of this diagnostic aid to physical examination are listed in Table 8-1. Doppler examination may suggest the need for additional testing, but is especially helpful as an inexpensive screening tool if a duplex ultrasound exam is not to be initially performed.

The purposes of the CWD examination are multiple: to identify or rule out reflux at the saphenofemoral and saphenopopliteal junctions, to trace the course of varicosities, and to identify other points of reflux through incompetent perforating veins in the thigh, calf, and ankle (Table 8-2).

Table 8-1
Guidelines for Use of Doppler

Physical Finding	Suspected Etiology
Varicosity > 3 mm into groin region	Saphenous or pudendal reflux
Varicosity > 3 mm into popliteal fossa	Saphenous or posterior thigh perforator reflux
Varicosity > 3 mm, coursing over majority of calf or thigh	Branch varicosities of saphenous system
Grouped reticular (as small as 1.5 mm)	Major reflux of LSVS
	Saphenous tributary reflux associated with LSVS
Any varicosity or reticular vein causing pain	Reflux associated with saphenous system
Ankle telangiectasias (corona phlebectasia)	Reflux of GSV when medial
	Reflux of LSV when lateral

CWD also gives an approximate sense of the speed and phasicity of venous flow at the saphenofemoral junction.

All physicians are familiar with the rapid pulsatile sound of CWD as used for the detection of fetal heart sounds and faint arterial sounds. In general, higher velocities of flow produce higher-pitched Doppler sounds, and higher volumes of flow produce louder sounds. Venous flow produces a nonpulsatile fairly low-pitched ghostly blowing sound ("wind in the rigging") that often is heard as a background to arterial sounds.

Principles of Doppler Ultrasound

Doppler ultrasound is named after the famed Austrian physicist Johann Christian Doppler, who in 1842 explained an apparent increase or decrease in the frequency of waves emitted or reflected from an object that is moving toward or away from the observer. The essence of the principle is this: when the object is moving toward the observer, each wave is emitted or reflected from a position a little closer than the one before, thus each wave comes back a little sooner than expected, and the frequency appears to be higher. When the object is moving away from the observer, each wave comes back a little later than it would if the object were not moving, so the frequency appears to be lower.

The Doppler principle applies to all types of wave phenomena in all types of media. The principle is familiar for its use in radar speed detection: when a radar gun is pointed at

Table 8-2
Purpose of CWD Examination

Identify or rule out reflux at the saphenofemoral and saphenopopliteal junctions
Identify most proximal point of reflux through branches off the saphenous system
Trace course of varicosities
Identify other points of reflux through incompetent perforating veins in the thigh, calf, and ankle

a stationary object, the reflected (returning) radar waves have the same wavelength and frequency as the emitted (outgoing) waves, but when the signal is reflected from a moving object (such as a car) the reflected waves have a wavelength and frequency that are different from those of the emitted waves. If the car is moving away from the radar gun, the reflected waves are farther apart than the emitted waves. If the car is moving toward the radar gun, the reflected waves are closer together than the emitted waves.

Doppler ultrasound probes use piezoelectric crystals to emit high-frequency (ultrasound) waves and to detect reflected waves returning to the probe. Ultrasound waves are reflected from many structures, but all the waves that return with the same frequency are ignored. When sound waves are reflected from blood cells that are moving relative to the probe, the frequency of the emitted waves is compared to that of the reflected waves, and the difference between the two (the Doppler shift) is an indication of the speed and direction of flow *(Figure 8-1)*.

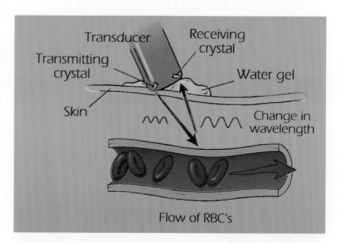

Figure 8-1. Schematic of Doppler ultrasound operation. The application of water-based gel allows a continuous medium for transmission of ultrasound. Red blood cells flowing away from the probe cause a decreased frequency reflected to the receiving crystal. This frequency shift is detected by the receiving crystal and causes an audible sound.

Handheld Doppler units use the Doppler shift frequency to modulate an audible sound that is lowest in pitch when there is slow flow and highest in pitch when there is high flow. The volume of a pitch depends on the number of cells flowing at a given velocity. The sound produced by a Doppler unit is a mixture of many different sound frequencies, because not all of the blood cells flow through the vessel at the same speed. Turbulence causes abrupt variations in flow velocity and direction, while friction produces a smooth gradient of velocity from the slowest-moving layers of fluid adjacent to the vessel walls to the fastest-moving layers in the middle of the stream. Each point of signal reflection makes a separate contribution to the aggregate sound reflecting the overall flow conditions within the vessel.

Many units can also produce a printed tracing of the speed, direction, and relative amount of flow. Unidirectional Doppler measures the speed of flow relative to the probe without regard to the direction, while bidirectional graphing Doppler can identify movement as being either toward or away from the transducer. Bidirectional Doppler is primarily used for waveform analysis of arterial pulses and is less useful for the analysis of venous reflux. In the venous system, the timing of flow sounds relative to various maneuvers that are performed best assesses the direction of flow.[2] Phlebologists have come to prefer bidirectional Doppler in recent years principally because most third-party payors will reimburse a patient for Doppler examination only if there is a printed bidirectional tracing.

Doppler probes of different frequencies are used depending on the depth of the vessels to be examined, because lower frequency ultrasound penetrates deeper through tissues before being reflected back to the transducer. A Doppler probe that emits frequencies of 8–10 MHz is best suited to examining vessels that are less than 2 cm deep, although we find it difficult to hear reflux greater than 1 cm below the skin surface with these frequencies. Vessels up to 4 cm in depth may be examined using a 5 MHz probe.[3]

To prevent signal loss, a coupling gel must be applied between the skin and the Doppler probe to eliminate any air between the two surfaces. Good results will only be obtained with a liberal amount of gel and a very light touch where the probe makes contact with the skin. The Doppler probe angle is also very important in obtaining a good quality signal: the Doppler effect detects only movement towards or away from the probe, so if the Doppler probe is at right angles to a vessel, there will be no net Doppler shift of the reflected signal, and thus no flow will be detected. A probe angle of 45 degrees relative to the vessel gives the most consistent signal with the least variation due to changes in the direction of unseen vessels.[4]

CW Doppler Ultrasound in Phlebology

Although Doppler ultrasound is useful in the assessment of any condition in which arterial or venous flow dynamics are altered, the primary phlebological purpose of venous Doppler ultrasound examination is the detection of retrograde venous flow (venous reflux) due to absent or malfunctioning venous valves.

To use CWD for venous diagnosis, one must be familiar with a standard examination and with the usual findings in a normal patient. Under normal conditions, spontaneous and respirophasic forward (cephalad) flow may be recorded in the common femoral vein, at the saphenofemoral junction, and occasionally at the popliteal vein. Doppler ultrasound is relatively insensitive to slow flow, thus detection of forward flow in other veins usually requires manual augmentation (squeezing the distal extremity in order to increase the volume and velocity of antegrade flow at the point of auscultation).

Abnormal spontaneous flow is detectable in areas of stenosis, where the normal flow velocity speeds up as it passes through the narrowed channel. Abnormal spontaneous flow may also be heard in any vein when the legs are extremely congested due to significant venous reflux. Retrograde venous flow is always abnormal: the detection of more than a half second of retrograde flow at any level always indicates incompetence of the valves in the vein being examined, whether the retrograde flow occurs spontaneously, upon Valsalva, or with reverse augmentation (*Figure 8-2*).

The Doppler examination is usually performed with the patient standing or sitting, because gravitational hydrostatic pressure enhances the volume and velocity of retrograde flow and makes it easier to detect. To perform this test, the non-dominant hand gently squeezes the leg well below (distal compression) or above (proximal compression) the point of auscultation, while the dominant hand holds the Doppler transducer lightly against the skin. Under normal circumstances, flow should be heard only during active distal compression. Flow that is heard during proximal compression or immediately after the release of distal compression is retrograde flow—a clear sign of incompetent valves.

FLOW PATTERNS WITH COMPETENT VALVES

In veins with normally competent valves, distal compression (augmentation) increases the amount and velocity of forward flow, producing an audible signal during compression. After manual compression is released, the sound normally ceases within a half-second as venous valves close to prevent reflux. In normal veins, proximal compression (reverse augmentation) causes a brief reflux of less than a half second duration while the valves float closed, after which there is no further reflux.

FLOW PATTERNS WITH INCOMPETENT VALVES

In veins with incompetent valves, distal compression initially causes a normal forward flow signal. When compression is released, instead of a cessation of flow, there is a new abnormal flow sound due to retrograde (downward) flow of the same blood that was initially propelled upward by compression. When venous valves are incompetent, proximal compression causes prolonged reflux as blood flows unhindered backwards through an incompetent valve. As proximal compression is released, reverse flow stops. If the legs

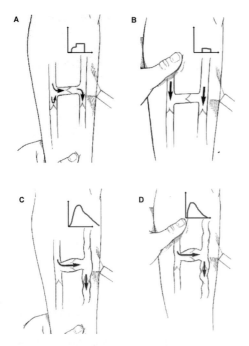

Figure 8-2. Proximal and distal compression Doppler ultrasound examination. *Competent Perforator Valve.* **(A)** During distal compression, brief normal forward flow is heard (inset). As distal compression is released, blood flows backwards under gravity but is rapidly stopped by competent valves. **(B)** During proximal compression, a brief sound is heard (inset), which rapidly concludes as blood movement is stopped by competent valves. *Incompetent Perforator Valves.* **(C)** During distal compression, a brief normal upward flow is heard; however, as distal compression is released, blood flow continues backwards with a prolonged sound (inset) as incompetent valves are unable to prevent continued flow propelled by hydrostatic pressure (gravity) *This is the most reliable way to measure for reflux.* **(D)** During proximal compression, a long sound is heard (inset) as blood movement is detected through a wide-open incompetent valve. The sound continues as long as compression is applied. As compression is released, flow stops. Deflections of the sound graph are shown here as a unidirectional Doppler tracing. Bidirectional Dopplers will show sound forward and reversed above and below the baseline.

are very congested with blood, low-velocity spontaneous forward flow may be detected shortly after the cessation of reflux.

RECOGNITION OF FLOW CHARACTERISTICS
The mixture of pitches in the Doppler sound changes depending on the velocities with which red cells are flowing, and the volume of each pitch in the mixture changes depending on the number of red cells flowing at any given velocity. Characteristic changes in the sound accompany anatomic and physiologic changes in the underlying vessels. The recognition of such sound characteristics requires much experience, but with practice, much more can be learned by

Doppler auscultation than by simple examination of a printed Doppler tracing. For example, when the transducer is moved along a superficial vein, incompetent perforating veins may be located by a characteristic increase in sound volume together with a rumbling quality produced by turbulent flow due to mixing. This evaluation is somewhat subjective and is highly dependent on the experience of the examiner. A range of accuracy for Doppler diagnosis from 49–96% has been reported, which probably reflects the wide range of examiner experience.[5,6]

Venous Doppler Examination in Detail
A rational approach to the Doppler examination of the venous system of the lower extremity is important. One begins proximally, proceeding downward from the saphenofemoral junction to the ankles *(Table 8-3, Figure 8-3)*. It is difficult to perform an adequate Doppler examination with the patient recumbent because without gravitational hydrostatic forces it may not be possible to elicit detectable amounts of reflux through incompetent valves. A comfortable position is essential, as any fidgeting will activate the calf muscle pump to cause increased flow and leg emptying. The ambient temperature will also affect the examination, as veins may be constricted in a cold environment. For best results, the patient should stand or sit in a warm room in a position permitting relaxed leg muscles. A sitting position may be used if the patient is unwilling or unable to stand.

First, the saphenofemoral junction and the saphenopopliteal junction are assessed for patency and valve competence. Any visible or palpable vessels are examined in order to document patterns of superficial reflux and to identify points of reflux from the deep system out into the superficial veins. A sample form on which to record Doppler examination findings is shown in Chapter 27. The therapeutic alternatives based on Doppler examination findings are outlined in Table 8-4.

SAPHENOFEMORAL JUNCTION
The Doppler transducer (8–10 MHz) is placed in the superior aspect of the groin crease at the level of the inguinal ligament, midway between the symphysis pubis and the anterior iliac crest. The rapid, pulsatile sound of flow in the

Table 8-3
Sequence of Doppler Examination

Femoral vein
Greater or long saphenous–femoral vein junction
Lesser or short saphenous–popliteal vein junction
Perforators
Saphenous branch veins
Reticular veins
Ankle–posterior tibial vein
Miscellaneous varicosities

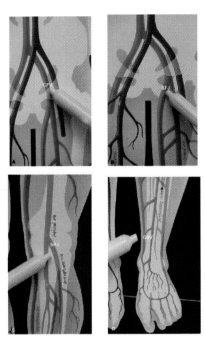

Figure 8-3. Key areas for Doppler examination. **(A)** Listen for normal flow sounds in the common femoral vein (CFV). **(B)** Listen for reflux at the saphenofemoral junction (SFJ). **(C)** Listen for reflux at the saphenopopliteal junction (SPJ). **(D)** Listen for reflux in the GSV at the medial ankle if there are telangiectasias or varicosities present (diagram courtesy of Julius Zorn Co., Cuyahoga Falls, OH).

femoral artery should be easily appreciated, and the transducer should be moved medially a millimeter at a time until the rapid, high-pitched arterial sounds start to fade, and a deeper rumbling or blowing sound is heard, indicating venous flow. Extremely rarely, absence of venous flow will indicate complete obstruction, while a continuous high-pitched sound indicating continuous high-velocity flow may indicate an area of partial obstruction due to deep vein thrombosis. When no sound is heard it is most likely due to

the inexperience of the examiner and improper positioning of the Doppler probe.

When the transducer is properly positioned in a patient without obstruction, spontaneously variable low-pitched blowing sounds are heard, waxing and waning as venous flow increases and decreases with inhalation and exhalation. Forward flow most often occurs during inhalation and ceases during exhalation, but this pattern may be reversed in patients who depend heavily upon abdominal accessory muscles for breathing. Examination findings should be symmetric bilaterally.

Once venous flow has been identified, augmentation and reverse augmentation maneuvers may be undertaken to test for reflux. Brief manual compression of the distal thigh should cause rapid augmentation of the venous forward-flow sounds, and cessation of compression should be met with cessation of the flow sounds, followed by gradual resumption of respirophasic flow sounds as the leg veins gradually become refilled. It is not possible to perform manual compression proximal to the saphenofemoral junction, but the same effect can be obtained by asking the patient to perform a Valsalva maneuver.

In the normal patient, a Valsalva maneuver (increasing intrabdominal pressure by taking a deep breath and "bearing down" with the abdominal muscles as if trying to defecate) causes forward flow to cease within a half-second as the valve shuts at the saphenofemoral junction. Because the veins are large at this level, reflux appears as a "hurricane" or "windstorm" sound, indicating the reverse flow that appears during Valsalva, or as "rebound reflux" immediately after cessation of distal compression. If the transducer is positioned directly over the saphenofemoral junction, reflux at this level indicates incompetent valves at the junction. If the transducer is positioned over the femoral vein, the saphenofemoral junction itself may be competent, and the reflux may be due to incompetent valves within the deep veins. Repositioning the transducer more proximally over the femoral vein and more distally over the greater saphenous vein permits the two conditions to be distinguished.

Up to 15% of asymptomatic individuals may have 1–5 seconds of "mild" reflux into the greater saphenous vein be-

Table 8-4
Therapeutic Decisions Based on Doppler Examination[a]

Saphenofemoral reflux	Ligation and/or short stripping
	RF endovenous occlusion
	Duplex guided sclerotherapy
Saphenopopliteal reflux	Ligation and/or short stripping
	RF endovenous occlusion
	Duplex guided sclerotherapy
Incompetent major perforators or branch varicosities	Ambulatory phlebectomy
	Sclerotherapy and/or duplex guided sclerotherapy
Minor reflux, e.g., lateral venous system	Sclerotherapy
	Ambulatory phlebectomy

[a]Confirmation by duplex recommended.

fore the valves of the SFJ close completely.[3] Any doubt over the Doppler findings, with suspicion of reflux through the saphenofemoral junction or into the deep venous system, is an indication for two-dimensional (2-D) ultrasound duplex imaging to better assess the anatomic abnormalities and to confirm the precise pattern of reflux.

GREATER SAPHENOUS VEIN

From the saphenofemoral junction, the Doppler transducer is gradually moved several centimeters below the inguinal ligament following the course of the greater saphenous vein. If the vein can be seen or palpated in this region, the probe can be placed by feel. Otherwise, the probe should be moved along the vein by following the sound of flow (whether spontaneous flow or augmented flow with compression). As the transducer passes distally to the valve of the junction, spontaneous phasic flow may no longer be heard. As before, distal compression and release should produce a transient increase in signal followed by a rapid cessation of flow as competent valves snap shut. Flow during proximal compression or after release of distal compression is a sign of valvular incompetence and reflux.

SAPHENOPOPLITEAL JUNCTION

The saphenopopliteal junction is best examined with the patient standing and supporting weight on the opposite leg. The rapid arterial pulsation sound of the popliteal artery is identified in the lateral mid-popliteal fossa between the two heads of the gastrocnemius muscle, and the Doppler transducer is moved laterally in the knee crease until the arterial sounds begin to diminish. In most patients, spontaneous flow at this level is too slow to be identified, but distal compression will produce an augmented venous flow signal within the popliteal and lesser saphenous veins that can be heard clearly. Although this is the "normal" location of the termination of the lesser saphenous vein (LSV) in the popliteal fossa, the anatomy of this region is highly variable. The LSV terminates well above the popliteal fossa in a significant number of patients. In order to detect flow in the LSV without hearing flow in the popliteal vein, the lateral retromalleolar region may be compressed, or the posterior surface of the calf may be gently stroked upwards from below.

If the LSV is visible or palpable, it may be followed directly until it terminates in the deep venous system at some level. In many patients it is not possible to appreciate the anatomy of the LSV in the popliteal fossa without the aid of a 2-D ultrasound duplex imaging study (see Chapter 10). When the LSV can be located, brief manual compression distal to the Doppler probe should lead to a brief augmentation of forward flow in the lesser saphenous system, followed by immediate cessation of flow after release of compression. If the anatomy is normal, reverse augmentation by proximal compression should cause immediate cessation of flow, but no reflux. If valves at the saphenopopliteal junction (or other adjacent perforating vein valves) are incompetent, then a long reflux sound will be heard during proximal compression and after release of distal compression.[7]

Even when valves at this level are incompetent, Valsalva usually has no effect on Doppler flow signals, because intact venous valves somewhere above this level prevent the transmission of backpressure from the abdomen, while venous capacitance of the thigh continues to permit antegrade flow even during a brief Valsalva maneuver.[8] Reflux in the popliteal vein itself can be distinguished from reflux through the junction into the saphenous vein by the following maneuver. Because the saphenous vein is superficial, pressure with the hand or probe will compress it, obliterating superficial reflux, while moderate external pressure will not easily obliterate reflux in the popliteal segment of the femoral vein, which is a deep structure. To master this technique of distinguishing reflux of the LSV from underlying popliteal vein takes some experience.

Not all varicose veins in the popliteal fossa arise from reflux at the saphenopopliteal junction. Hidden reflux from the greater saphenous system will often lead to varicosities of the posterior lower leg. Figure 8-4 illustrates such a case and highlights both the limitations of Doppler examination and the extraordinary value of duplex evaluation for accurate diagnosis. While some varicosities in the popliteal fossa arise from that lateral venous system (also referred to as the lateral subdermic venous system or LSVS), in these cases the reflux sites are usually more superficial and easily found by Doppler examination.

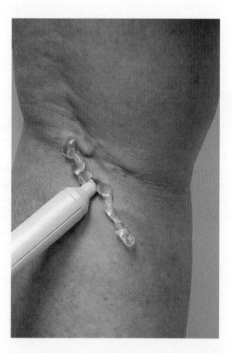

Figure 8-4. Handheld Doppler detects reflux in a branch varicosity below the point of origination. Duplex ultrasound is the only certain way to precisely locate the site of origin. This varicosity derived from reflux in a branch off the GSV, not the LSV, despite the popliteal location. This highlights the importance of supplementing Doppler with duplex in unclear situations. The fatty tissue of this patient's leg obscured the true source of reflux, making duplex necessary.

When a patient has fully occluding deep venous thrombosis at or above the level of the popliteal vein, no flow is detectable at any time. As in the thigh, incomplete obstruction or partially recanalized thrombus causes an increased velocity of flow through the narrowed venous channels. When this happens, spontaneous flow may be appreciated in the popliteal vein of the affected leg, but not in the normal leg. In theory, distal augmentation by squeezing below the site of obstruction should produce less augmentation of flow as compared to the unaffected side, but this finding is unreliable due to the large numbers of accessory veins that may bypass an area of thrombosis.

LARGE PERFORATING VEINS

If incompetent perforating veins are present, reflux at the level of the incompetent perforating vein will be detected even if superficial reflux from above is absent or has been controlled with a Penrose drain or other tourniquet placed immediately above. To demonstrate this, place a tourniquet immediately above the area to be examined and perform distal and proximal augmentation while the Doppler probe is held over the varicosity immediately below the tourniquet. As before, reflux through incompetent perforating veins is manifest as the presence of a flow sound during proximal (reverse) compression, and as the presence of a prolonged "rebound" flow sound immediately after the cessation of distal (forward) compression. Although fascial defects may sometimes be palpated at the sites of perforating veins, most palpable fascial defects do not contain perforating veins and most perforating veins do not join the peripheral venous system at the site of fascial defects. When perforating veins do emerge through palpable fascial defects there is often an artery or arteriole lying in close proximity to the perforating vein.

LARGE SAPHENOUS BRANCH VEINS

If reflux originates at a branch point from the greater saphenous vein, particularly in the medial thigh, reflux is often heard in the location at which the branch vein arrives 1 cm below the skin's surface. The location from which the branch vein emerges through the superficial fascia may be palpated as a small fascial defect. The value of palpation in diagnosis is discussed in detail in Chapter 6. The origin of the reflux at the level of the saphenous vein may be too deep to hear with the 8 Mhz transducer. Duplex ultrasound is often indicated to pinpoint the location at which the branch varicosity originates.

RETICULAR VEINS

Superficial venectasias and telangiectasias often are associated with an incompetent subcutaneous feeder vein of 3 mm or more in size. Because such veins usually are connected together in a netlike pattern, they have been referred to as reticular veins. If a high-frequency probe is used with an extremely light touch, it often is possible to locate an incompetent perforator or some other source of reflux into the telangiectatic veins. The technique for identifying reflux into reticular veins by distal and proximal compression (augmentation and reverse augmentation) is the same technique that has been previously described for identifying reflux into varicosities. Several common patterns of refluxing reticular veins arising from incompetent perforators have been mapped, and can serve as a guide to the clinician.[9]

POSTERIOR TIBIAL VEIN

The Doppler transducer is placed posterior to the medial malleolus near its superior aspect. The rapid, pulsatile sound of flow in the posterior tibial artery should be easily appreciated, and the transducer should be moved posteriorly a millimeter at a time until the rapid, high-pitched arterial sounds fade away. Spontaneous flow is never detected in the normal posterior tibial vein, nor does Valsalva exert any audible effect at this level. Augmentation by squeezing the foot produces temporary forward flow, but if deep vein valves are intact, reverse augmentation by squeezing the calf should have no effect. An increase in flow with reverse augmentation suggests some degree of deep venous insufficiency. Occlusion of other deep veins may produce spontaneous continuous forward flow within the posterior tibial vein.

VARICOSITIES

The examination thus far has covered all the principal superficial veins of the upper and lower leg. If there remain any areas of varicosity that have not been identified as tributaries of one of the veins already examined, these veins must be investigated directly. Each variceal system should be examined with compression–decompression maneuvers, starting at its most distal extent and following the path of reflux proximally until all incompetent perforating veins and all truncal feeders of the refluxing system have been identified.

Summary

Detection of the amount, direction, and timing of flow using Doppler ultrasound is an essential part of the examination of the venous system whenever there is evidence of macroscopic reflux. Because abnormal flow patterns in subsurface vessels may not be suspected on the basis of history and physical examination alone, many phlebologists feel the Doppler exam should be performed as a routine part of every examination, regardless of the presence or absence of other clinical signs and symptoms. Typical patterns of flow in response to manual compression and release of compression are reliable indicators of reflux at every level.

References

(1) Weiss RA. *Evaluation of the venous system by Doppler ultrasound and photoplethysmography or light reflection rheography before sclerotherapy.* Semin Dermatol 1993; 12:78–87.

(2) Weindorf N, Schultz-Ehrenburg U. *Der wert der photoplethysmographie (Licht reflexions rheography) in der phlebologie.* Vasa 1986; 15:397–401.

(3) O'Donnell TF, Jr., McEnroe CS, Heggerick P. *Chronic venous insufficiency.* Surg Clin North Am 1990; 70:159–180.

(4) Weiss RA. *Vascular studies of the legs for venous or arterial disease* [review]. Dermatol Clin 1994; 12(1):175–190.

(5) Evans DS, Cockett FB. *Diagnosis of deep-vein thrombosis with an ultrasonic Doppler technique.* Br Med J 1969; 2(660):802–804.

(6) Milne RM, Gunn AA, Griffiths JM, Ruckley CXV. *Postoperative deep venous thrombosis. A comparison of diagnostic techniques.* Lancet 1971; 2(7722):445–447.

(7) Partsch H. *Primary varikose der vena saphena magna und parva.* In: Kriessman A, Bollinger A, Keller H, editors. Praxis der Doppler Sonographie. Stuttgart: Thieme, 1982: 101–103.

(8) Schultz-Ehrenburg U, Hubner H-J. *Reflux diagnosis with doppler ultrasound* (monograph). Stuttgart: Schattauer, 1989.

(9) Weiss RA, Weiss MA. *Painful telangiectasias: diagnosis and treatment.* In: Bergan JJ, Weiss RA, Goldman MP, editors. Varicose Veins and Telangiectasias: Diagnosis and Treatment, 2nd ed. St. Louis: Quality Medical 1999: 389–406.

CHAPTER 9

Physiologic and Other Tests for Venous Evaluation

Blood Tests

Functional Tests

    Ambulatory Venous Pressure

    Plethysmography

    Calf Muscle Pump Expulsion Fraction

    Venous Refilling Time

    Tourniquet Refilling Time

    Maximum Venous Outflow

Summary

When symptoms of venous pathology are recognized or suspected, the underlying etiology is rarely immediately apparent. A careful diagnostic evaluation is necessary if one is to understand the particular venous hemodynamics of an individual patient. Although continuous-wave Doppler ultrasound can identify sites of valvular incompetence, photoplethysmography (PPG) and other forms of plethysmography offer a simple, reproducible technique to examine the physiologic significance of those findings, and to correlate them with the patient's symptoms. It has been said that the continuous-wave Doppler is analogous to the stethoscope, the plethysmographic test analogous to an EKG, and the duplex ultrasound equivalent to an echocardiogram.

The performance and interpretation of diagnostic tests must be guided by knowledge of the pathophysiology underlying a patient's clinical problem. For example, if a patient has signs and symptoms of pulmonary embolism (PE), failure to demonstrate deep vein thrombus (DVT) (by any means) carries little clinical weight. In contrast, for a patient without signs of PE but with clinical signs of proximal DVT (pain and swelling of the leg extending well above the knee), the demonstration of a normal color-flow duplex exam is a reasonably reliable indicator of some other, non-thrombotic etiology.

Blood Tests

Blood tests are rarely helpful in the evaluation of venous pathology. Most patients with deep venous thrombosis and pulmonary embolism have normal protime (PT) and activated partial thromboplastin time (APTT) studies. A low white blood cell (WBC) count lowers the likelihood of an infectious process and raises the likelihood of DVT or PE, but an elevated WBC count is nonspecific because both normal and elevated WBC counts are common in patients with deep venous thrombosis.[1] Both chronic venous insufficiency (venous congestion due to reflux) and deep vein thrombosis can mimic leg cellulitis, and true cellulitis is a frequent complication of both conditions.[2]

Since D-dimer is a breakdown product of the lysis of cross-linked fibrin clots, plasma D-dimer levels are now under investigation as potential aids to the diagnosis of DVT and PE. However, it is unlikely that D-dimers will prove dramatically helpful in the evaluation of venous disease. Recent literature suggests that about 10% of patients with symptoms of PE and a negative D-dimer screen (level less than 500 ng/ml) will have a positive pulmonary angiogram, while about 30% of similar patients with a positive D-dimer screen will have a positive angiogram.[3] The positive and negative predictive values for non-embolic venous thrombosis have not been established.

Functional Tests

Several important functional tests prove extremely useful in helping to assess the condition of the superficial and deep venous systems *(Table 9-1)*. Most important of these is the *venous refilling time* (VRT). The VRT is the time required for the leg to refill with blood after being emptied. A short VRT indicates early refilling. Early refilling most often occurs when valve damage in the deep or superficial veins allows venous blood to reflux downward into the extremity from retrograde venous flow, but it can also result from outflow obstruction or from increased arterial inflow due to arteriovenous malformations.

Two other commonly performed functional tests are of secondary importance. The fraction of blood that is pumped out of the calf with each exercise of the calf muscle is called the *muscle pump ejection fraction* (MPEF). The MPEF is decreased when there is failure of the calf muscle pump mechanism, which can reflect muscle wasting, outflow obstruction, or widespread valve failure. When venous outflow from the lower leg is temporarily obstructed with a tourniquet, the fraction of blood that exits in the first second after tourniquet removal is the *maximum venous outflow* (MVO). A reduced MVO indicates venous outflow obstruction.

AMBULATORY VENOUS PRESSURE

All of these functional parameters can be measured using a variety of different methods. The gold standard for functional testing of the lower extremity venous system is *ambulatory venous pressure (AVP)* monitoring. Ambulatory venous pressure tracings are obtained by placing a catheter into a superficial vein of the lower leg. Pressure changes are recorded while the patient exercises the calf muscle pump by walking, rising up on tiptoe, or performing ankle dorsi-

flexion movements. The recorded pressure tracings reflect the functional condition of the venous system *(Figure 9-1)*. In a normal leg, each pumping cycle lowers the pressure, as blood is pumped inward and upward. Under normal conditions, six to ten pumping cycles are sufficient to achieve a maximal reduction in pressure. With rest, the pressure normally rises again slowly as the leg is refilled, reaching a maximum in a healthy leg within 2–5 minutes. Direct measurement of the AVP is the most reliable means to detect abnormal venous function, but is rarely used in clinical practice because of its invasive nature. Instead, a variety of plethysmographic methods are used to approximate the results of AVP monitoring.

PLETHYSMOGRAPHY

The term "plethysmography" describes a number of techniques used to measure pressure or volume changes directly or indirectly. A plethysmograph consists of a mechanism to sense a change within the lower leg and a modifying unit (transducer), which translates changes from a displacement-sensing device into electrical energy that is then recorded. Each type of unit measures a different physical parameter in order to detect increased inflow or reduced outflow in the extremity being tested *(Table 9-2)*. Impedance plethysmography (IPG) records changes in the characteristic impedance (electrical resistance) of the extremity. Strain-gauge plethysmography (SGPG) measures a change in the circumference of the calf by sensing tension changes in a wire or strap encircling the leg. Photoplethysmography (PPG) and the minor variant of PPG known as light reflection rheography (LRR) measure changes in light absorption within dermal capillaries.[4] Pneumoplethysmography (PNPG) and air plethysmography (APG) depend upon direct measurement of changes in calf circumference or calf volume using an air bladder. The VRT and the MPEF can be measured using PPG or any other plethysmographic method, but the measurement of MVO requires a direct volumetric or pressure-sensing method, such as SGPG, IPG, PNPG, or APG.

Despite the fact that it cannot be used to measure maximum venous outflow, PPG remains the most popular method for assessing venous function because it is inexpensive, easy to perform, and can be used even by an examiner of limited experience.[5,6] With PPG, a single photoelectric light source illuminates a small area of skin, and an adjacent photoelectric sensor measures the reflectance of light.[7] Near-infrared (940 nm) is well suited for optimal measure-

Table 9-1
Physiologic Venous Measurements of Plethysmography

VRT	Venous refilling times	Time for complete refilling of the venous compartment of the leg after emptying by calf muscle pump activity
MVO	Maximum venous outflow	Venous emptying in the first second after artificial outflow obstruction is released
MPEF	Muscle pump ejection fraction	Fraction of emptying caused by a single contraction of the calf muscle pump when the venous compartment of the leg is nearly full

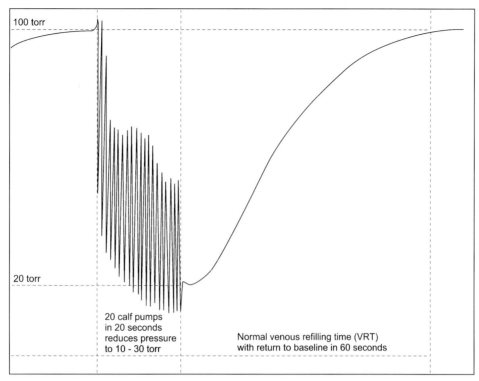

100 torr

20 torr

20 calf pumps
in 20 seconds
reduces pressure
to 10 - 30 torr

Normal venous refilling time (VRT)
with return to baseline in 60 seconds

A

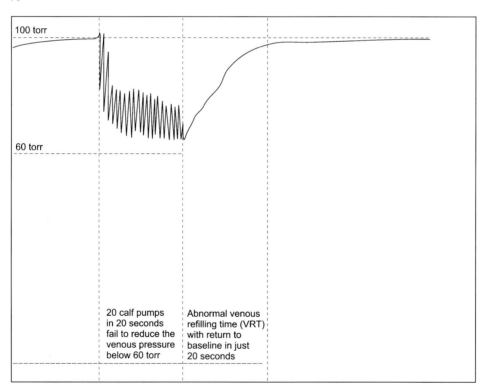

100 torr

60 torr

20 calf pumps
in 20 seconds
fail to reduce the
venous pressure
below 60 torr

Abnormal venous
refilling time (VRT)
with return to
baseline in just
20 seconds

B

Figure 9-1. **(A)** Normal ambulatory venous pressure tracing. **(B)** Ambulatory venous pressure in a patient with venous insufficiency.

Table 9-2
Different Forms of Plethysmography

Types of Plethysmography	Method of Volume Change Measurement
Ambulatory venous pressure (AVP)	Direct invasive manometric measurement of absolute venous pressure
Strain gauge (SGPG)	Expansion of spring loaded tension sensor
Impedance (IPG)	Electrical resistance in the extremity
Photo (PPG)	Changes in reflected 940 nm light
Light reflectance rheography (LRR)	Changes in reflected 940 nm light (averaged value from three emitters)
Digital photo (D-PPG)	Microprocessor controlled light emission to adjust for absorption
Pneumo	Pressure sensor measures changes in pressure within an air bladder inflated around one segment of the leg. The bladder is not calibrated, so that only relative changes are measured.
Air	Pressure sensor measures changes in pressure within an air bladder inflated around the entire length of the leg. The bladder is calibrated to measure the absolute volume change as the leg goes from empty to full.

ment of skin blood content because epidermal melanin absorption at this wavelength is limited to 15% of emitted light.

For any type of PPG examination, the patient sits on a chair in a relaxed position with the knees bent at a 110–120 degree angle. A small probe containing light-emitting and sensing diodes is taped to the medial aspect of the lower leg about 8–10 cm above the medial malleolus. The leg is allowed to fill for several minutes, and the patient then dorsiflexes the foot eight to ten times, activating the calf muscle pump to empty the venous system. As the skin venous plexus empties, it causes increased reflectance of light because less hemoglobin remains to absorb light. A tracing is made of the changes in reflected light from the skin under the probe. After the calf muscle pumping ceases, blood refills the skin plexus, increasing amounts of light are absorbed as blood fills venules, and the PPG tracing returns to its initial resting value. The surface vessel filling time (PPG refill time) correlates very well with direct invasive pressure measurements of venous refilling.[8] False negative readings are obtained when ankle joint mobility is reduced or when arterial occlusive disease prevents normal inflow to the skin.[9] False positives can occur due to sensor movement during testing, but are less common with modern equipment such as the digital-PPG (D-PPG).

Light reflection rheography (LRR) is a variant form of photoplethysmography that uses three light diodes rather than one, and was intended to decrease variation due to surface reflection or external light.[10] Commercially available LRR units also include a sensor that shuts the machine off if the skin temperature is too cold for reliable rheography.[11]

A more valuable new form of photoplethysmography is D-PPG (ELCAT GmbH, Wolfratshausen, Germany). D-PPG differs from ordinary PPG in that it uses a dedicated microprocessor to standardize the signal received by the photoelectric sensor,[12] allowing a standard baseline regardless of skin thickness or pigmentation. This allows semi-quantitative venous pump measurements without the need for cumbersome apparatus or extensive calibration.[13] The D-PPG unit measures the same physiologic parameters that other PPG units measure, but has two advantages. Besides providing a baseline that is standardized across patients, the D-PPG machine calculates the venous refilling time (VRT) and the muscle pump ejection fraction (MPEF) automatically *(Figure 9-2).*

CALF MUSCLE PUMP EXPULSION FRACTION

The muscle pump expulsion fraction test (MPEF) is used to detect failure of the calf muscle pump to expel blood from the lower leg. MPEF results are highly repeatable, but do re-

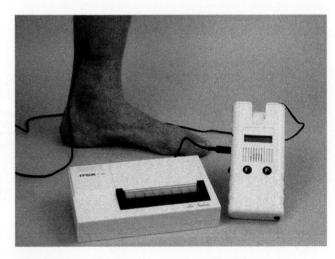

Figure 9-2. The digital PPG unit is compact and reliable. (Courtesy of Elcat GmBH, Wolfratshausen, Germany.)

quire a skilled operator to obtain "clean" meaningful tracings. The test is performed with the patient sitting and the feet flat on the floor. The patient is asked to perform 10–20 tiptoes or dorsiflexions at the ankle, and the change in some physical parameter that reflects calf blood volume is recorded as the calf muscle is pumped *(Figure 9-3 top)*. A stepwise tracing is obtained if the calf muscle pump is functional and the deep outflow tracts are patent with competent valves. A low-amplitude sinusoidal or sawtooth tracing that fails to move much from the baseline indicates calf muscle pump failure, severe distal outflow obstruction, or completely incompetent deep vein valves both in the calf and in the distal thigh *(Figure 9-3 bottom)*.

Venous Refilling Time

The venous refilling time (VRT) is used to assess the competence of venous valves in the leg. The test is virtually always performed in conjunction with the muscle pump expulsion fraction test discussed earlier. Results of VRT measurements are highly repeatable, but environmental factors can interfere with the test, and only a skilled operator can obtain clean meaningful tracings.

The test is performed with the patient sitting and the feet flat on the floor. The patient is asked to perform 10–20 tiptoes or dorsiflexions at the ankle, and the change in a physical parameter that reflects calf blood volume is recorded. The main parameter of interest is the refilling time

(VRT) after the ankle dorsiflexions are stopped. Although published international standards define any refill time greater than 25 seconds as "normal," this is an oversimplification, as venous reflux may be minimal, mild, moderate, or severe *(Table 9-3)*.

A normal-amplitude tracing that slowly returns back to the baseline over a period of 2–5 minutes is evidence of perfectly competent valves in both the deep and superficial venous systems, so that all venous refilling is due to arterial inflow *(Figure 9-4)*.

A normal-amplitude tracing that returns to the baseline in 40–120 seconds is typical of most adults with clinically healthy legs. This more rapid refilling reflects a small degree of venous reflux through failed valves in small perforating veins or small superficial veins, but because this small amount of reflux is so common and because it is not associated with obvious clinical symptoms, it is generally considered to be functionally normal.

A normal-amplitude tracing that returns to the baseline in 25–40 seconds is somewhat abnormal, reflecting retrograde venous flow through failed valves in superficial and/or perforating veins. This degree of reflux may or may not be associated with the typical symptoms of venous insufficiency. Such patients rarely have severe disease, but often complain of nocturnal leg cramps, restless legs, leg soreness, burning leg pain, and premature leg fatigue.

A normal-amplitude or low-amplitude tracing that returns to the baseline in less than 25 seconds is markedly ab-

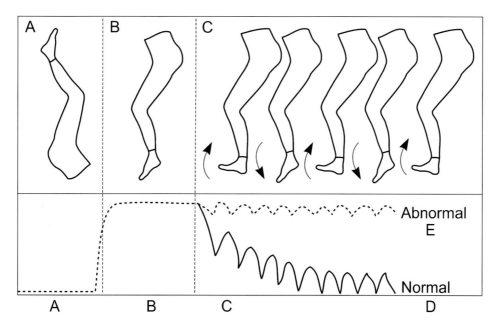

Figure 9-3 (top).   The calf muscle pump and venous volume. **(A)** Patient supine with leg elevated; calf veins empty. **(B)** Patient standing with leg down; calf veins full. **(C)** Foot is dorsiflexed 10 times to exercise calf muscle pump. **(bottom).** Normal and abnormal muscle pump tracings. **(A)** Veins empty, pressure and volume at a minimum. **(B)** Veins full, pressure and volume at a maximum. **(C)** Calf muscle pump active, pressure and volume changing. **(D)** Normal ejection empties veins and approaches baseline rapidly. **(E)** Calf muscle problems, severe reflux, or outflow obstruction prevent effective pumping, causing ambulatory venous hypertension.

Table 9–3
Interpretation of Venous Refilling Time

Grade	Refill Time (T_0)	Interpretation
Normal	Greater than 120 seconds	All refilling is through arterial inflow
Normal	40–120 seconds	Minimal venous reflux
Normal	25–40 seconds	Mild small-vessel venous reflux (often asymptomatic)
Grade I	24–20 seconds	Mild venous insufficiency
Grade II	19–10 seconds	Moderate venous insufficiency
Grade III	Under 10 seconds	Severe venous insufficiency (often involving deep veins)

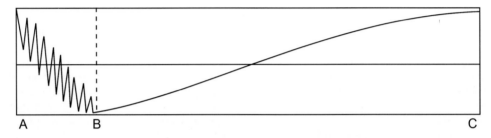

Figure 9-4. Venous pressure at the ankle over time. **(A)** Calf muscle pumped 10 times to empty leg veins. **(B)** Relaxation of muscle pump. **(C)** As leg refills, venous pressure returns to baseline. The time from B to C is the VRT. A short VRT means that ambulatory venous hypertension exists.

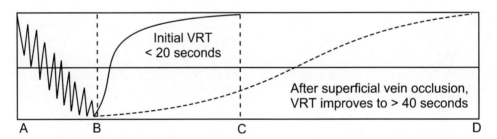

Figure 9-5. Short VRT due to correctable superficial venous reflux. **(A)** Calf muscle pumped 10 times to empty leg veins. **(B)** Relaxation of muscle pump. **(C)** As leg refills via reflux, venous pressure returns rapidly to baseline. **(D)** After tourniquet occlusion of superficial incompetent (varicose) veins, reflux is obliterated and the leg refills normally.

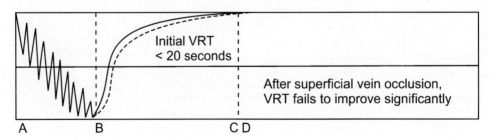

Figure 9-6. Short VRT due to uncorrectable deep venous reflux. **(A)** Calf muscle pumped 10 times to empty leg veins. **(B)** Relaxation of muscle pump. **(C)** As leg refills via reflux, venous pressure returns rapidly to baseline. **(D)** Tourniquet occlusion of superficial veins fails to correct VRT, suggesting deep venous reflux.

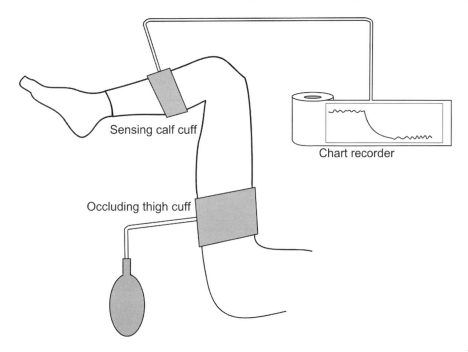

Figure 9-7. Maximum venous outflow (MVO). After the leg is congested with blood, the thigh cuff is suddenly deflated and the venous outflow pattern is recorded.

normal, and is due to high volumes of retrograde venous flow either in the superficial veins, in large perforators, or in the deep veins. This degree of reflux is nearly always symptomatic. If the refilling time is shorter than 10 seconds, venous ulcerations are so common as to be considered virtually inevitable.

TOURNIQUET REFILLING TIME

With the addition of a tourniquet test, plethysmography can help distinguish between superficial and deep venous insufficiency. If reflux is principally through the superficial system, then tourniquet occlusion of the superficial venous system (but not of the deep veins) should yield marked improvement or even normalization of the measured VRT *(Figure*

9-5). Failure to improve the VRT with occlusion of the superficial veins strongly suggests venous reflux due to failed valves in the deep venous system *(Figure 9-6).* Actual worsening of the VRT after application of a tourniquet suggests the possibility that the superficial veins are serving as a bypass pathway due to obstruction in the deep venous system.

To perform the tourniquet test on a patient with a short VRT, plethysmography is repeated with a tourniquet inflated to 80–100 mm Hg around the mid to lower thigh. The refilling time should return to normal if the source of reflux is the superficial system above the tourniquet. If the VRT remains shortened with a tourniquet above the knee, the test is repeated with a tourniquet below the knee, to eliminate reflux from perforator-fed varicosities lower on the leg.

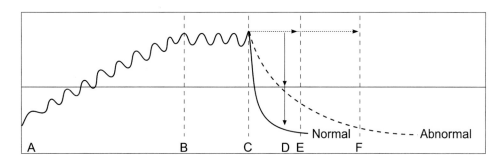

Figure 9-8. Normal and abnormal maximum venous outflow (MVO). **(A)** Venous tourniquet occludes deep and superficial venous outflow at the thigh, while still permitting arterial inflow. **(B)** Leg veins are completely congested with blood. **(C)** Thigh tourniquet is suddenly released. **(D)** Fraction of venous outflow from the calf in 1 second should be greater than 80%. **(E)** The normal time to 90% outflow is less than 2 seconds. **(F)** Venous obstruction prolongs outflow time.

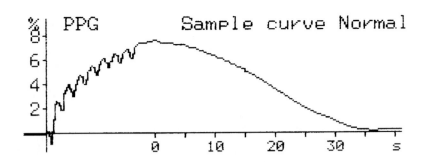

Quantitative parameters:

Venous refilling time   : To =   34   s
Venous pump power   : Vo =   7.7 %

A

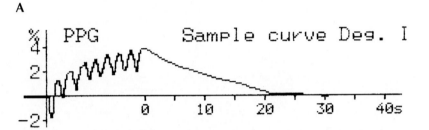

Quantitative parameters:

Venous refilling time   : To =   22   s
Venous pump power   : Vo =   4.0 %

B

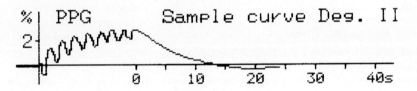

Quantitative parameters:

Venous refilling time   : To =   15   s
Venous pump power   : Vo =   3.0 %

C

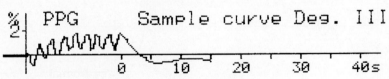

Quantitative parameters:

Venous refilling time   : To =   6   s
Venous pump power   : Vo =   1.9 %

D

Figure 9-9. Digital PPG is easy to use and provides automatic calculation of results. **(A)** D-PPG output showing a normal result, with a VRT of 34 seconds and a normal MPEF of 7.7%. **(B)** D-PPG output showing mild to moderate venous reflux with a VRT of 22 seconds and a normal MPEF of 4%. **(C)** D-PPG output showing moderate to severe venous reflux, with a VRT of 15 seconds and a borderline MPEF of 3%. **(D)** D-PPG output showing severe venous impairment, with a VRT of 6 seconds and an MPEF of 1.9%, demonstrating failure of the calf muscle pump.

Duplex ultrasound evaluation is always indicated whenever a shortened VRT is not correctable with placement of a tourniquet. Although in theory the VRT should always be correctable when reflux is predominantly from the superficial system, in practice there are many reasons why purely superficial reflux may not be controlled with the tourniquet test. For this reason, these authors often proceed directly to a duplex ultrasound examination when an abnormal VRT is detected.

MAXIMUM VENOUS OUTFLOW

The maximum venous outflow test (MVO) detects obstruction to venous outflow from the lower leg. MVO results are highly repeatable, and are not operator dependent. The test is performed using a plethysmograph that is functionally equivalent to a pair of ordinary blood pressure tourniquets, a pressure sensor, and a strip chart recorder. The advantage of MVO testing is that it is a functional test, rather than an anatomic one, and is sensitive to significant intrinsic or extrinsic venous obstruction from any cause, at almost any level. It can detect obstructing thrombus in the calf veins, the iliac veins, and the vena cava, sites where ultrasound and venography are insensitive. It also detects venous obstruction due to extravascular hematomas, tumors, and other extrinsic disease processes. The disadvantage of the test is that it is sensitive only for significant venous obstruction, and will not detect partially obstructing thrombus. It is *not* useful for detection of venous insufficiency states. A normal MVO absolutely does not rule out deep vein thrombosis.[14,15]

The study is performed with the patient supine, the hip flexed, and the lower leg horizontal. A sensing device (a venous catheter, an external impedance sensor, or an air tourniquet connected to a pressure sensor) is placed at the level of the calf to measure volume changes, and a proximal thigh tourniquet is inflated to occlude the superficial and deep veins while permitting continued arterial inflow. Within a few minutes, a volume of blood is accumulated in the venous capacitance system of the calf. The occluding thigh tourniquet is suddenly released, and the time necessary for venous outflow from the calf is measured on a chart recorder *(Figure 9-7)*. Both legs should be studied for comparison. If the deep veins are normal, 90% or more of the blood that had been trapped in the calf veins will exit in the first second *(Figure 9-8)*. If there is significant occlusion of the deep veins, the outflow will be delayed, so that less than 60% of the total outflow will occur in the first 2 seconds. The test may be nondiagnostic if the leg is excessively swollen or excessively obese.

Summary

Venous imaging is very important in the diagnosis of venous disease, but there are many disturbances of venous function that cannot be detected or elucidated by venous imaging alone. Physiologic testing of venous function adds an important dimension to the evaluation of venous insufficiency, and can guide therapeutic considerations *(Table 9-4)*. When used as an initial investigative tool, physiologic tests such as the PPG can alert the clinician to unseen and unsuspected venous problems that will cause poor response to

Table 9-4
Therapeutic Considerations after Plethysmography

Refill > 25 seconds
   Sclerotherapy of superficial varicosities
Refill 10–25 seconds, but correctable with tourniquet
   Sclerotherapy or ambulatory phlebectomy
Refill < 10 seconds or not corrected with tourniquet
   Duplex ultrasound mandatory
   Treatment based on anatomic findings
   Sclerotherapy rarely helpful in presence of deep venous insufficiency
Poor muscle pump ejection fraction
   Duplex ultrasound mandatory
   Treatment based on anatomic findings
   Sclerotherapy is contraindicated in presence of deep obstruction
Diminished maximum venous outflow
   Deep vein obstruction is likely
   Duplex ultrasound mandatory
   Sclerotherapy is contraindicated in presence of deep obstruction

simple sclerotherapy. Medical assistants and other staff personnel can easily be trained to perform these tests, particularly when automated equipment such as the D-PPG is available *(Figure 9-9)*. In this modern era, proper diagnosis and treatment planning requires both an anatomic and a functional assessment of the venous system, especially when complex, difficult, or resistant cases are encountered.

References

(1) Schonell ME, Crompton GK, Forshall JM, Whitby LG. *Failure to differentiate pulmonary infarction from pneumonia by biochemical tests.* Br Med J 1966; 5496:1146–1148.

(2) Quartey-Papafio CM. *Lesson of the week: importance of distinguishing between cellulitis and varicose eczema of the leg.* BMJ 1999; 318(7199):1672–1673.

(3) Goldhaber SZ, Simons GR, Elliott CG, Haire WD, Toltzis R, Blacklow SC et al. *Quantitative plasma D-dimer levels among patients undergoing pulmonary angiography for suspected pulmonary embolism* [see comments]. JAMA 1993; 270(23):2819–2822.

(4) Rosfors S. *Venous photoplethysmography: relationship between transducer position and regional distribution of venous insufficiency.* J Vasc Surg 1990; 11:436–440.

(5) Weindorf N, Schultz-Ehrenburg U. *Der wert der photoplethysmographie (licht reflexions rheography) in der phlebologie.* Vasa 1986; 15:397–401.

(6) McMullin GM, Coleridge Smith PD. *An evaluation of Doppler ultrasound and photoplethysmography in the investigation of venous insufficiency.* Aust N Z J Med 1992; 62:270–275.

(7) Hertzman AB. *The blood supply of various skin areas as estimated by the photoelectric plethysmograph.* Am J Physiol 1938; 33:498–499.

(8) Abramowitz HB, Queral LA, Flinn WR, et al. *The use of photoplethysmography in the assessment of venous insufficiency: a*

comparison to venous pressure measurements. Surgery 1979; 66:434–441.

(9)   Schroeder PJ, Dunn E. *Mechanical plethysmography and Doppler ultrasound. Diagnosis of deep-venous thrombosis.* Arch Surg 1982; 117(3):300–303.

(10)   Wienert V, Blazek V. *Eine neue methode zur unblutigen dynamischen venendruckmessung.* Hautarzt 1982; 33:498–499.

(11)   Neumann HAM, Boersma I. *Light reflection rheography. A non-invasive diagnostic tool for screening of venous disease.* J Dermatol Surg Onc 1992; 18:425–430.

(12)   Blazek V, Schmitt HJ, Schultz-Ehrenburg U, Kerner J. *Digitale photoplethysmographie (D-PPG) fur die beinvenendiagnostik. medizinisch-technische grundlagen.* Phlebol Proktol 1989; 18:91–97.

(13)   Kerner J, Schultz-Ehrenburg U, Lechner W. *Quantitative photoplethysmographie bei gesunden erwachsenen, kindern und schwangeren und bei varizenpatienten.* Phlebol 1992; 21: 134–139.

(14)   Ginsberg JS, Wells PS, Hirsh J, Panju AA, Patel MA, Malone DE et al. *Reevaluation of the sensitivity of impedance plethysmography for the detection of proximal deep vein thrombosis.* Archives of Internal Medicine 1994; 154(17):1930–1933.

(15)   Anderson DR, Lensing AW, Wells PS, Levine MN, Weitz JI, Hirsh J. *Limitations of impedance plethysmography in the diagnosis of clinically suspected deep-vein thrombosis* [see]. Ann Intern Med 1993; 118(1):25–30.

Venous Imaging/ Duplex Ultrasound

Proper diagnosis of venous system disease often requires both functional and anatomic information about the venous circulation. Functional tests such as the maximum venous outflow (MVO), the venous refilling time (VRT), and the calf muscle pump ejection fraction (MPEF) (see Chapter 9) are extremely useful as measures of whole-leg or regional venous function, but can detect only regionally significant reflux or a significant impediment to venous outflow. Anatomic imaging of the venous system does not assess overall hemodynamic function, but can detect even very small amounts of local and regional reflux, and can visualize both obstructing and nonobstructing thrombus.

Successful imaging of the deep venous system requires a thorough knowledge of venous anatomy and physiology, as well as meticulous attention to detail. The most useful modalities available for venous imaging are contrast venography, magnetic resonance imaging (MRI), and the present day duplex ultrasound, which has become the "gold standard"[1–3] *(Table 10-1)*. Superficial venous imaging is primarily performed by duplex ultrasound. A detailed protocol for its use is described in this chapter.

Contrast Venography

Contrast venography is neither absolutely sensitive nor specific in the diagnosis of venous pathology but prior to the introduction of duplex ultrasound, it had been the standard to which all other diagnostic tests have been compared. Deep and superficial venous thrombosis and venous insufficiency can be evaluated.

Superficial veins and varices are imaged by direct injection of a radiopaque contrast material into the veins of interest. After a tourniquet is placed around the lower leg in order to occlude the superficial, but not the deep, veins, contrast material is injected into a superficial dorsal foot vein. The contrast passes through perforating veins into the deep venous system. Thrombus appears either as a filling defect outlined by contrast, or as a "cutoff" lesion stopping the flow of contrast *(Figure 10-1)*. Reflux is detected when contrast flows backwards through failed valves into a more distal segment of the vein.

If whole-leg deep vein reflux is suspected, it may be confirmed by injection of contrast into the common femoral vein with the patient in the standing position. A complete reflux exam of the deep system is laborious, requiring pas-

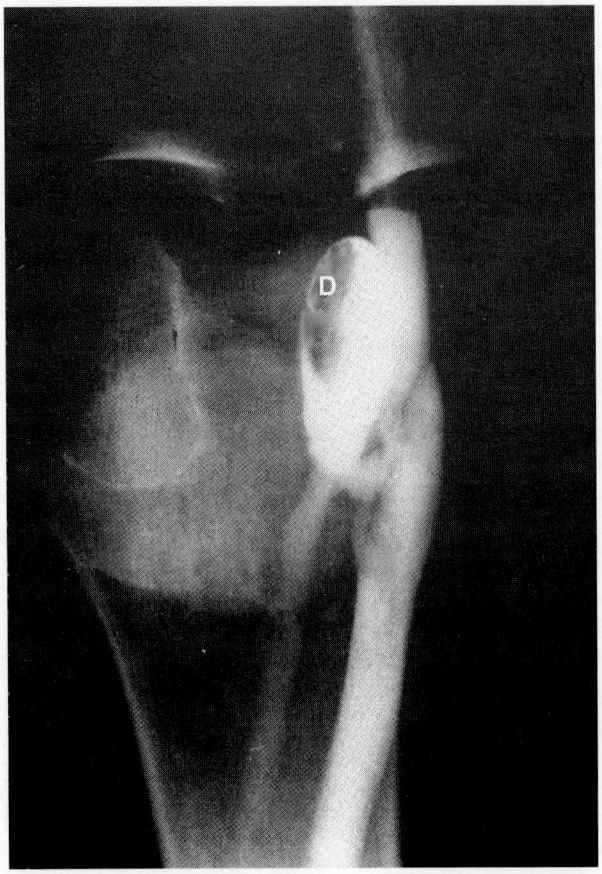

Figure 10-1. Contrast venography demonstrating a filling defect (D) typical of a thrombus.

sage of a catheter proximally from the saphenopopliteal junction all the way to the groin. With the patient standing, contrast is injected into each venous segment.

Contrast venography is an invasive technique, with a significant morbidity and mortality. Besides being painful, there is risk that extravasation of dye into the dorsum of the foot may cause sloughing of tissue.[4] At least 4% of patients develop venous thrombosis after venography.[5] Anaphylactic reactions to contrast material occur in 3% of patients, and are associated with a substantial mortality.[6]

Magnetic Resonance Imaging

Magnetic resonance imaging (MRI) offers great promise as it becomes increasingly available for the evaluation of venous pathology. Spin-echo and gradient-recalled acquisition in steady state (GRASS) images can reliably detect thrombus in deep veins of the calf, thigh, and pelvis.[7] MRI is particularly useful because unsuspected non-vascular causes for leg pain and edema often may be seen on the MRI scan when the clinical presentation erroneously suggests venous insufficiency or venous obstruction.

Radionuclide Venography

The radiolabelled substances used in scintigraphic lung scanning may be injected into the foot in the manner usually employed for contrast venography. The leg, thigh, and pelvis may be scanned as the radionuclide ascends through the venous circulation to the lungs. The resulting images are of low contrast and are sometimes difficult to read, but at some institutions they are routinely performed as a part of every scintigraphic lung perfusion scan. If positive, the nuclear venogram is nearly as reliable as a standard contrast study. A negative nuclear venogram cannot rule out deep venous thrombosis (DVT), and should rarely be trusted as evidence against the diagnosis.

Spiral CT Scan

The spiral CT scan can provide very high-resolution images of vascular structures, and gives early promise for peripheral venous imaging, but the need for contrast material makes it a less attractive modality than MRI.

Radiolabeled Fibrinogen

If fibrinogen labeled with radioactive iodine (I-131) is injected into a patient with acute DVT, radiolabeled fibrinogen is incorporated into the developing thrombus. Radioactive "hot spots" may be imaged with a gamma camera, or a simple counter may be used to demonstrate the localization of radioactivity at sites within the legs and pelvis. Radiolabeled fibrinogen can detect both acutely forming thrombus and subacute fully-formed thrombus, but cannot detect chronic thrombus that has been in place for several months. The technique is of limited modern value for two major reasons: several days are required to incorporate detectable amounts of radioisotope within a developing thrombus, and fibrinogen is a human blood product that comes with an unavoidable risk of infection. It is not possible to distinguish between superficial and deep venous thrombosis using this method, as even a superficial chemical phlebitis due to sclerotherapy gives a positive fibrinogen scan.[8]

Radiolabeled Monoclonal Antibody to Fibrin

Radiolabeled fibrinogen scanning is primarily of historical interest, but radiolabeled monoclonal antibodies to mature and immature thrombus have shown promise as a more rapid and more reliable test for venous thrombosis and pulmonary thromboembolism.[9] The technique has recently become available for clinical use.

Duplex Imaging

The availability of inexpensive ultrasound equipment has made it much easier to diagnose and treat venous pathology in the office. B-mode (or time-delay) ultrasound forms a gray-scale picture based upon the time delay of ultrasonic pulses reflected from deep structures. Structures that absorb, transmit, or scatter ultrasonic waves appear as dark areas, while structures that reflect the waves back to the transducer appear as white areas in the image. Vessel walls reflect ultrasound, while blood flowing in a vessel absorbs and scatters ultrasound in all directions, thus the normal vessel appears as a dark-filled white-walled structure. Nonflowing blood and thrombus are somewhat ultrasonically reflective, although less so than the vessel wall, thus they appear as heterogeneous areas of gray echogenicity within the vessel.

A duplex scanner is the combination of a B-mode ultrasound machine with a continuous-wave (CWD) Doppler probe built in. The scanner screen can be set to display just the B-mode image, or just a time plot of the Doppler flow velocity, or both at the same time. The Doppler information can also be heard through the speakers, exactly like the sound from a handheld Doppler probe. More expensive machines offer "color-flow" imaging, which converts the Doppler information to visually colorize areas of the B-mode image in which flow has been detected. Vessels with flow are colored red for flow in one direction and blue for flow in the other, with a graduated color scale to reflect the speed of the flow (*Figure 10-2*). Color-flow systems are significantly easier to use than gray-scale systems, and can help the examination go much faster, but most skilled examiners are of the opinion that color does not really increase the intrinsic sensitivity or specificity of the B-mode duplex scan. Incompetent small perforating veins, however, may be nearly impossible to detect without color flow

Modern color-flow duplex ultrasound equipment can provide flow information at the same time that it gives sur-

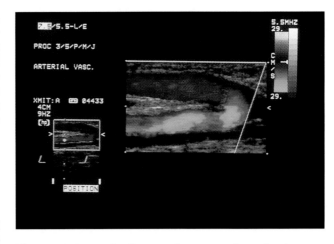

Figure 10-2. Color-flow Duplex image of A–V fistula showing flow in opposite directions as represented by red and blue coloration. (Courtesy Agilent Technologies.)

prisingly high-resolution views of both deep and superficial venous systems, including delicate valves, small perforating veins, and even reticular veins as small as 1 mm in diameter. Using the duplex scanner, it is possible to elucidate venous pathophysiology with great confidence. Venous thrombosis is readily detected, and the anatomic pathways of normal and aberrant flow in the deep and superficial venous systems lie fully exposed.

Lower-extremity examinations are best performed using solid-state linear array transducers, which have no moving parts within the transducer. Older models have a fluid-filled head in which the transducer mechanically rotates. Most modern ultrasound machines have two different transducers that are appropriate for vascular examinations: one with a frequency of approximately 7.5 MHz, used for superficial vessels, and one with a frequency of approximately 4.5 MHz, used for deeper vessels and for obese patients. Two frequencies are necessary because the depth at which clear images can be seen is a function of the frequency. Low transducer frequencies permit the sound to reach deeper structures, but also yield poorer near-field images of superficial structures. Newest high-resolution machines utilize a 10 Mhz transducer to allow examination of veins as small as 0.75 mm.

TECHNIQUE FOR IDENTIFICATION OF THROMBUS

Although thrombus sometimes is clearly seen within the veins, it may be present without being directly visible. The diagnosis of intravascular thrombus depends upon the fact that a direct downward pressure readily collapses normal veins. This pressure is placed on the vein with the ultrasound transducer. For a normal vein, walls will coapt (compress together completely) and the vein will disappear on the scan display, indicating the absence of thrombus. This is often referred to as the vein "winking" at the examiner. A vein that does not compress completely along with echogenic signals in the lumen usually indicates the presence of thrombus (*Figure 10-3*). This is the hallmark of test-

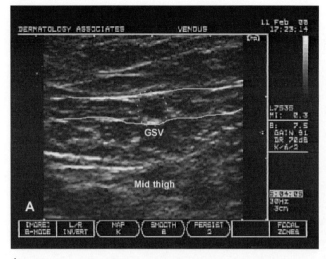

A

B

Figure 10-3. Detection of thrombus by duplex ultrasound. **(A)** A vein in cross-section. The superficial fascia surrounding the greater saphenous vein (GSV) is enhanced in white, showing as two parallel white lines above and below the GSV (*round dark circle in middle*). **(B)** Compression of that vein shows disappearance; therefore no thrombus is present. **(C)** Compression of a deep vein shows inability to compress with an echogenic lumen. This is a sign of thrombus. The tip of the thrombus is indicated with an *arrow*. This is a longitudinal view, which would be confirmed by a transverse view.

C

ing for thrombus by duplex ultrasound. Compression to observe complete collapse in a normal vein is performed repeatedly along the entire course of the vein with the transducer held in a transverse plane. When the transducer is held longitudinally, some areas of thrombus may be missed since the vein may not be visualized in its entirety.

TECHNIQUE FOR DIAGNOSIS OF REFLUX

Reflux is diagnosed by placing the transducer over the vessel in a longitudinal plane and observing the Doppler signal in the vessels while the distal leg is momentarily compressed and released (with the free hand) to increase the cephalad movement of blood *(Figure 10-4)*. Functional valves permit flow only in the antegrade direction, but normal vessels can demonstrate brief retrograde flow due to slow closing of valves. Retrograde flow of duration greater than one-half second is considered pathologic reflux, and reflux that lasts more than 2 seconds is hemodynamically significant. Reflux can also be seen in the transverse view, however, this requires an expert examiner. Quantification of reflux volume and flow velocity requires measurement of cross-sectional flow, and is beyond the scope of this text.

THE COMPLETE DUPLEX EXAMINATION

The complete venous duplex scan uses both longitudinal and transverse imaging planes and often requires both high- and low-frequency transducers. The scan is predominately done in the transverse plane because as the transducer slides along the vein, it provides a stepwise picture of the entire vein in cross section, giving a more complete picture of the anatomy. When needed, measurements of vessel diameters are taken from the transverse plane. As the transverse scan progresses, the transducer is used to compress the vein walls every few centimeters to be sure there is no thrombus within the veins. Periodically, the transducer is turned into the longitudinal plane and Doppler signals are obtained with distal augmentation. For detection of reflux, the patient must be positioned a minimum of 30 degrees reverse Trendelenburg all the way to a fully standing position.

PATIENT POSITIONING

Three patient positions are used for the examination of each leg. The patient begins in a lateral semi-supine position with the hip and knee slightly abducted. Gel is applied to the medial aspect of the thigh and calf from the inguinal ligament to the medial malleolus. All of the deep and su-

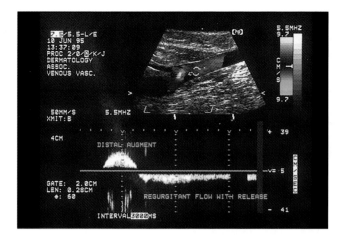

Figure 10-4. Testing for reflux at the saphenofemoral junction. A spectral sound image is added, which shows the CWD signal of flow. The exact location of reflux testing is targeted perfectly at the SFJ, shown by the *blue circle*. Distal compression shows forward flow, release demonstrates a long flow sound in the opposite direction (*below the line*). Unlike the handheld Doppler, this method allows exact visual assessment of reflux location.

perficial veins on the medial aspect of the lower extremity are scanned in this position. The patient then turns slightly more supine to permit scanning of the anterolateral aspect of the leg below the knee, just lateral to the tibia. The patient then rolls to a lateral semi-prone position with weight on the opposite hip, to allow a relaxed leg with access to the posterior aspect of the thigh, the popliteal fossa, and the posterior calf. The three positions are then repeated for the other leg.

The entire scan is performed with the patient on a tilt-table in reverse Trendelenburg (with the head up and the feet down) at an angle of 30–45 degrees. This tilt position increases pooling in the distal veins, and the resulting vasodilatation facilitates visualization of venous structures. If a tilt table is not available, most of the scan can be completed with the patient supine and the head slightly elevated. Because reflux often is not detectable with the patient horizontal, mapping of reflux often requires that the patient stand for portions of the examination.

THE EXAMINATION

The complete examination is illustrated in Figure 10-5 and outlined in Table 10-2. The examination begins with the vessels of the medial leg. On the tilt-table the patient is supine and assumes a semi-lateral position with weight on the hip and with the hip and knee slightly abducted. Gel is applied to the medial aspect of the thigh and calf from the inguinal ligament to the medial malleolus.

Deep veins from the groin to the knee

The scan is started with the transducer at the inguinal crease. This is the level of the saphenofemoral junction, where the greater saphenous vein communicates with the

Table 10-2
Sequence of the Duplex Examination

Deep veins from the groin to the knee
   Common femoral vein
   Confluence of the superficial and deep femoral veins
   Distal femoral vein at the level of the popliteal segment
   Each deep vein must be demonstrated to be compressible along its entire length
Greater saphenous vein and tributaries
   Inguinal crease: saphenofemoral junction
   Two valves visualized in greater saphenous vein
   Competence assessed with distal augmentation and Valsalva maneuver
   Major tributaries at S-F junction—most commonly visualized is epigastric
   Identify any perforating veins and communicating veins
   Identify sizeable superficial tributaries in communication with GSV
   Check for reflux with distal compression at all levels
Posterior tibial veins
   Anteromedial aspect of the calf
   Check for reflux with distal compression at all levels
Anterior tibial veins
   Lateral aspect of the tibia from mid-ankle to the knee
   Join the popliteal vein in the posterior popliteal fossa
   Check for reflux with distal compression at all levels
Popliteal vein
   Posterior thigh into popliteal fossa
   Check for reflux with distal compression at all levels
Tibial and peroneal veins
   Popliteal vein divides at level of popliteal crease
   Medial branch becomes the paired posterior tibial system
   Lateral branch becomes the peroneal system
   Check for reflux with distal compression at all levels
Lesser saphenous vein (LSV)
   Easy to find as the dominant superficial vein on the posterior calf
   Subcutaneous layer sandwiched between two fascial layers
   Extends to lateral posterior malleolar region
   At LSV termination: examine for anatomic variations, reflux, and gastrocnemius veins from calf
   Check for reflux with distal compression at all levels
Remaining varices
   Start at the most distal portion and follow path of reflux proximally to origin

common femoral vein. In a longitudinal plane, obtain a Doppler sample in the proximal and distal common femoral vein with a distal augmentation just distal to the probe. At the confluence of the superficial and deep femoral veins, obtain a Doppler signal with a distal augmentation at the origin of both femoral veins while in a longitudinal plane. The probe is then turned into the transverse position. The deep system is examined from the inguinal crease distally to the

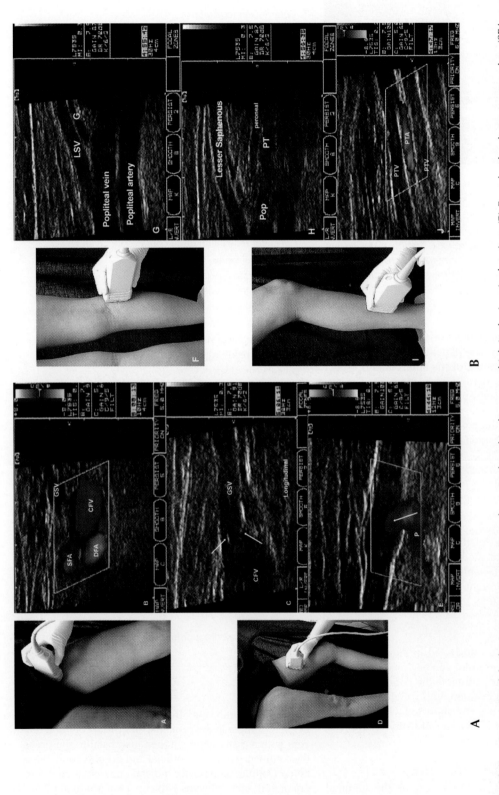

Figure 10-5. Sequence of duplex examination: **(A)** Transducer is placed in the upper thigh in the inguinal region. **(B)** Examination in transverse view (SFA, superficial femoral artery; DFA, deep femoral artery; CFV, common femoral vein; GSV, greater saphenous vein). This is the so-called lateral "Mickey Mouse" view. **(C)** The transducer is rotated into the longitudinal position showing the saphenofemoral junction. *Arrows* indicate terminal valves (CFV, common femoral vein; GSV, greater saphenous vein). **(D)** The transducer is moved down the thigh to examine the GSV. Diameter, branch points, perforators, and reflux in these structures are recorded. **(E)** An example of a mid-thigh Hunterian perforator with reflux (*arrow*) back into the GSV. Note the deforming bulge in the GSV above the "jet" of reflux. The perforator would be difficult to find without the assistance of color-flow imaging. **(F)** The transducer is moved to the popliteal fossa slightly to the lateral of midline. **(G)** In location F, a view of the terminal area of the lesser saphenous vein (LSV) can be found. The LSV empties into the popliteal vein that connects more proximally with the femoral vein. A gastrocnemius vein (G) is seen directly under the LSV. The popliteal artery (a vessel to always avoid) is seen beneath the popliteal vein. The compressed and complex anatomy of the popliteal fossa demonstrated by this ultrasound view is the reason for the increased risks associated with injections attempted here. **(H)** As the transducer is moved slightly distally, the division of the popliteal vein (Pop) into the peroneal and posterior tibial (PT) can be seen. **(I)** The transducer is then placed near the medial ankle where the paired posterior tibial veins (PTV) can be seen surrounding the posterior tibial artery (PTA). **(J)** This site is excellent for looking for deep venous reflux.

area just above the knee, beginning with the common femoral vein and ending with the distal femoral vein at the level of the popliteal segment, where the vessel passes posteriorly. In order to comment on the presence or absence of deep vein thrombosis, each deep vein must be demonstrated to be compressible along its entire length: when pressure is applied with the transducer, the veins walls must coapt (come together) completely to assure that there is no intraluminal thrombus.

Greater saphenous vein and tributaries

Once the proximal portion of the deep system has been examined for thrombus, the transducer is again placed in the inguinal crease at the saphenofemoral junction for examination of the medial superficial system. In the longitudinal view, the origin of the greater saphenous vein is identified as it courses off the common femoral vein. Two valves can be visualized in the greater saphenous vein. The first of these is the terminal valve, which lies at the vein origin. Distal augmentation for Doppler flow reveals competence or incompetence of this valve. The second, the subterminal valve, is examined in the same fashion. Valsalva maneuver may also show incompetence of these valves. Major tributaries that empty into the region of the saphenofemoral junction can be identified here. These include the circumflex, pudendal, epigastric, and others. Most commonly seen is the epigastric because of its size and position in the same plane as the termination of the greater saphenous vein.

The transducer is then turned to the transverse plane to examine the full length of the superficial system from proximal to distal. Doppler signals are identified in all of the branches and tributaries of the greater saphenous vein down to the level of the medial malleolus. An effort is made to identify any perforating veins and communicating veins, as well as any sizeable superficial tributaries that are in communication with the greater saphenous system. During the investigation, pulsed Doppler signals are obtained with distal augmentation at regular intervals to assess the presence or absence of reflux at every level. Color flow should also be used to observe color changes in distal augmentation flow.

Posterior tibial veins

Beginning at the level of the medial malleolus and moving proximally, examine the distal portion of the deep venous system. The posterior tibial veins are deep veins that are located within the anteromedial aspect of the calf, lying medial to the tibia all the way up the leg from the malleolus up to the tibial-peroneal trunk just below the knee. This portion of the exam is performed with the transducer in the transverse plane and using distal augmentation to increase flow so that Doppler signals can be obtained along the course of the vessel. Color flow is used to search for perforating veins connecting superficial veins to the deep posterior tibial system. When a perforating vein is identified, a directed Doppler signal is obtained, with distal augmentation to check for regurgitant flow.

Anterior tibial veins

The paired anterior tibial veins lie along the lateral aspect of the tibia from mid-ankle to the knee. To examine these vessels, the leg must be repositioned into a slightly more supine position and gel must be applied to the anterolateral aspect of the calf. The transducer is held in the transverse plane to image the vessels from the lateral malleolus up to the knee, where the vessels pass under the fibula to join the popliteal vein in the posterior popliteal fossa.

Popliteal vein

Examination of the remaining deep and superficial veins requires a posterior approach. Rotate the patient to the opposite hip with the leg placed directly on the table and the knee slightly bent. The leg must be completely relaxed. Apply gel to the distal posterior thigh and down the posterior calf. Beginning in the posterior distal thigh, locate the distal femoral vein and use a transverse plane with compression maneuvers to examine the deep system all the way down to the popliteal fossa and the trifurcation of the vein. Return to the posterior thigh, turn the transducer longitudinally, locate the distal superficial femoral vein, and obtain a Doppler signal with distal augmentation. Follow the vessel down into the popliteal fossa and obtain another Doppler signal with distal augmentation at that level.

Tibial and peroneal veins

As the femoral vein becomes the popliteal vein and passes distally into the popliteal fossa, it first gives rise to the anterior tibial veins, which immediately pass anteriorly below the fibula. The anterior tibial vein is not well visualized with the ultrasound probe on the posterior leg, but has already been examined along its course in the anterolateral leg. As the popliteal vein reaches the medial fossa at the level of the popliteal crease it again divides into two veins. One travels medially and becomes the paired posterior tibial system, which has already been examined along its course in the anteromedial leg. The other branch of the popliteal vein travels laterally and becomes the peroneal system. The peroneal veins course downward in the lateral calf medial to the fibula, and a transverse examination with compression is carried out along this path from proximal to distal. The transducer is then turned longitudinally and reflux is assessed with augmentation using color-flow, as well as Doppler, signals.

Lesser saphenous vein

The lesser saphenous vein is the dominant superficial vein on the posterior calf. Like the greater saphenous vein, it lies in a subcutaneous layer sandwiched between two fascial layers. It can be located at the ankle in the posterior malleolar region along the lateral aspect of the Achilles tendon.

Starting in the distal segment of the vein, obtain a Doppler signal with augmentation by squeezing the foot. Examine the vein along its entire course as it passes proximally, assessing reflux in any perforating veins, communicating veins, or branch tributaries. Follow the vein proximally to its termination, which may be into the Giacomini vein in the posterior thigh, into the distal femoral vein, into the popliteal segment of the femoral vein, or (less commonly) into some other venous structure in the upper or lower leg. At the termination of the lesser saphenous vein, look for reflux by obtaining a Doppler signal with distal augmentation.

Remaining varices

The examination thus far has covered all the principal deep and superficial veins of the upper and lower leg. If there remain any areas of varicosity that have not been identified as tributaries of one of the veins already examined, these veins must be investigated directly. Each variceal system should be examined starting at its most distal extent and following the path of reflux proximally until all incompetent perforating veins and all truncal feeders of the refluxing system have been identified. Once the entire leg has been scanned, the entire process is repeated on the opposite leg.

Summary

Contrast venography and magnetic resonance venography are useful imaging techniques that can reliably identify causes of outflow obstruction and can elucidate unusual venous anatomy. For the evaluation of patients with venous insufficiency, however, color-flow duplex ultrasound is the technique of choice because it is inexpensive, noninvasive, and gives both anatomic and hemodynamic information at the same time. Duplex ultrasound is indicated whenever treatment decisions depend on precise knowledge of the structure and function of the venous system.

References

(1) Labropoulos N, Leon M, Nicolaides AN, Giannoukas AD, Volteas N, Chan P. *Superficial venous insufficiency: correlation of anatomic extent of reflux with clinical symptoms and signs.* J Vasc Surg 1994; 20:953–958.

(2) Nicolaides A. *Quantification of venous reflux by means of duplex scanning.* J Vasc Surg 1990; 10:670–677.

(3) Thibault P, Bray A, Wlodarczyk J, Lewis W. *Cosmetic leg veins: evaluation using duplex venous imaging.* J Dermatol Surg Onc 1990; 16:612–618.

(4) Bettmann MA, Paulin S. *Leg phlebography: the incidence, nature and modification of undesirable side effects.* Radiology 1977; 122(1):101–104.

(5) Hull R, Hirsh J, Sackett DL, Powers P, Turpie AG, Walker I. *Combined use of leg scanning and impedance plethysmography in suspected venous thrombosis. An alternative to venography.* N Engl J Med 1977; 296(26):1497–1500.

(6) Shehadi WH. *Contrast media adverse reactions: occurrence, recurrence, and distribution patterns.* Radiology 1982; 143(1):11–17.

(7) Vukov LF, Berquist TH, King BF. *Magnetic resonance imaging for calf deep venous thrombophlebitis.* Ann Emerg Med 1991; 20(5):497–499.

(8) Partsch H, Lofferer O, Mostbeck A. *Diagnosis of established deep-vein thrombosis in the leg using 131-I fibrinogen.* Angiology 1974; 25(11):719–728.

(9) Alavi A, Palevsky HI, Gupta N, Meranze S, Kelley MA, Jatlow AD, et al. *Radiolabeled antifibrin antibody in the detection of venous thrombosis: preliminary results.* Radiology 1990; 175(1):79–85.

PART III

Treatment

CHAPTER 11

Patient Education and Informed Consent

Introduction

A good outcome means both a good medical response to therapy and a satisfied patient. Patient satisfaction depends not so much on the technical success of the procedure as it does on the patient's expectations before the procedure. The best way to ensure a good outcome is to make sure that the expectations of both the patient and the doctor are the same before beginning any treatment. Patient education is an important first step. There are risks associated with every procedure, and no procedure guarantees an excellent medical outcome every time. The patient must understand that medicine is not an exact science, and that there is no guarantee that he or she will be satisfied with the improvement in his or her varicose veins after treatment. To ensure consistency, a list of standard topics for discussion should be adopted. Each topic should be explained carefully, preferably with pictures, in such a way that the patient is able to understand. Each patient must have ample opportunity to ask any questions and to receive complete answers. One should not proceed with treatment until one feels comfortable with the patient's understanding and expectations. It is difficult to establish the appropriate physician–patient relationship with patients who are unreasonable, overly demanding, or unable to comprehend the basics. These types of patients are also the most likely to complain about any or all aspects of their treatment.

Topics for Discussion

Typical topics for *(Table 11-1)* discussion include reasonable patient expectations, underlying causes of venous disease, the medical and cosmetic benefits of treatment, the risks of unsucchealal treatment and of complications, the types of treatments available, the alternatives to treatment, the reasons for requiring a complete examination with testing where indicated, the medications that may be used in treatment and their potential side effects, and any temporary problems that may arise during the course of treatment and the healing phase. Only after such a discussion can an informed consent document reasonably be signed.

PATIENT EXPECTATIONS

Improvement of pain and other symptoms *if* caused by abnormal veins

Complete closure of any particular vein to be treated

80% clearing of overall areas treated for cosmetic reasons: *no* promises of complete clearance

Length of time for clearance is typically 6 months

Only the veins will change, the underlying legs will remain the same

Excellent cosmetic results, but not "perfect legs"

Ability to wear shorts without embarrassment

CAUSES OF VARICOSE VEINS AND SPIDER VEINS

High pressure converting normal veins into varicose veins

Heredity resulting in weak vein walls or malformed vein valves

Hormones making vein walls and valves more elastic

Trauma injuring vein valves in a local area

Professions involving much standing (if genetically susceptible)

Table 11-1
Topics for Discussion with the Patient

Patient expectations

Causes of venous disease

Medical benefits of treatment

Cosmetic benefits of treatment

Risks of unsuccessful treatment

Risks of complications or side effects

Types of treatments available

Alternatives to treatment

Reasons for requiring a complete examination with vascular testing where indicated

Medications that may be used in treatment and their potential side effects

Temporary problems that may arise during the course of treatment

What to expect during the healing phase

BENEFITS OF TREATMENT

Symptoms improved (if due to diseased veins)

Improved appearance

Prevent worsening of, and hopefully avoid, ultimate nonhealing stasis ulcers

Prevent the spread of disease to other connected veins (high-pressure effects)

TREATMENTS AVAILABLE AND TECHNIQUES USED

Injection-compression sclerotherapy (with or without duplex guidance)

Laser treatments for small vessels without high pressure

Minimal surgery–ambulatory phlebectomy

RF endovenous occlusion (Closure™ VNUS Medical Technologies, Sunnyvale, CA)

Surgical stripping

Surgical ligation (usually in combination with stripping or sclerotherapy)

Watchful waiting

Compression stockings alone

NEED FOR COMPLETE EXAMINATION AND POSSIBLE TESTING

To make a correct diagnosis before considering treatment

To identify any potentially correctable cause for vein problems

To give a prognosis for recurrent or new vein problems after treatment

To measure the severity of the problem quantitatively, (for later comparison)

To identify possible contraindications for treatment:
- Deep vein blockage by blood clots, malformation, or scarring
- Deep vein valve leakage

To develop an appropriate treatment plan for each individual patient

MEDICATIONS USED

More than 30 different medications are available for sclerotherapy, but only a few are considered truly safe and effective in the United States today. Sodium morrhuate and ethanolamine oleate are FDA-approved sclerosants, but are rarely recommended because of a reportedly high incidence of serious side effects, including anaphylaxis and death. Polidocanol, Sotradecol, and hypertonic saline are widely considered to be safe and effective sclerosing agents (see Chapter 14).

Polidocanol (Laureth-9)

Polidocanol is a European drug, not yet approved by the FDA but believed by many specialists to be the safest agent with the least side effects. Originally developed in 1931 and sold as a local anaesthetic agent, polidocanol has been used as a sclerosant for more than 50 years. It is used regularly for sclerotherapy by many vein specialists in the United States and worldwide, especially for small veins where a good cosmetic result is important. The U.S. phlebology community hopes that the FDA will approve polidocanol for sale by 2001. A foam version of this sclerosing agent is in development.

Sotradecol

Sotradecol also dates from the 1930s, and was "grandfathered" by the FDA for approval as a sclerosant. Sotradecol is safe and effective, and has a low incidence of problems such as anaphylaxis, ulcer scars, and staining. Most specialists in the United States use sotradecol for larger vessels, and many use it for vessels of all sizes in the appropriate dilutions.

Hypertonic saline

Hypertonic saline is approved by the FDA for use as an abortifacient, so its use in sclerotherapy is considered "off-label." Its use was taught in vascular surgery and dermatology residencies for many years, and many older practitioners still use it regularly. Hypertonic saline is a relatively weak, but effective, sclerosant that can be very painful on injection and can cause severe muscle cramps lasting some time after a treatment session. Hypertonic saline is not usually the best choice where cosmetic outcome is important,

because it can cause a very high incidence of ulcer scars and permanent staining (larger vessels).

POTENTIAL COMPLICATIONS (SEE CHAPTER 24)

Poor results due to persistent high pressure

Staining, especially where large veins have been present for a long time

Swelling of foot if treated

Skin ulceration and "freckle" scar formation

Telangiectatic matting (new tiny "blush" vessels, usually temporary)

Allergy to medications, tape, or stockings

Fainting from nervousness

Known risk of blood clots after vein surgery

Theoretical (but unproven) increased risk of blood clots after sclerotherapy

Risk of blood clots from untreated varicose veins

TREATMENT CAVEATS

Areas treated with any agent may look temporarily inflamed, with tiny red "blush" vessels

Temporary bruising will occur at treatment sites

Patient consent for treatment

I understand that medicine is not an exact science, and that even though the vast majority of patients are satisfied with their results, there is no guarantee I myself will be satisfied with the improvement in my varicose veins after treatment. I acknowledge that the following topics have been explained to me, and that I understand the explanations I was given. I have had the opportunity to ask any questions. In particular, I am familiar with the following information:

☐ The various techniques that can be used for treating diseased veins
☐ The option to do nothing about my vein problem
☐ Benefits of treatment
☐ Risks & potential complications
☐ Bruising & discoloration
☐ Inflammation or trapped blood
☐ Fainting from nervousness
☐ Allergic reaction to medication or tape
☐ Skin staining (hyperpigmentation)
☐ Skin ulcers
☐ Telangiectatic matting
☐ Recurrence of varicosities
☐ Theoretical risk of thrombosis, embolism, and death

I recognize that even though any particular problem may be extremely rare, it is always possible that any patient may have one of these problems. I accept that possibility for my own treatment.

I understand that ultimately I am responsible for my own medical bills. I understand that unless otherwise agreed in writing, I must pay my bill in full at the time of each visit. If this medical practice agrees to accept initial insurance assignment for some portion of my medical care, I authorize this medical practice to submit bills to my insurance company and to receive reimbursement directly from my insurance company.

*Signed:*_____   *Date:*_____   *Witness:*_____

Figure 11-1.   Patient consent for treatment.

Trapped blood may cause local soreness until it is reabsorbed or released

Results will not usually be visible until several treatments have been completed

Some eventual recurrence or development of new veins is inevitable unless the cause can be removed

Informed Consent

Obtaining informed consent before a procedure is a legal duty owed to the patient. Informed consent need not be obtained in writing—a simple conversation may be sufficient—but a written document offers many advantages for the physician. It is a way for the patient to demonstrate an informed willingness to accept the risks of treatment and to share in the responsibility for the outcome. It is also a way to identify a patient who doesn't want to sign because he or she does not truly accept the intrinsic risks of treatment. An informed consent document does not offer legal protection for the physician, but the absence of such a document can be an important deficiency in the defense against any future complaint. Figure 11-1 is a sample consent document for patients who will undergo sclerotherapy for superficial venous insufficiency (see also Chapter 27).

Summary

Patient education and informed consent are the most important way of enhancing overall patient satisfaction with a normal range of outcomes. Presentation of a standard list of topics, followed by open discussion, will provide the best opportunity to fully understand a patient's needs and wishes. Equally important is the opportunity to communicate a reasonable expectation of what can and cannot be achieved. Informed consent will not prevent a lawsuit from an unreasonable patient, but the entire process of education and consent can diminish the overall likelihood of a lawsuit being filed or of having an adverse outcome for the physician.

CHAPTER 12

Treatment of Large Varicose Veins

General Principles

Make a Correct Diagnosis

General Principles

No matter what the size, all varicosities result from pressures too high for the vein walls to withstand. To correct the problem, all abnormal sources of high pressure must be found and eliminated. In treating veins of any size by any method, the best results are obtained when the treatment plan is based on a complete understanding of the anatomy of the refluxing circuit. Main high-pressure reflux points should be treated first, even though more distal areas may be more visually disturbing to the patient.

When a correct underlying diagnosis has been made and an appropriate treatment plan developed, sclerotherapy can be an effective therapy for veins of any caliber. How-

Table 12-1
Principles of Large Vein Sclerotherapy

> Identify and treat specific reflux points
> The order of treatment is proximal to distal
> Treat larger veins before smaller veins
> Empty vein of blood by various maneuvers
> Treat entire varicosity at one time
> Compress immediately and adequately
> Patient ambulates following treatment

ever, the larger and more proximal the reflux entry point, and the higher the pressure at that point, the greater the likelihood of early recurrences. There is evidence that the initial success rate can be higher and that any recurrences can be delayed several additional years when surgery is used to treat the most proximal sites of reflux, such as the saphenofemoral junction.[1,2]

Although there is a widespread preference for surgery in patients with junctional incompetence, successful sclerotherapy of the saphenofemoral junction is possible.[3] Many experienced practitioners do use sclerotherapy for junctional incompetence, but sclerosis of truncal varices with high-grade junctional reflux often requires special techniques and high-potency sclerosants that are not part of the basic armamentarium. The inexperienced phlebologist is unlikely to have success in such efforts. A reasonable rule of thumb is that if maneuvers such as Valsalva can elicit reflux through the saphenofemoral junction with the patient supine, the junction probably will be resistant to basic methods of large-vessel sclerotherapy.

Varicosities that arise from perforator incompetence usually are amenable to sclerotherapy, no matter how large and convoluted they may appear.[4] Large varices can be as much as 30 mm or more in diameter, but the same basic approach is useful for all vessels in which reflux can be identified. Principles of large vein sclerotherapy are listed in *Table 12-1*.

Make a Correct Diagnosis

It is possible to have a certain amount of short-term success with the occasional patient simply by injecting sclerosants into any visible spider veins and varicose veins. This haphazard approach will not lead to a successful phlebology practice, however, because the number of treatment failures and of complications will be much too high. Long-term success depends upon first making the correct diagnosis, that is, identifying the sources of reflux that have caused the problem and that will cause it to recur if not properly treated.

STEPS PRIOR TO TREATMENT

When patients present for treatment of varicose veins, history and physical examination are very important. (See Chapter 27 for appropriate questionnaires and forms.) The

patient's legs must be thoroughly examined with the patient standing so that more subtle varicosities may become visible. Noninvasive testing (see Chapters 6, 8, 9, and 10) is critical to establish the abnormal anatomy, since this is what dictates possible treatments. As discussed above, a malfunctioning saphenofemoral junction must be corrected before distal associated varicosities are treated.

Education and consent of the patient are also important (see Chapter 11). After photographs are taken and pre- and posttreatment instructions reviewed, one may proceed with a first treatment "test" injection. The first treatment session is usually limited to a small number of sites of telangiectasias rather than varicosities, for several reasons. One can thus observe the patient for any allergic reactions, judge the effectiveness of a particular concentration and class of sclerosing agent, and observe any reactions to the tape or foam pads used for compression. It also serves to familiarize the patient with sclerotherapy, the treating physician, clinic surroundings, and the sensation of the fine needle. The test site also complies with the recommendation of the manufacturer's (Wyeth-Ayerst) package insert for sodium tetradecyl sulfate. In two of these authors' practices, Doppler examination and D-PPG are commonly also done at this first visit. The patient returns separately for complete or limited duplex examination, as necessary, prior to his or her first full treatment session.

Adopt an Appropriate Treatment Plan

Large vessels (and smaller vessels fed by identifiable sources of reflux) are best treated either by surgical removal or by ablation using injection-compression sclerotherapy. Older approaches, such as thermocoagulation and electrocoagulation, should be avoided because they rarely are able to address the underlying reflux, and usually cause excessive collateral tissue damage and scarring. Photocoagulation using laser or intense pulsed-light treatment is effective primarily for small vessels without identifiable sources of reflux (see Chapter 20).

START WITH REFLUX ENTRY POINTS

Whether the treatment of larger veins is by surgery or by sclerotherapy, if the principal site of high-pressure reflux is not controlled, the patient will nearly always suffer the early reappearance of spider veins and varicose veins, either as newly recruited vessels, or as treated vessels that have reopened. Every treatment plan is aimed first at the ablation of high-pressure reflux, and only secondarily at the ablation of superficial vessels that may be of more concern to the patient.

TREAT PROXIMAL VARICES BEFORE DISTAL TELANGIECTASIA

Proximal vessels and larger vessels are most often conduits that deliver high pressure to smaller, more distal vessels, thus treatment generally should move from proximal to distal and from larger to smaller vessels. Patients often try to insist that the most visible vessels be treated first, even if they are smaller and more distal, but the temptation to yield must be resisted.

Pitfalls of beginning treatment distally

There are several problems that often arise when an area of distal branch varicosities or spider veins is treated without first addressing the principal site of reflux. Once the most obvious vessels are gone, the patient may consider the treatment complete, and may fail to return for treatment directed at the site of reflux. This leads to early recurrence in nearly every case. In some cases, distal varicosities serve as a "runoff" conduit that reduces the pressure in the refluxing circuit by allowing reflux to re-enter the deep veins at a more distal location. When this is the case, closing the distal veins before addressing the proximal reflux causes an immediate rise in static pressure in the circuit. This often causes a very rapid appearance of large numbers of new exuberant telangiectasia, which are very distressing to the patient (Figure 12-1). Sclerotherapy beginning with distal vessels may cause secondary thrombosis of more proximal segments, making it impossible to inject the proximal segments later. Lacking a sufficient endothelial injury, the thrombosed vessel will recanalize and the original problem will recur.

TREAT AN ENTIRE VESSEL AT ONE TIME

When one portion of a varicosity is treated and another is not, the untreated segment often becomes thrombosed and feels hard and tender. Since there has been no real endothelial destruction, however, that portion of the vessel recanalizes quickly and appears as a treatment failure.

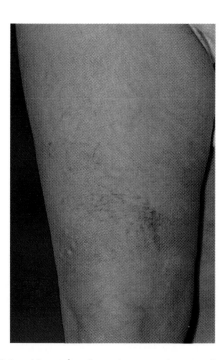

Figure 12-1. New telangiectasias occurring at a site of previous treatment in which a distal outflow vein has been sclerosed. Treatment of the proximal refluxing vein might have prevented this.

EMPTY VEINS OF BLOOD BEFORE INJECTING

Any blood remaining in the vein will serve to dilute the injected sclerosant, rendering it less effective. Maneuvers that can reduce the amount of blood in the vein will lead to a better result with a lower initial concentration of sclerosant. Reducing the amount of blood also theoretically reduces the risk of postsclerosis pigmentation.

MAINTAIN COMPRESSION AFTER TREATMENT

Effective ablation of a treated varix is much more likely when collagen microfibrils can span the entire vessel from wall to wall, and this is more likely when the vessel is kept compressed after treatment. Compression also reduces the amount of intravascular coagulum (posttreatment thrombus) in the treated vessel, thus reducing pain, inflammation, bruising, and hemosiderin deposition in the tissues. Compression is also desirable because it is an effective form of prophylaxis against deep vein thrombosis in the posttreatment period.

KEEP THE PATIENT AMBULATORY

Injection sclerotherapy produces local endothelial injury and alteration of circulating coagulation and fibrinolytic factors, increasing the theoretical risk of deep venous thrombosis. To prevent this complication, it is extremely important that venous stasis be avoided after sclerotherapy. Together with compression, increased ambulation is an important way to prevent or reduce venous stasis.

REASSESS THE DIAGNOSIS WHEN NECESSARY

Whenever a patient fails to respond to treatment as expected, the underlying diagnosis should be questioned. Although some patients can be very resistant to treatment, most treatment failures result because previously unrecognized high-pressure points have been left untreated. Duplex ultrasound examination is extremely helpful in reassessing a patient who has failed treatment or who has had an early recurrence after apparently successful treatment.

Techniques for Sclerotherapy of Large Varices

Many different techniques for large-vein sclerotherapy have been described historically, and different methods have found popularity in different countries at different times. Aside from injection under direct ultrasound visualization (see Chapter 19), there are two principal techniques for large-vein sclerotherapy that have gained widespread popularity in the United States at this time, both derived from techniques that were originally popularized by Tournay in France[5], Sigg in Germany[6], Hobbs in England[7], and Fegan in Ireland[8]. The classic schools are summarized in Table 12-2.

The two principal techniques of large-vessel sclerotherapy that are currently popular in the United States differ primarily in their method of vein cannulation. Experienced practitioners employ many variations. In all cases, the goal

Table 12-2
Classic Schools of Large Vessel Sclerotherapy

Physician	Country	Method	Compression
Tournay	French	Proximal to distal	No compression
Sigg	Swiss	Entire varicosity at one time	Compression
		Totally "empty" vein technique	
Fegan	Ireland	Perforating veins targeted	Compression
		Slight leg elevation during treatment	

Table 12-4
Main Steps for Supine Direct Cannulation (SDC) Technique

Primary sites of reflux identified

Every 3–4 cm along each vein to be treated is marked or noted with patient standing

Patient in supine or prone position for actual treatment

27–30 G needle on a 3 cc syringe utilized

Needle is advanced while aspirating

Aspiration of blood indicates penetration of the lumen

0.5 to 1.5 cc (safer to be closer to 0.5 cc) sclerosant injected at each site

Move to next site 3–4 cm away

Endpoint: vein completely contracted

Placement of cotton roll and tape over vein, then support hose

is the sclerosis of proximal, large, high-pressure vessels. However the varicose vein is cannulated, the concentrations and dosages of sclerosants are similar (*Table 12-3*).

SUPINE DIRECT CANNULATION (SDC) TECHNIQUE

In this technique (*Table 12-4*), the patient stands at first, causing the varices to bulge and become more visible. Injection points are marked at primary sites of reflux into the system and approximately every 3–4 cm along each vein to be treated (*Figure 12-2*). The patient is then placed in a supine or prone position as necessary, and a syringe and needle are used to inject a small volume of sclerosant at each one of the marked points along the veins to be treated. A 27–30 Gauge needle on a 3 cc syringe is often employed for this technique. The needle is advanced while aspirating the syringe until aspiration of dark venous blood indicates penetration of the lumen. At this point 0.5–1.5 cc of concentrated sclerosant is injected at the site. The needle is withdrawn and redirected to the next site. At the conclusion of treatment the vein should be visually contracted. This is a rapid and efficacious technique that is used by the majority of phlebologists treating large veins in the United States today.

When this technique is used, it must be recognized that the vessels being injected are not fully empty of blood, thus the sclerosant being injected must be more concentrated to allow for dilution by the blood remaining in the vessel. The

largest vessels contain more blood and therefore require higher concentrations of sclerosant, and possibly higher volumes, to produce effective sclerosis after dilution.

In experienced hands this technique has proven safe, rapid, convenient, and effective. Patients are more comfortable and much less likely to faint receiving treatment lying down. Millions of patient treatment sessions have been safely performed with this technique. The principal disadvantages of this approach are that it requires a concentrated sclerosant to withstand dilution by blood that remains within the vessels. Needle-tip control is maintained by resting the syringe against the non-dominant hand. A steady hand is still necessary to avoid rare extravasation of the concentrated sclerosant. Inexperienced phlebologists sometimes have been said to extravasate up to half of the volume injected (the so-called "50-50 injection") due to unexpected vasospasm or poor needle-tip control. Extravasation of highly concentrated sclerosants can cause neuritis, arteritis, and periostitis, besides the more obvious complications of soft tissue necrosis. A secondary concern is that this approach carries the extremely remote possibility of inadvertent arterial injection, because the color of aspirated blood is not a totally reliable guide to distinguish venous from arterial cannulation. Perforating arteries often accompany perforating veins, and injection into an artery nearly always leads to substantial tissue necrosis, and sometimes even loss of the entire limb. Finally, there is a concern that if a concentrated sclerosant is inadvertently injected directly into a perforat-

Table 12-3
Dosage of Sclerosants for Large Vein Sclerotherapy

Sclerosant	Concentration	Volume
Sodium tetradecyl sulfate (Sotradecol)	0.5–3%	Maximum 10 cc of 3%
Polidocanol (Aethoxysklerol, Laureth-9)	1–5%	Maximum 20 cc of 3%
Variglobin (polyiodinated iodine salt)	1–6%	Maximum 2 cc of 6%
Sclerodex (only reticular)	Undiluted	Maximum 20 cc per session
Hypertonic 23.4%	Undiluted	Maximum 20 cc per session

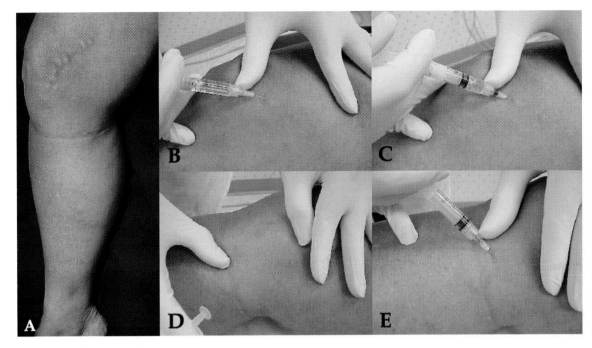

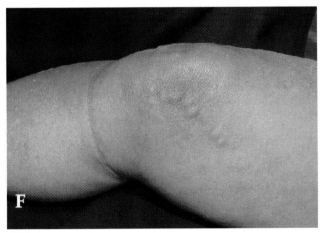

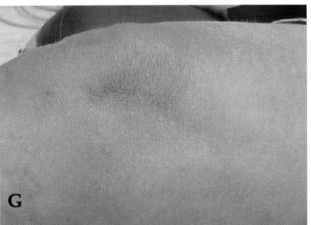

Figure 12-2. Method of large-vein injection by the supine direct cannulation technique. **(A)** Entire leg is examined and evaluated. A large GSV branch varicosity without SFJ reflux is seen. Early stasis dermatitis changes are noted on ankle. **(B)** Needle cannulation (30 gauge) with patient in supine position. **(C)** Trendelenburg position increased to flatten vein with flashback of dark blood into the needle hub or syringe. Injection then proceeds. **(D)** After 1 cc of injection volume, pressure is applied for one minute and solution is spread to neighboring branches. **(E)** Additional branches are then treated with treatment spaced at 3–4 cm intervals. **(F)** View before treatment. **(G)** Proper endpoint of treatment with total collapse and contraction of the targeted vein. Compression is then applied with cotton rolls and overlying compression stockings.

ing vessel, it may pass directly into the deep venous system and cause deep system injury or thrombosis before it is diluted below the threshold of efficacy.

A commonly used modification of this technique reduces the amount of dilution with intravascular blood by using the fingers of the non-injecting hand to "milk" blood from the area to be injected. Although the vein is not truly empty after being "milked," this approach does decrease the volume of dilution, and is referred to as an empty-vein technique. After the injection, finger pressure is maintained several centimeters above and below the injection point to

confine the sclerosing solution as long as possible.[9] This finger pressure is maintained for 30–60 seconds, and is followed by compression with a cotton roll or foam pad.

MULTIPLE PRECANNULATION SITES (MPS) TECHNIQUE

Some practitioners believe that the multiple precannulation sites (MPS) technique, although less convenient and slower, may offer greater precision with a greater margin of safety *(Table 12-5)*. For this technique, the patient initially stands,

Table 12-5
Main Steps for Multiple Precannulation Sites
(MPS) Technique

Patient standing for varices to bulge

Injection points are marked at proximal and distal sites

Sites to be treated are cannulated with a butterfly needle or an intravenous cannula

Connected tubing briefly opened to air to confirm no arterial pressure

Butterfly needles or cannulae firmly secured

Patient moved to treatment table, leg elevated

Small volume of normal saline solution is injected into the cannula

It is not possible to withdraw blood to confirm intravascular placement

If no swelling at tip, then 2–3 cc of sclerosant is infused into the cannula

Endpoint: vein completely contracted

Placement of cotton roll and tape over vein, then support hose

---

encouraging the varices to bulge and become more visible. Injection points are marked at proximal and distal sites along the bulging varices (*Figure 12-3*). With the veins distended, sites to be treated are cannulated with a butterfly needle and tubing, or a plastic intravenous cannula and extension tubing, at both proximal and distal sites, and the tubing is opened to air to ensure that there is no evidence of arterial pressure and that no pulsations are evident within it. The butterfly needles or cannulas must be firmly secured, as the patient then moves to the treatment table and elevates the leg well above the level of the heart. One pitfall of this technique is dislodgement of the well-placed intravascular needle or cannula with the patient's movement.

If the legs are properly elevated, the superficial varices usually are completely collapsed, and it usually is not possible to withdraw blood to confirm the position of the needle or cannula. Instead, a small volume of normal saline solution is injected into the cannula and the surrounding area is observed for swelling or other evidence of extravasation. In many cases, the infusion of saline causes a "thrill" that may be palpably appreciated more proximally along the cannulated vein. After intravascular position has been verified, 2 cc–3 cc of sclerosant is infused into the cannula. Since the vein is nearly empty, the amount of dilution will be small, and the sclerosant injected need not be extremely concentrated. In this position, limited dilution also allows the sclerosant to travel more proximally before it drops below the threshold of efficacy. In most cases, a single proximal and a single distal injection point are sufficient to sclerose a large, tortuous vessel.

While used much less often worldwide than the SDC approach, the principal advantages of the MPS approach are that dilute sclerosants may be extravasated with less risk of collateral injury to adjacent tissues, that dilute sclerosants will not cause deep venous injury even if infused directly into the deep veins (which contain large volumes of diluting blood), and that the open butterfly or intravenous cannula

reliably protects against inadvertent arterial injection. The great disadvantages of the technique are that it is very time-consuming, requires more supplies, and that the butterfly needles or cannulae may be dislodged as the patient reclines and the legs are elevated. Also, patients are more likely to experience vasovagal reactions to the venipunctures while in a standing position. These disadvantages may be offset by the greater control offered to the inexperienced phlebologist. RW and MW prefer the SDC technique, while CF favors the MPS technique.

VARIATIONS

There are many widely used variations on these common approaches to large-vessel sclerotherapy.

In the "air-block technique," 0.5–1.0 ml of air is injected initially to "clear" the varix of blood.[10] This technique is of unproven efficacy, but despite its alternate moniker as the "air embolism" technique, it is probably safe, because the bolus of air becomes trapped in the pulmonary vascular bed and is absorbed without sequelae.

Detergent sclerosants may also be injected using a "foam technique," in which foam is produced by shaking the sclerosing agent vigorously or by drawing tiny bubbles of air through the sclerosant using a glass syringe.[11,12] When injected, such foams are diluted less rapidly than a dissolved sclerosant would be, and so they remain in longer contact with the vessel wall. This foam also maximizes the fraction of sclerosant that is in the bioactive micellar form, and is believed to permit a lower volume and a lower concentration of sclerosant. Recent reports have claimed far greater efficacy for sclerosant foamed into a mousse,[13] but for most clinicians the clinical efficacy of a non-commercially prepared foam has not been proven. In some cases the tiny foam bubbles have been blamed for several cases of visual disturbances and temporary blindness that may have been caused by the passage of tiny foam aggregates through a patent foramen ovale and into the retinal circulation.

A power table permits needles or cannulae to be introduced with the patient in slight reverse Trendelenberg, after which the table can be tipped until the legs are in a neutral or elevated position. The table also facilitates elevation of the leg immediately after injection, believed by some to improve the response to treatment.

An older European approach uses an open needle (with no syringe) to drain venous blood from the varix into a basin, in an effort to obtain a vein that is truly empty (the open needle also guards against inadvertent arterial cannulation).[14] After the flow of venous blood from the varix has diminished, a syringe is affixed and the sclerosant is infused. It is difficult to comply with OSHA bloodborne pathogen guidelines (US) utilizing this technique.

Treatment of Reticular Varicose Veins

In treating reticular veins, the concentration, strength, and volume of sclerosing solution are decreased with decreasing vein diameter. The sclerosing solutions most commonly used

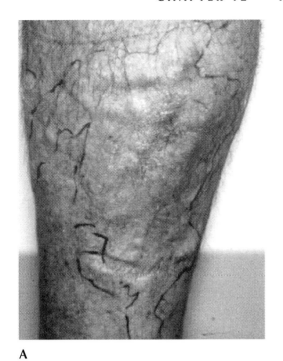

A

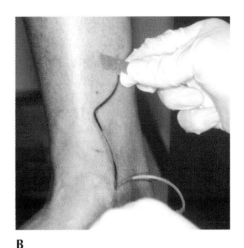

B

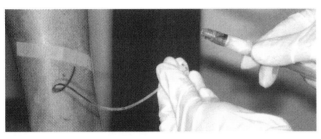

D

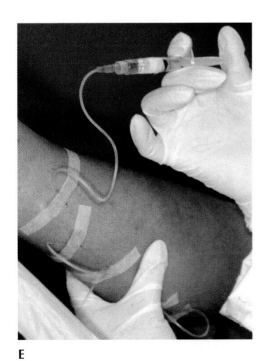

E

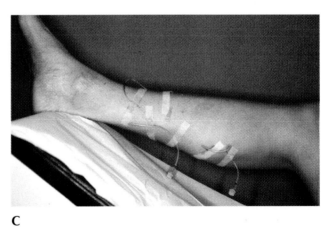

C

Figure 12-3.   Method of large-vein injection by the multiple precannulation sites technique. **(A)** Marking. **(B)** Cannulation of bulging vein. **(C)** Patient placed on treatment table with legs elevated. **(D)** Syringe attached to butterfly. **(E)** Sclerosing solution injected into empty vein.

for reticular veins are sodium tetradecyl sulfate (Sotradecol) in concentrations of 0.2–0.5%, and polidocanol (Aethoxysclerol) in concentrations of 0.5%–1%. These veins usually are quite superficial and visibly blue, and usually do not require marking by pen.

Subdermic reticular veins and their associated telangiectasias should be treated only after all recognized sources of reflux have been treated by sclerotherapy and/or surgery. If telangiectasias are to be treated, feeding reticular veins should also be treated, because treatment of reticular veins greatly reduces the rates of recurrence of telangiectasias and side effects.[15]

SUPINE DIRECT CANNULATION (SDC) TECHNIQUE FOR RETICULAR VEINS

With the patient recumbent, a 3 cc syringe with a 27- or 30-gauge needle is inserted into the vessel. Bending the needle to allow placement parallel to the skin surface eases cannulation. When the sensation of piercing the vein is felt, the plunger is pulled back gently until blood begins to back up into the transparent hub. This is possible even with a 30-gauge needle, although a 27-gauge is most commonly employed. The volume injected should be just sufficient to perfuse the reticular vein in question, and rarely exceeds 0.5 cc per injection site.

MULTIPLE PRECANNULATION SITES (MPS) TECHNIQUE FOR RETICULAR VEINS

With the patient recumbent, a 27-gauge butterfly needle is used to cannulate a visible reticular vein in the usual fashion. The blood flow into the butterfly tubing is observed to ensure the absence of arterial pulsations, and a 3 cc syringe is attached and used to infuse approximately 0.5 cc of sclerosant at the site. If the reticular vein is long, additional injections may be made every 4–6 cm along its length.

Compression

After any of these techniques, a compression bandage of some sort is usually applied to the treated vessels. There are a number of experienced and well-recognized phlebologists who do not use compression at all in their practice, but the majority of practitioners have come to agree that compression leads to better, faster outcomes, with fewer side effects. Cotton rolls, cotton pads, cotton balls, or specially manufactured foam pads are applied along the entire course of the treated vessel and are held there by a compression garment. In the United States, compression usually is applied using 30–40 mm Hg gradient compression hose. European phlebologists prefer firm rolls of cotton wool, which are fixed over the course of the entire vein, with additional compression given by a combination of a class I (daytime and nighttime) and class II (daytime only) medical compression hosiery.[16] Some European phlebologists still prefer compression bandaging alone, although its application is more difficult.

The optimum duration of compression was shown in a recent study to be a minimum of 3 weeks, although 3 days demonstrated better results than no compression.[17] After a treatment, some physicians recommend 72 hours of uninterrupted compression, during which time patients may bathe or shower by securing a large plastic bag over the compression bandage or stocking. After the first 72 hours, any compression pads or cotton rolls are discarded, and patients are thereafter permitted to remove the stocking as needed for bathing and sleeping. Continuous compression (interrupted only for bathing and sleeping) is recommended for a period of 3 weeks because patients poorly accept longer regimens.

An alternative approach, used by two of the authors, is the application of Medi-Rip™, Conco Medical Company, Bridgeport, CT, bandages over the linearly taped cotton balls when the treated varicose vein is greater than 1 cm in diameter. Compression hose (30–40 mm) are worn over these. At bedtime of the day of treatment, the hose are removed and the patient sleeps with the Medi-Rip™ in place. The next morning, the patient removes the Medi-Rip™ and cotton balls, and wears the compression stockings daily for 2–3 weeks, removing only for sleeping and bathing.

Many patients routinely wear a pair of normal pantyhose or tights in a dark shade or color over their compression hose. This is an effective way of maintaining a normal appearance in a patient who has just undergone treatment. For a "dressier" look, women may wear sheer black hose over their compression hose.

Treatment Intervals and Progress

Typically, patients are seen for follow-up treatment at 2–4 week intervals until the treated veins appear to be satisfactorily sclerosed. At these follow-ups, it is not uncommon to find firm areas of almost nodular hyperpigmentation along the track of the treated varicose and reticular veins. On follow-up sessions, these areas are typically "nicked" with an 18-gauge needle to release the dark, liquid blood trapped in the developing fibrosis. This allows faster resolution of the pigmentation (see Chapter 24). Two to three sessions of sclerotherapy are commonly needed to resolve an area of varicose veins.

When patients have had a poor response to the initial series of treatments, a hidden or unresolved source of reflux may be present. Evaluation with handheld Doppler and color-flow duplex ultrasound is indicated to elucidate the patterns and sources of reflux that have led to a treatment failure. A higher concentration of sclerosant may be necessary. Patient compliance with compression must be stressed. Duplex-guided sclerotherapy may become necessary.

Contraindications to Sclerotherapy

Although generally safe and effective in most situations, sclerotherapy should be avoided when varices carry antegrade flow and when there is a high risk of complications (Table 12-6) (see Chapter 18).

Table 12-6
Contraindications to Sclerotherapy

Bedridden patient
Severe arterial obstruction
Diabetes (severity dependent)
History of deep venous obstruction with antegrade flow in varicosities
Allergy to sclerosing agent or urticaria after previous treatment
Hypercoagulable states—may predispose thrombosis extending into the deep system
Pregnancy (compression is treatment of choice)
Massive obesity
Poor tolerance of support hose

PRIOR HISTORY OF DEEP VENOUS THROMBOSIS

If there is an obstruction of the deep venous system, secondary varicose veins may serve as an important "bypass" conduit to carry blood around the obstruction and back to the central circulation. When this is the case, flow through the varicosities is not retrograde, but rather antegrade. Because of this possibility, patients with a history of deep thrombophlebitis must be fully evaluated by duplex ultrasound before sclerotherapy is considered. "Bypass" varicosities carrying antegrade flow are hemodynamically useful, and must not be ablated.

INABILITY TO AMBULATE

A bedridden patient is not a good candidate for sclerotherapy because ambulation is necessary following treatment to clear the sclerosant from the legs, and thus to decrease the possibility of deep vein thrombosis.

ARTERIAL INSUFFICIENCY

Patients with severe arterial obstruction to the legs are very poor candidates for venous sclerotherapy because they cannot tolerate compression and cannot ambulate freely. Such patients may nonetheless benefit dramatically from treatment to correct major venous reflux, which may be undertaken if the benefits are believed to outweigh the risks. Patients with mild proximal or distal arterial disease, including those with arteriolar sequelae of diabetes, may be treated cautiously.

ALLERGY

Previous allergy to a particular sclerosing agent is a relative contraindication to its further use.

HYPERCOAGULABLE STATES

Sclerotherapy should be avoided in hypercoagulable states that may predispose thrombosis extending into the deep system.

PREGNANCY

Early practitioners did not consider pregnancy to be a contraindication for sclerotherapy, and many thousands of pa-

tients have undergone sclerotherapy during pregnancy. Nonetheless, sclerosing solutions do cross the placental barrier, and their effects on fetal development are unknown. Pregnancy and the postpartum period are hypercoagulable states, and the risk of DVT is elevated in these patients. Finally, many varicosities and telangiectasias that appear or

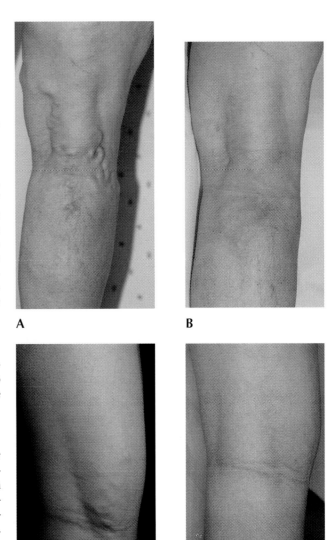

Figure 12-4. Successful varicose vein sclerotherapy **(A)** Vein of Giacomini before sclerotherapy. **(B)** Vein of Giacomini after 3 sessions of sclerotherapy spaced 3 weeks apart. The first utilized 1 cc of 2% sotradecol proximally, with 5 other sites of 0.5 cc of 1% sotradecol, and 0.1% sotradecol into the associated distal telangiectasias; the second two sessions used only 1% sotradecol. **(C)** Typical large posteromedial branch varicosity off of the greater saphenous vein (in the so-called Dodd's region). **(D)** Three months after one session utilizing 1% sotradecol, 1 cc into each of 3 spaced sites (3 cc total) showing excellent resolution.

worsen during pregnancy will resolve spontaneously within a few months postpartum. For all of these reasons, the current recommendation is to utilize compression alone as the treatment of choice during pregnancy, and to defer treatment for 3–6 months thereafter.

MASSIVE OBESITY

It is extremely difficult to obtain or maintain adequate compression on severely obese legs. Whenever possible, sclerotherapy of larger varicosities should be postponed until weight reduction is achieved.

UNWILLINGNESS TO TOLERATE COMPRESSION

During hot summer months, some patients cannot tolerate heavy compression hose. For these patients, cooperation is assured by postponing treatment of larger varicosities to winter months, when the warming effect of compression hose can be appreciated.

Summary

Successful treatment of large varicose veins and reticular veins depends not on pure technical ability, but on careful pretreatment planning. The most important factors are appropriate patient selection, careful evaluation, correct diagnosis, and an appropriate treatment plan. With good preparation, the technical approach to these patients is not difficult, and many variations in technique are possible. Results of properly done varicose vein sclerotherapy can be excellent, and patients very gratified (*Figure 12-4*).

References

(1) de Groot WP. *Treatment of varicose veins: modern concepts and methods.* J Dermatol Surg Onc 1989; 15:191–198.

(2) Neglen P, Einarsson E, Eklof B. *The functional long-term value of different types of treatment for saphenous vein incompetence.* J Cardiovasc Surg (Torino) 1993; 34:295–301.

(3) Kanter A, Thibault P. *Saphenofemoral incompetence treated by ultrasound-guided sclerotherapy.* Dermatol Surg 1996; 22(7):648–652.

(4) Thibault PK, Lewis WA. *Recurrent varicose veins. Part 2: Injection of incompetent perforating veins using ultrasound guidance.* J Dermatol Surg Onc 1992; 18:895–900.

(5) Tournay R, Caille JP, Chatard H, et al. *La sclerose des varices,* 3 ed. Paris: Expansion Scientifique, 1980.

(6) Sigg K. *The treatment of varicosities and accompanying complications.* Angiology 1952; 3:355–379.

(7) Hobbs JT. *The treatment of varicose veins: a random trial of injection/compression versus surgery.* Br J Surg 1968; 55:777–780.

(8) Fegan WG. *Continuing uninterrupted compression technique of injecting varicose veins.* Proc R Soc Med 1960; 53:837–840.

(9) Fegan WG. *Continuous compression technique of injecting varicose veins.* Lancet 1963; 2:109–112.

(10) Orbach EJ. *Sclerotherapy of varicose veins: utilization of intravenous air block.* Am J Surg 1944; 66:362–366.

(11) Orbach EJ, Petretti AK. *Thrombogenic property of foam synthetic anionic detergent (sodium tetradecyl sulfate, N.N.R.).* Angiology 1950; 1:237–243.

(12) Fluckiger P. [*Intraoperative obliteration of varicose veins with sodium tetradecysulfate foam in Babcock's operation*]. Zentralbl Phlebol 1967; 6(4):514–518.

(13) Sadoun S, Benigni JP. *Bonnes pratiques cliniques et mousse de sclérosant: propositions pour une étude randomisée contrôlée, prospective, multicentrique, comparative, en aveugle, sur le traitement sclérosant par la mousse d'aetoxisclérol à 0,20 %.* Phlebol 1999;(3):291–298.

(14) Bernbach HR. [*Sigg's sclerosing therapy*]. Phlebologie 1991; 44:31–32; discussion 33–36.

(15) Weiss RA, Weiss MA. *Painful telangiectasias: diagnosis and treatment.* In: Bergan JJ, Weiss RA, Goldman MP, editors. Varicose Veins and Telangiectasias: Diagnosis and Treatment, 2nd ed. St. Louis: Quality Medical, 1999: 389–406.

(16) Tazelaar DJ, Neumann HA, De Roos KP. *Long cotton wool rolls as compression enhancers in macrosclerotherapy for varicose veins.* Dermatol Surg 1999; 25(1):38–40.

(17) Weiss RA, Sadick NS, Goldman MP, Weiss MA. *Post-sclerotherapy compression: controlled comparative study of duration of compression and its effects on clinical outcome.* Dermatol Surg 1999; 25(2):105–108.

Treatment of Small Veins

Introduction

Sclerotherapy is a useful adjunct to large-vein surgery as well as a highly effective primary treatment for telangiectasia. Patients with axial varicosities often also have large numbers of small reticular veins and telangiectasia. Although these may be surgically removed by stab avulsion, sclerotherapy presents a rapid, effective, and cosmetically acceptable alternative that is particularly attractive in patients with very extensive networks of small abnormal veins (Figure 13-1).

Isolated small reticular veins and telangiectasia often cause severe symptoms that are worsened by prolonged standing or sitting, and that may be relieved by wearing support hose or by elevation of the legs.[1] Vein size alone does not predict the presence of symptoms. Vessels causing symptoms may be as small as 1 mm in diameter or less.[2]

Besides symptoms of pain, burning, and fatigue, the appearance of the telangiectatic veins may be so disturbing that patients curtail their activities and modify their lifestyles to avoid situations in which their legs may be seen. Sclerotherapy not only offers the possibility of remarkably good cosmetic results, but also has been reported to yield an 85% reduction in symptoms (Figure 13-2).[1]

Developing Expertise

A substantial investment of time and effort is required to develop expertise in sclerotherapy of veins of any size. Prior experience with venipuncture helps very little with treatment of larger veins, and is completely irrelevant in the treatment of the smallest veins. Successful treatment requires the correct technique, the correct diagnosis, and the

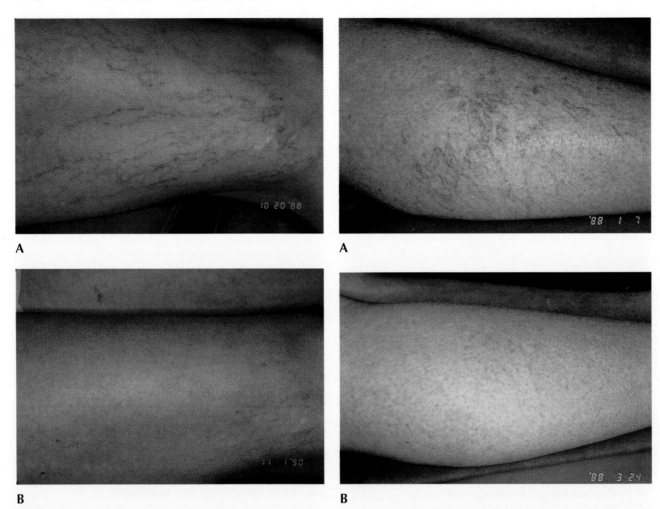

Figure 13-1. Extensive network of protuberant telangiectatic webs, most efficiently treated by sclerotherapy. **(A)** Before sclerotherapy with 0.1% and 0.2% sotradecol **(B)** After three sessions, two years later good results persist.

Figure 13-2. Good cosmetic results and symptomatic improvement after sclerotherapy of painful telangiectasias. **(A)** Before treatment **(B)** After 2 sessions using 0.1% sotradecol in the telangiectasias, and 0.5% sotradecol in the feeding reticular vein.

correct treatment plan for the type and size of vein to be treated. The procedure is mastered by reading written descriptions of proper technique and by observing and emulating the fastidious technique of skilled physicians. Many different techniques have been used in the treatment of small veins, but certain basic principles are universal.[3–8]

Classification and Anatomy

In order to diagnose and treat telangiectasias in a logical way, a classification scheme is helpful *(Table 13-1)*. A discussion of painful telangiectasia includes telangiectasias (type I), venulectases (type II), and associated blue reticular veins (type III). For the purposes of sclerotherapy of telangiectasias, it will be assumed that the major primary varicose veins of types IV and V have already been eliminated or are absent.

TELANGIECTASIA FROM AXIAL REFLUX

Telangiectatic webs may be the result of axial reflux due to junctional or large perforator incompetence.[7] It is crucial to realize that axial reflux does not always result in large visible varicosities. Therefore a detailed history and physical examination, including continuous-wave Doppler (CWD) ultrasound, is essential to identify patients who require further non-invasive diagnostic evaluation prior to treatment. All large sources of reflux must be detected and eliminated before any treatment of telangiectasias. Failure to do so will cause a high rate of failures and complications, including telangiectatic matting, hyperpigmentation, and early recurrence.[7]

TELANGIECTASIA FROM RETICULAR VEINS

Telangiectasia can develop due to reflux from reticular veins, thin-walled blue superficial venules that are part of an extensive network of subcuticular veins. This network

Table 13-1
Classification of Veins

Type I	Telangiectasia (spider veins) 01.–1 mm diameter, usually red
	IA - telangiectatic matting (red network)
Type II	Venulectasia 1–2 mm diameter, violaceous
	IIA - venulectatic matting (violaceous network)
Type III	Reticular Varicosities (feeder veins) 2–4 mm diameter, cyanotic blue to blue green
Type IV	Varicosities (secondary saphenous branch or perforator related) 3–8 mm, blue to blue-green or colorless if deeper
Type V	Saphenous varicosities (truncal or axial varicosities including main saphenous trunks and first generation branch varicosities) 5 mm or greater, blue to blue-green, colorless if deeper, may be palpable and not visible

Adapted from Weiss RA, Weiss MA: Sclerotherapy. In Wheeland RG (ed): *Cutaneous Surgery*. Philadelphia, W.B. Saunders, 1994:951–981.

usually has direct connections to the saphenous systems and also through small perforating veins to the deep system, particularly in the calf. Reticular veins associated with telangiectasia are commonly called "feeder" veins. With careful Doppler technique, free reflux with augmentation can be heard through these reticular veins, and ultra-high-resolution duplex ultrasound has been used to map the path of transmission of venous hypertension from small reticular veins into telangiectasias *(Figure 13-3)*.[9,10]

ISOLATED ARBORIZING WEBS

High-pressure reflux through failed valves is at the root of nearly all telangiectatic webs. When diagnostic tests fail to identify a large vessel or a reticular network as a source of reflux, localized small-vein valve failure usually is the culprit. Flow within even the smallest of venules is normally regulated by valves,[11] and localized valve failure can produce arborizing networks of dilated cutaneous venules that are direct tributaries of underlying larger veins.[12] Arborization

occurs through a recruitment phenomenon in which high pressure causes dilatation of a venule, failure of its valves, and transmission of the high pressure across the failed valves into an adjacent vein. Treatment of an arborizing system must be directed at the entire system, because if the point source of reflux is not ablated, the web will rapidly recur.

Steps Prior to Treatment

HISTORY AND PHYSICAL EXAMINATION

No matter how small and how localized the telangiectasia, every patient must initially be evaluated by detailed history and physical examination, with non-invasive diagnostic vascular tests performed as necessary. Even when the physical examination is normal, historical factors may make further testing necessary. Previous venous surgery is an indication for more extensive evaluation, as is a family history of large varicose veins, since such patients are likely to have early axial reflux even when presenting with telangiectasias alone.[13–15]

EDUCATION AND CONSENT

Once a diagnosis is made and the patient is judged to be a candidate for sclerotherapy, it is necessary to obtain informed consent. Photographs or a videotape are shown, and possible complications such as hyperpigmentation, matting, and ulceration are discussed. The necessity for multiple treatment sessions is emphasized. If the treatment plan will include sclerosants that are used off-label or are not FDA-approved, this fact must be clearly communicated. After the patient understands the plan, risks, benefits, and alternatives, the consent form is signed.

PHOTOGRAPHS

It is impossible to overemphasize the importance of photographs. As treatment progresses, patients invariably forget the original appearance of the treated areas. Pretreatment photographs are absolutely essential to help the physician evaluate treatment progress and to allow the patient to recognize improvement (see Chapter 27).

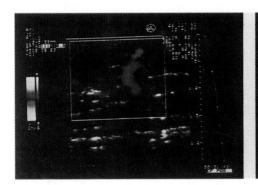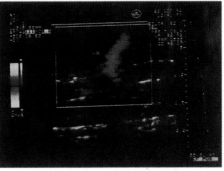

Figure 13-3. Duplex ultrasound (10 Mhz) showing reflux from reticular vein back to surface in region of bridge of telangiectasias. **(A)** Calf compression. **(B)** Calf release. Blue indicates surface to deep flow. Red indicates deep to surface flow (reprinted with permission from the Dermatalogic Surgery Journal).

PRETREATMENT INSTRUCTIONS

Patients are told to wear shorts and not to use moisturizers or shave their legs on the day of treatment. Shaving the leg may cause erythematous streaks, making it difficult to visualize patterns of reticular and telangiectatic veins. Use of moisturizers causes poor adhesion of tape used to secure compression following injections and causes slower evaporation of alcohol used to prep the leg. Patients are encouraged to eat at least a small meal beforehand in order to minimize vasovagal reactions (see Chapter 27).

FIRST TREATMENT "TEST"

The first treatment session is usually limited to a small number of sites in order to observe the patient for any allergic reactions, ability to tolerate the burning or cramping of a hypertonic solution, judge the effectiveness of a particular concentration and class of sclerosing agent, and to observe any reactions to the tape or foam pads used for compression. It also serves to familiarize the patient with the treatment, treating physician, clinic surroundings, and the sensation of the fine needle. This allows more extensive treatment on the second visit, as the patient is typically more relaxed. The test site also complies with the suggestion in the package insert for sodium tetradecyl sulfate.

When the patient returns in 2–6 weeks, the "test" site or limited treatment area is compared with pretreatment photographs. Any side effects such as matting and pigmentation can be explained to the patient. Reasonable time intervals for clearance of treated vessels can be reinforced. At each session, all sites treated are noted in anatomic diagrams in the chart.

Treatment of Small Reticular "Feeder" Veins

The same basic principle of treatment from the largest to the smallest varicosities holds true no matter what the size being treated. Sclerotherapy of telangiectasias begins with injection of the feeding reticular veins, then venulectases, then telangiectatic webs or networks, and finally the smallest and most isolated telangiectasias.

TREATMENT PLAN

Use of continuous-wave Doppler during each treatment session is helpful when first beginning to treat reticular feeders and telangiectatic webs, because when a high point of reflux into a telangiectatic web can be identified, the injections are initiated at that point. When no clear feeder vessel is seen or identified by Doppler, injections begin at the point at which the telangiectasias begin to branch out.

With increasing experience and recognition of common patterns, injection sites are based increasingly on known patterns of reflux, with treatment-session Doppler reserved for unusual cases and for patients who fail to respond to sclerotherapy. For example, reticular veins usually feed a group of telangiectasias on the lateral thigh from a varicose lateral subdermic venous system. Similar common sites of reflux include: lateral knee, posterior thigh perforating vein,

lateral thigh perforating vein, and arising from gluteal system. At the time of initial diagnostic evaluation, this pattern of telangiectasias and feeder veins would have been recognized and confirmed with CWD. The treatment session would begin with reticular veins from which reflux is suspected to arise and would proceed along the course of the reticular vein, with injections every 3–4 cm along the feeder. **It is neither possible nor advisable to treat every reticular vein of the thigh; only those reticular veins visibly connected to a telangiectatic web should be targeted.** The "arrowhead" sign may be helpful in tracing the associated reticular vein back from a telangiectatic web *(Figure 13-4)*.

As sclerosing solution flows away from the point of injection, it is diluted by blood and becomes less potent. At some distance from the point of injection, the volume and concentration of sclerosing solution will be insufficient to produce irreversible endothelial injury. When injecting a reticular vein, the sclerosing solution sometimes is seen flowing into the telangiectasia. When this happens, the telangiectasias often do not need to be injected directly. Similarly, sclerosing solution injected into a telangiectasia may be seen flowing into the feeder vein, but reticular veins usu-

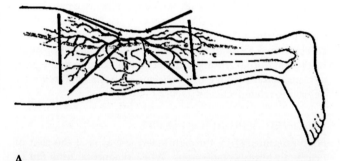

A

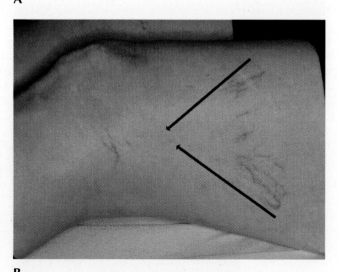

B

Figure 13-4. Arrowhead sign. **(A)** Schematic: When lines are drawn from the outermost telangiectasias of a telangiectatic web, they intersect over the reticular vein which is connected to the telangiectatic group. **(B)** Clinical application.

ally still need to be injected directly, as it is difficult to deliver an effective volume and concentration of sclerosant to the reticular vein indirectly.

Until the reticular vein has been adequately treated, telangiectasia will be resistant to treatment and will demonstrate early recurrence. For this reason, some prefer to treat reticular veins first, to wait and assess the results of treatment after a few weeks, and to treat remaining telangiectasia at a later time.[16, 17, 18] Others prefer to treat the entire refluxing system at one time, although the method of treating reticular veins first theoretically minimizes pigmentation and matting in telangiectatic webs.[6, 18]

TECHNIQUE

The technique used for injection of small reticular "feeder" veins is very similar to the supine direct cannulation technique used for the injection of larger, deeper reticular veins and varicose veins. Reticular feeder veins usually are quite superficial and visibly blue, and unless the physician is color-blind, these veins usually do not require preliminary marking by pen.

The patient is recumbent in a position that allows convenient access to the reticular veins to be treated. A 3 cc syringe with a 27- or 30-gauge needle is used, which is bent to an angle of 10–30 degrees to facilitate cannulation (rather than transfixion) of the vein. The syringe is held in the dominant hand, which rests on the patient's leg, and the needle is advanced at a shallow angle through the skin and into the reticular vein. When the physician feels the typical "pop-through" sensation of piercing the vein, the plunger is gently pulled back until blood return is seen in the transparent plastic hub *(Figure 13-5)*. Typically one injects up to 0.5 cc of sclerosant and then massages the solution toward any associated telangiectasias. Injection must stop immediately if any signs of leakage occur or if a bleb or bruising is noted. As the needle is withdrawn, pressure is applied immediately either with a cotton ball and tape or compression bandaging.

The cannulation of a reticular vein can be quite difficult at times because reticular veins can go into spasm, and may virtually disappear during an attempt at cannulation. When this occurs, another injection site must be sought. During the injection of sclerosant, extravasation will result from the slightest movement of the injecting hand, and can also occur when the vessel goes into spasm and pulls away from the cannulating needle. Until the physician gains experience with reticular veins, cautious injection with the gentlest sclerosants should be the rule, in order to avoid tissue necrosis

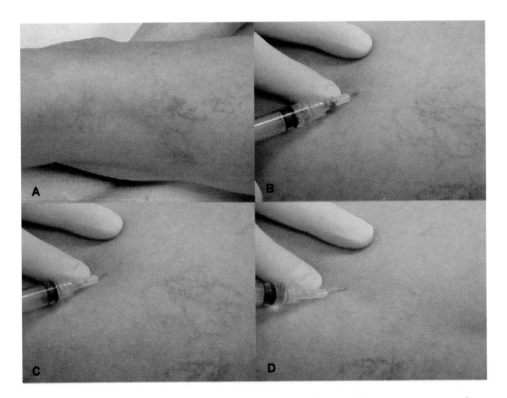

Figure 13-5. Sequence of reticular vein injection. **(A)** The reticular vein is seen extending from the popliteal fossa to feed posteriolateral telangiectasias. **(B)** The needle, bent to an angle of 10–30 degrees to facilitate cannulation, is advanced at a shallow angle through the skin and into the reticular vein. The plunger is pulled back gently until blood return is seen in the transparent plastic hub. **(C)** Up to 0.5 cc of sclerosant is injected at one site, causing the reticular vein to disappear as it fills with clear sclerosant. **(D)** The telangiectasias visually clear as the sclerosant reaches them. Pressure is applied immediately afterwards with cotton balls and tape.

Table 13-2
Advantages and Disadvantages of Treatment
of Reticular Veins

Advantages
  Lower recurrence rate
  Fewer numbers of treatments
  Less puncture sites per treatment session
  May cover more territory
  Decreased matting and pigmentation
  Less likelihood of bleb formation
  Necrosis risk decreased
Disadvantages
  Fragile wall—more easily torn
  Bruising at injection site
  Extravasations more likely
  Harder to visualize than telangiectatic webs
  Spasm with decreased lumen size may occur
  Patients can tolerate only detergent sclerosing solution

and ulceration. Any resistance to injection means the needle tip is not inside the vein. When this happens, the injection should be terminated immediately and the needle withdrawn. Failed cannulation will rapidly produce a bruise at the site of injection *(Table 13-2)*.

SCLEROSANT

The smaller the vein, the lower the initial volume and concentration of sclerosant needed for effective treatment. This is because smaller veins contain less blood to dilute the injected sclerosant. Table 13-3 shows suggested volumes and concentrations of sclerosants for treating small reticular veins.

The volume injected should be only as much as necessary to flush clear of blood the visible segment of vein that is being treated. Usually no more than 0.5 cc of sclerosing solution per injection site is necessary, although some larger or longer reticular veins may require up to 1 cc of solution. In many cases, spasm may be observed after injection of sclerosant. When this occurs, it is a desirable endpoint.

Table 13-3
Sclerosant Concentrations for Small Reticular Veins

Recommended starting concentration	Maximum recommended concentration	Sclerosant
0.2%	0.5%	Sodium tetradecyl sulfate (Sotradecol™, Fibrovein™)
0.5%	1.0%	Polidocanol (Laureth-9) (Acthoxysklerol™)
20%	23.4%	Hypertonic saline
10% Hypertonic saline and 25% dextrose	Unchanged	Hypertonic saline and dextrose (Sclerodex™)

Injection of Telangiectasias

Injection of telangiectasias is performed after all sites of reflux, larger varicosities, and feeding vessels have been injected. Chapter 27 further details supplies, equipment, forms, and distributors.

EQUIPMENT

- Cotton balls soaked with 70% isopropyl alcohol
- Protective gloves
- 1 cc or 3 cc disposable syringes
- 30-gauge ½-inch disposable transparent hub needles
- Cotton balls or foam pads for compression
- Hypoallergenic tape (synthetic silk or paper)
- Nitrol ointment (2%)
- Sclerosing solutions (sequestered from other injectables in the clinic)
- Magnifying loupes or lenses (2–3 X)

The choice of syringe is a personal one. Some phlebologists believe that a 3 cc syringe allows optimal control. Others feel that a 1 cc syringe is preferable because the smaller plunger offers reduced plunger friction and allows smoother control with less jerkiness; however, less resistance may induce quicker vessel rupture. Still others insist that the best results require use of a glass syringe offering the minimum possible friction and allowing the maximum control over the plunger. It is worth the effort to try a variety of syringes, as there is a marked difference in plunger friction between different kinds of syringes and between syringes from different manufacturers.

When using sodium tetradecyl sulfate (STS), it is recommended to use latex-free syringes. In high enough concentration (0.5% and above), STS will dissolve the rubber from the plunger, thereby releasing rubber and rubber products into solution (data on file, Wyeth-Ayerst Laboratories). There is a relatively high and increasing incidence of latex allergy in the general population.[19] Theoretically, the risk of a severe allergic reaction may be increased with latex-containing syringes. We have not yet seen allergic reactions to STS in over 100,000 injections since switching to latex-free syringes in 1994.

PATIENT PREPARATION

The patient is recumbent in a position that allows convenient access to the telangiectasias to be treated. If available, a motorized table with height adjustment will facilitate easy access to all regions of the leg. The areas to be treated are repeatedly cleansed with cotton balls saturated with 70% isopropyl alcohol, temporarily allowing better visualization of the vessels by increasing light transmission through reflective white scale on the epidermal surface. The alcohol is allowed to evaporate completely to minimize pain of the needle pushing alcohol into the skin. Use of double-polarized lighting (Syris v600, Syris Scientific, Gray, ME) has also proven to be helpful. Neck and back position of the treating physician must be optimal to avoid injury over the long term to the physician. Indirect lighting is best, as harsh halogen surgical lights bleach out reticular veins and some telangiectasias.

HAND POSITION

A syringe of sclerosant is prepared with a 30-gauge needle that has been bent to an angle of 10–30 degrees with the bevel up. The needle is placed flat on the skin so that the needle is parallel to the skin surface. Some prefer to inject tiny vessels with the needle pointing towards the clinician. In this case, the syringe is held between the thumb and the last three fingers, and the index finger is used to control the plunger (*Figure 13-6A*). Others prefer to inject with the needle pointing away from the clinician. In this case, the syringe is held like a cigarette between the index and middle fingers, and the thumb is used to control the plunger (*Figure 13-6B*).

In both cases, the hand rests on the patient's leg, with the fourth and fifth fingers providing stabilization in a fixed position to facilitate controlled penetration of the vessel. The non-dominant hand is used to stretch the skin around the needle and may offer additional support for the syringe. The firmly supported needle is then slowly moved 1–2 mm forward, piercing the top of the tiny vein just enough to allow infusion of solution with the most minimal pressure on the plunger (*Figure 13-7*).

CANNULATION OF THE VESSEL

The technique requires a gentle, precise touch, but with practice the beveled tip of the 30-gauge (0.3-mm diameter) needle may be used to cannulate vessels as small as 0.1 mm. The bevel of the needle usually can be seen within the lumen of the telangiectasias with use of 1.75x–2x magnification. Needles smaller than 30 gauge or longer than ½ inch are difficult to use because they tend to veer off course when advanced through the skin. Depending on the patient's skin type, needles can become dull rather quickly, and should be replaced whenever resistance to skin puncture is noted. This typically occurs within 3 to 10 punctures. In the U.S., one must follow OSHA bloodborne pathogen guidelines when changing needles.

Once the needle tip is seen in the lumen of the vessel, a tiny bolus of air (<0.05 cc) may be injected to help demonstrate that the needle is within the vein. Some phlebologists recommend an "air block" technique in which a larger bolus of air is used to clear the arborizing vessels of blood before the sclerosing solution is infused.[20] Future foam based sclerosants will achieve this as well.

INJECTION OF SCLEROSANTS

Concentrations of sclerosants used for telangiectasias are less than those used for reticular veins (*Table 13-4*). When sclerosing solutions are injected into telangiectasia, blood is usually flushed out of the vessel ahead of the solution, thus the sclerosant usually is not diluted at all. For this reason, the initial treatment of telangiectatic webs begins with the minimal effective concentration of sclerosant.[21] At the next visit, the same concentration is used if sclerosis was effective, and a higher concentration is used if sclerosis was ineffective.

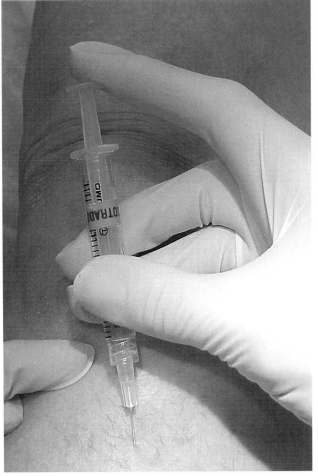

A

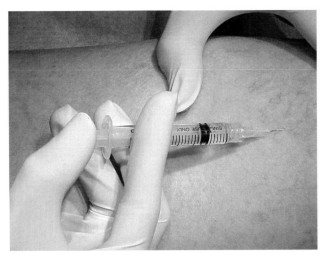

B

Figure 13-6. Hand positions for injection of telangiectasias. **(A)** Index finger controls plunger. **(B)** Thumb controls plunger.

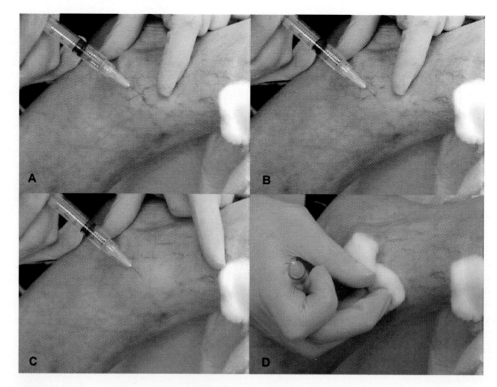

Figure 13-7. Sequence of telangiectatic web injection. **(A)** A 30-gauge needle (bent to an angle of 10–30 degrees, bevel up) is placed flat on the skin so that the needle is parallel to the skin surface. **(B)** The firmly supported needle pierces the top of the tiny vein just sufficiently to allow infusion of solution with the most minimal pressure on the plunger. **(C)** The amount slowly infused is approximately 0.1 cc–0.2 cc per site, leading to visible blanching of the connected telangiectasias. **(D)** Cotton balls and tape are applied.

The injection of telangiectasias is performed very slowly, with minimal pressure on the syringe. A few drops of sclerosant are sufficient to fill the vein and maintain contact with the vessel wall for 10–15 seconds. The amount infused is approximately 0.1–0.2 cc per site, which is often sufficient to produce blanching in a radius of 2 cm from the site of injection. Rapid flushing of the vessels with larger volumes of sclerosant or with higher pressures leads to problems with extravasation, tissue necrosis, and ulceration, as well as an increased incidence of telangiectatic matting and hyperpigmentation.[22]

If a hypertonic solution is being used, cramping and burning can be minimized if the injection of sclerosant is stopped when blanching in a radius of 2 cm has occurred, or when 15 seconds have elapsed. When painless detergent sclerosants are used, small volumes and small areas of short duration blanching are still important to minimize side effects such as telangiectatic matting. Sometimes there is no blanching at the site of injection, but the sclerosing solution flows easily through the telangiectasia or can even be seen flowing through adjacent telangiectasias or reticular veins several centimeters away from the injection site. In this case the injection is stopped after no more than 0.5 cc of sclerosant has been injected. Immediately after injection, the treated area is gently massaged in the desired direction of further spread of sclerosant.

To minimize skin necrosis, extravasation must be avoided. If there is resistance to the flow of sclerosant, or if a "bleb" begins to form at the injection site, the injection must be stopped immediately. Extravasation of low concentrations of polidocanol does not cause tissue necrosis, but significant extravasation of higher concentration (>0.1%) sodium tetradecyl sulfate or of hypertonic saline will cause necrosis and ulceration. A randomized study in animals found the incidence of ulceration to be greater when attempts were made to dilute the extravasated sclerosant by the injection of nor-

Table 13-4
Sclerosant Concentrations for Telangiectasia

Minimum effective concentration	Maximum recommended concentration	Sclerosant
0.1%	0.5%	Sodium tetradecyl sulfate (Sotradecol™, Fibrovein™)
0.25%	0.6%	Polidocanol (Laureth-9) (Acthoxysklerol™)
11.7%	23.4%	Hypertonic saline
10% Hypertonic saline and 25% dextrose	Unchanged	Sclerodex™

mal saline into the area.[23] Vigorous massage of any blebs is recommended to minimize the chance of necrosis.

COMPRESSION

Compression will speed vessel clearance and reduce staining from any vessel that protrudes above the surface of the skin.[24-26] After treatment of telangiectasias, compression is provided by ready-to-wear gradient compression hose (15–20 mm Hg) placed over cotton balls that are secured with tape at the sites of injection. If larger reticular veins (>3 mm) are treated at the same session, then compression consists of Class I 20–30 mm Hg compression (Table 13–5). Some authorities recommend that continuous compression be applied for as long as the patient will tolerate it (usually 1–3 days). The stockings are then removed and the cotton balls discarded; the patient bathes and puts the stockings back on, wearing them for the next two weeks except when bathing and sleeping. Two of the authors do not use continuous compression for telangiectasia treatment, but rather have the patient remove both stockings and cotton balls at bedtime of the day of treatment. Compression hose are then worn daily for two weeks, except when bathing and sleeping.[26-28] Patients are encouraged to walk, and the only restrictions on activity are those that result in sustained forceful muscular contraction and venous pressure elevation, such as heavy weightlifting.

TREATMENT INTERVALS

Physician and patient preferences play a large role in determining treatment intervals. New areas may be treated at any time, but retreatment of the same areas should be deferred for several weeks because some telangiectasias will ultimately clear after exhibiting no initial response within the first two weeks.

Patients often are anxious to speed their course of treatment, but allowing a longer time between treatment sessions may minimize the number of sessions needed. Some physicians recommend waiting as long as 4–8 weeks between treatments, while others may see their patients at weekly intervals.

It is not uncommon for there to be small, firm areas of hyperpigmentation along the track of reticular veins and protuberant telangiectasias. On follow-up sessions, these areas are typically "nicked" with an 18-gauge needle to release the dark, liquid blood trapped in the developing fibrosis. This allows faster resolution of the pigmentation (see Chapter 24).

The number of treatments needed depends on the extent of the problem and the extent of areas treated at each session. Some patients are highly responsive to treatment, and can be treated with weak sclerosants in only a few sessions. Others are highly resistant, and may require more sessions and stronger sclerosants.

After the initial series of treatments, a "rest" period of 4–6 months will allow time for pigmentation and matting to clear, and for any remaining reticular veins to establish "new" routes of reflux or drainage. Approximately 80% of patients will clear to their satisfaction during the first course of treatment. Any remaining telangiectatic webs or new telangiectasias are then reassessed to determine the best approach for another round of treatment.

POOR RESPONSE TO TREATMENT

When patients have had a poor response to the initial series of treatments, the original diagnosis must always be called into question (Table 13-6). Failed treatment often means that a hidden source of reflux was overlooked. Evaluation with handheld Doppler and possibly color-flow duplex ultrasound is indicated to elucidate the patterns and sources of reflux that have led to a treatment failure. Unsuspected sources of reflux can include truncal varices, incompetent perforating veins, and unrecognized reticular vessels.

If no untreated source of reflux can be identified, the patient must be carefully questioned about proper compliance with compression. Many patients abandon compression immediately after sclerotherapy, and this can lead to treatment failures. The concentration and volume of sclerosant used should also be reexamined. It is not uncommon to find that the concentrations selected were ineffective for the size and type of vessel being treated.

If no explanation for the treatment failure is found, the concentration of sclerosant may be increased or another class of sclerosants may be used.[29] Some women taking high doses of estrogen and progesterone may improve the results of sclerotherapy by temporarily suspending hormonal supplementation.[30-32]

SCLEROSANT CONSIDERATIONS

For consistent results, detergent sclerosants should always be used in the same temperature range, as the bioactive effective strength of detergent sclerosing solutions is highly temperature dependent. Some physicians prefer to work with solutions at room temperature, while others prefer refrigerated solutions. The consistent use of either tempera-

---

Table 13-5
Guidelines for Compression

Telangiectasias only: over-the-counter ready-to-wear 15–20 mm Hg
Telangiectasias and reticular veins: 20–30 mm Hg
Reticular and small varicose: 20–30 mm Hg
Truncal varicose: 30–40 mm Hg
All compression for two to three weeks, most critical first three days

---

Table 13-6
Considerations when Patients have Poor Response

Was Doppler exam adequate and accurate?
Reticular vein adequately treated?
Is duplex required?
Change the solution type—Hyperosmolar vs. detergent
Did the patient comply with compression?
Is patient on hormonal therapy?

ture range will allow a consistent and predictable response to treatment.

Solutions of STS greater than 0.5% are stored in glass vials until just prior to injection, because concentrated STS will dissolve some of the rubber of the syringe plunger, causing difficulty moving the plunger and contaminating the sclerosing solution with rubber breakdown products (data on file, Wyeth-Ayerst Laboratories). Latex-free syringes are recommended for injection to reduce to the incidence of inadvertent latex injection with STS. STS in concentrations greater than 0.5% should not be predrawn and stored in syringes containing rubber of any kind.

Summary

When based upon a correct diagnosis and an appropriate treatment plan, sclerotherapy is a highly effective method of treatment for telangiectasias. Formulating an effective treatment plan requires a detailed knowledge of venous anatomy, a thorough understanding of the principles and patterns of reflux, and an intimate familiarity with a range of volumes and concentrations of sclerosing solutions. The results obtained depend greatly on the experience of the clinician, but with care and attention to detail, clearing rates of 90% can be achieved in many patients.

Patient satisfaction is enhanced through education and informed consent, photographic documentation, and a measured approach to treatment. When the basic principles of diagnosis and treatment are followed meticulously, a successful outcome is highly likely. It is important to educate the patient that telangiectasias may be a lifelong problem. Development of new veins within a few years after successful treatment does not constitute treatment failure; rather, it demonstrates the chronicity of venous insufficiency.

References

(1) Weiss RA, Weiss MA. *Resolution of pain associated with varicose and telangiectatic leg veins after compression sclerotherapy.* J Dermatol Surg Onc 1990; 16:333–336.

(2) Weiss RA, Heagle CR, Raymond-Martimbeau P. *The Bulletin of the North American Society of Phlebology. Insurance Advisory Committee Report.* J Dermatol Surg Onc 1992; 18:609–616.

(3) Duffy DM. *Small vessel sclerotherapy: an overview.* Adv Dermatol 1988; 3:221–242.

(4) Duffy DM. *Sclerotherapy.* Clin Dermatol 1992; 10:373–380.

(5) Goldman MP, Bennett RG. *Treatment of telangiectasia: a review.* J Am Acad Dermatol 1987; 17:167–182.

(6) Weiss RA, Weiss MA. *Sclerotherapy.* In: Wheeland RG, editor. Cutaneous Surgery. Philadelphia: W.B. Saunders, 1994: 951–981.

(7) Weiss RA, Weiss MA. *Painful telangiectasias: diagnosis and treatment.* In: Bergan JJ, Weiss RA, Goldman MP, editors. Varicose Veins and Telangiectasias: Diagnosis and Treatment, 2nd ed. St. Louis: Quality Medical, 1999: 389–406.

(8) Goldman MP, Weiss RA, Bergan JJ. *Diagnosis and treatment of varicose veins— a review.* J Am Acad Dermatol 1994; 31(3:Part 1):393–413.

(9) Weiss RA, Weiss MA. *Doppler ultrasound findings in reticular veins of the thigh subdermic lateral venous system and implications for sclerotherapy.* J Dermatol Surg Onc 1993; 19(10):947–951.

(10) Somjen GM, Ziegenbein R, Johnston AH, Royle JP. *Anatomical examination of leg telangiectases with duplex scanning.* J Dermatol Surg Onc 1993; 19(10):940–945.

(11) Braverman IM, Keh-Yen A. *Ultrastructure of the human dermal microcirculation. IV. Valve- containing collecting veins at the dermal-subcutaneous junction.* J Invest Dermatol 1983; 81(5):438–442.

(12) deFaria JL, Moraes IN. *Histopathology of telangiectasias associated with varicose veins.* Dermatologica 1963; 127:321–329.

(13) Thibault P, Bray A, Wlodarczyk J, Lewis W. *Cosmetic leg veins: evaluation using duplex venous imaging.* J Dermatol Surg Onc 1990; 16:612–618.

(14) Komsuoglu B, Goldeli O, Kulan K, Cetinarslan B, Komsuoglu SS. *Prevalence and risk factors of varicose veins in an elderly population.* Gerontology 1994; 40(1):25–31.

(15) Schultz-Ehrenburg U, Weindorf N, Matthes U, Hirche H. *New epidemiological findings with regard to initial stages of varicose veins (Bochum study I-III).* In: Raymond-Martimbeau P, Prescott R, Zummo M, editors. Phlebologie '92. Paris: John Libbey Eurotext, 1992: 234–236.

(16) Guex JJ. [*The treatment of microvarices, varicosities and telangiectasis in 1992*]. Phlebol 1992; 45:401–404; discussion 405–407.

(17) Guex JJ. *Indications for the sclerosing agent polidocanol (aetoxisclerol dexo, aethoxisklerol kreussler).* J Dermatol Surg Onc 1993; 19:959–961.

(18) Guex JJ. *Microsclerotherapy.* Semin Dermatol 1993; 12:129–134.

(19) Cheng L, Lee D. *Review of latex allergy.* J Am Board Fam Pract 1999; 12(4):285–292.

(20) Bodian EL. *Sclerotherapy: a personal appraisal.* J Dermatol Surg Onc 1989; 15:156–161.

(21) Sadick NS. *Sclerotherapy of varicose and telangiectatic leg veins. Minimal sclerosant concentration of hypertonic saline and its relationship to vessel diameter* [see comments]. J Dermatol Surg Onc 1991; 17:65–70.

(22) Ouvry PA, Davy A. *The sclerotherapy of telangiectasia.* Phlebol 1982; 35:349–359.

(23) Zimmet SE. *The prevention of cutaneous necrosis following extravasation of hypertonic saline and sodium tetradecyl sulfate.* J Dermatol Surg Onc 1993; 19:641–646.

(24) Fegan WG. *Continuing uninterrupted compression technique of injecting varicose veins.* Proc R Soc Med 1960; 53:837–840.

(25) Goldman MP, Beaudoing D, Marley W, Lopez L, Butie A. *Compression in the treatment of leg telangiectasia: a preliminary report.* J Dermatol Surg Onc 1990; 16:322–325.

(26) Weiss RA, Sadick NS, Goldman MP, Weiss MA. *Post-sclerotherapy compression: controlled comparative study of duration of compression and its effects on clinical outcome.* Dermatol Surg 1999; 25(2):105–108.

(27) Struckmann J, Stange-Vognsen HH, Andersen J, et al. *Venous muscle pump improvement by low compression elastic stockings.* Phlebol 1986; 1:97–103.

(28) Partsch H. *Compression therapy of the legs.* A review. J Dermatol Surg Onc 1991; 17:799–805.

(29) Sadick NS. *Hyperosmolar versus detergent sclerosing agents in sclerotherapy—effect on distal vessel obliteration.* J Dermatol Surg Onc 1994; 20(5):313–316.

(30) Weiss RA, Weiss MA. *Incidence of side effects in the treatment of telangiectasias by compression sclerotherapy: hypertonic saline vs. polidocanol.* J Dermatol Surg Onc 1990; 16:800–804.

(31) Sadick NS, Niedt GW. *A study of estrogen and progesterone receptors in spider telangiectasias of the lower extremities.* J Dermatol Surg Onc 1990; 16:620–623.

(32) Davis LT, Duffy DM. *Determination of incidence and risk factors for postsclerotherapy telangiectatic matting of the lower extremity: a retrospective analysis.* J Dermatol Surg Onc 1990; 16:327–330.

Sclerosing Solutions

It is not always easy to sclerose a varicose vein. Even a small amount of damage will produce intravascular thrombus, but thrombosis alone usually does not obliterate the vessel. Intact endothelium contains tissue plasminogen activator that can dissolve thrombus. A thrombosed vessel with intact endothelium will simply recanalize.

Vascular fibrosis and obliteration only occurs in response to irreversible endothelial cellular destruction. If an injected sclerosant is too weak, the vessel may initially close, but recanalization will occur and an incompetent pathway for reflux then persists. If the injected sclerosant is too strong, the varicose vessel endothelium is destroyed, but the sclerosant will also affect adjacent normal vessels causing damage there as well. The goal is to deliver a *minimum* volume and concentration of sclerosant that will cause irreversible damage to the endothelium of the abnormal vessel to be sclerosed, while leaving adjacent normal vessels unaffected.

No single sclerosing agent can provide perfect results in every clinical setting. Not only are there significant differences between agents of different classes, but there are important subtle differences between agents of the same class that at first glance seem very similar. There is also a great deal of individual variability in response to sclerosing solutions. The clinician must be prepared to work with a variety of agents to meet the needs of circumstance. The choice of which sclerosing agent to use is based on a good understanding of the mechanism of action of each sclerosing solution.

The Ideal Sclerosant

Virtually any foreign substance can cause venous endothelial damage. Historical methods for producing venous endothelial trauma have included "a slender rod of iron" (reportedly used by Hippocrates himself), phenol, absolute alcohol, ferric chloride, anti-syphilitic mercurial drugs, and hundreds of other agents. These early sclerosing agents caused many deaths in addition to a high incidence of local tissue necrosis, pain, failed sclerosis, and allergic reactions.

An ideal sclerosing solution would have no systemic toxicity. It would produce local endothelial destruction extending all the way to the adventitia with a minimum of thrombus formation. Because all sclerosants eventually flow into the deep system, an ideal sclerosant would be rapidly inactivated by dilution. It would require a long period of contact to be effective, making it more effective in areas of stasis and safer in normal veins where there is high flow. It would be non-allergenic. It would be strong enough to sclerose even the largest vessels, yet it would produce no local tissue injury if extravasated. It would not cause staining or scarring, nor telangiectatic matting. It would be perfectly soluble in normal saline. It would be painless upon injection, inexpensive, and approved by the United States Food and Drug Administration (FDA).

The ideal sclerosant does not yet exist, but modern sclerosants can exhibit near-ideal behavior when used correctly. The degree of endothelial cell destruction can often be tempered by adjusting the concentration of the sclerosing solution.[1,2] Proper patient positioning allows the varicose veins to be treated in a nearly "empty" condition, so that a "minimum effective concentration" will disrupt the varicose veins, but will be diluted below the threshold of bioactivity immediately upon flowing into the deep veins. The type of sclerosant can be carefully matched to the type, size, and location of the vessel, and the volume used can be adjusted for optimum effect.

Many currently available sclerosants will cause cutaneous necrosis if extravasated. Even those that do not cause extravasation necrosis can still cause cutaneous necrosis if inadvertently injected into a telangiectasia that participates in an arteriovenous anastomosis. Sclerosant flow into the small end-arteriole causes immediate and persistent blanching of all the tissues in a roughly circular area. The problem is largely avoided by using very small injection volumes and slow injection rates under low pressure. If the typical pattern of blanching is observed, the local application of nitrol ointment has been reported to prevent or mitigate the ulceration.[3]

Sclerosant Categories

Sclerosing solutions often are artificially classified into three broad categories: hypertonic or hyperosmotic agents, detergent sclerosants, and chemical irritants, sometimes called "corrosives" or "toxins." All of these agents interfere with the function of endothelial and subendothelial cell-surface proteins that are necessary for survival of the cell, but each member of each class does so in a slightly different way. Table 14-1 lists the classification of some commonly available sclerosing agents. Each type has its own properties (Table 14-2).

HYPERTONIC SOLUTIONS

Hypertonic solutions cause several different types of injuries to the endothelium. Blood cells exposed to hypertonic saline undergo dehydration and cell wall disruption, but this probably is not the principal mechanism by which endothelial cells are affected. Instead, concentrated osmotic or ionic solutions may partially denature cell surface proteins *in situ*. Tight junctions between cells are immediately affected, exposing lower cell layers to the hyperosmotic substance.

The time sequence of the remainder of the destructive process is relatively slow, requiring minutes rather than seconds for endothelial destruction.[4] For effective sclerosis, the osmotic agent must be of sufficient strength to dis-

Table 14-1
Classification of Common Sclerosing Solutions

Solution (generic name)	Brand names	FDA approved for sclerotherapy?
Hyperosmolar solutions		
Hypertonic saline (HS)	None	No—but FDA approved for other uses
Hypertonic saline + dextrose (HSD)	Sclerodex™	No
Detergent solutions		
Polidocanol (POL)	Aethoxysklerol™, Sclerovein™ Aetoxysclerol™, Etoxisclerol™, Sotrauerix™, Laureth 9, AET	Pending
Sodium tetradecyl sulfate (STS)	Sotradecol™, FibroVein™, Trombovar™, Thromboject™	Yes
Ethanolamine oleate	Ethamolin™	Yes
Sodium morrhuate	Scleromate™	Yes
Chemical irritants		
Chromated glycerin	Scleremo™, Chromex™	No
Polyiodide iodine	Variglobin™, Sclerodine,	No
Sodium salicylate	Saliject™	No

Table 14-2
Properties of Sclerosing Solutions

Hypertonic	Detergent	Toxins
Dehydration and cell wall disruption	Micelles cause "protein theft denaturation" to disrupt cell surface membrane	Poisons cell surface proteins by affecting chemical bonds
Destructive process is slowest	Irreversible cellular morphological changes are seen within minutes	Full thickness vessel injury at the site of injection within seconds
Works very locally—rapid dilution rapidly diminishes the local concentration of the drug	Effects of a detergent solution can spread further	Consumed—limiting the concentration of cell injury remote from the injection site
Effective for smaller vessels and for low-flow vessels	Used for larger vessels	Largest or smallest vessels—few in between
Nerve endings in the vessel adventitia can be affected	Little stimulation of nerve endings	Destruction of nerve endings if contacted

rupt the full thickness of the vessel wall for complete destruction.[5] Because rapid dilution rapidly diminishes the local concentration of the drug, this class of sclerosing solutions is primarily effective for smaller vessels and for low-flow vessels such as a leg telangiectasia. There is a smaller amount of inflammation produced by this class of sclerosing agents. A side-by-side comparison will frequently show less hyperpigmentation with the hypertonic solutions (Figure 14-1).

Hyperosmotic solutions are nonselective in their effects, affecting all cells in the path of the osmotic gradient. Nerve endings in the vessel adventitia can be affected, causing a focal, often intense, burning pain upon injection. Changes in the ion gradient of the extracellular fluid of muscles can trigger severe cramping that can last for minutes at a time. Extravasation can cause extensive tissue necrosis and large ulcers that are slow to heal and can cause significant scarring.

DETERGENT SOLUTIONS

Long-chain fatty alcohol detergents with the right combination of lipophilic and polar hydrophilic regions have long been used in biochemistry labs to extract cell-surface proteins from otherwise intact cells *in vitro*. This is most likely the mechanism by which the detergent sclerosing solutions work *in vivo*, and has been called protein theft denaturation.

For each detergent sclerosant, there is some threshold concentration below which the agent causes no injury. At low concentrations, most detergent molecules are individually dissolved in solution. When the concentration reaches a threshold known as the critical micellar concentration (CMC) nearly all further detergent molecules added to the solution will enter into amphiphilic bilayers known as micelles. Individual detergent molecules have no toxicity to the vascular endothelium, but micelles can cause protein theft denaturation and can disrupt the cell surface membrane in other ways.

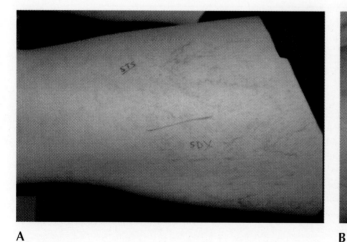

A

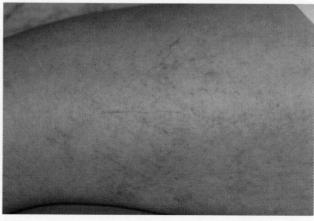

B

Figure 14-1. Comparison of a test site on the thigh of Sclerodex™ versus STS with similar concentrations. **(A)** Lateral venous system before treatment with 0.1% Sotradecol™ (STS) anteriorly and Sclerodex™ (SDX) laterally. **(B)** After 1 month, slightly more hyperpigmentation is present at the STS site, and slightly more matting at the SDX site. The patient was pleased with the results of both.

The loss of essential cell surface proteins causes delayed cell death. When vascular endothelium is exposed to detergent micelles, irreversible cellular morphological changes are seen within minutes by scanning electron microscopy, but the fatal cellular changes that are visible by normal light microscopy do not become apparent for many hours.[6] Unlike many other agents, the detergent sclerosants do not cause hemolysis, nor do they provoke direct intravascular coagulation.

As a practical matter, the effects of a detergent solution can spread further than the effects of osmotic solutions because it takes more time for bioactive aggregates to dissolve than for the osmotic gradient to disperse. The volume and concentration of these solutions must be carefully tailored to the situation. Varying the strength of the detergent solution and the amount of time the solution is trapped within the vessel changes the timing and the extent of damage.

Detergent sclerosants are potent agents that have a clearcut threshold below which they have absolutely no injurious effect on venous endothelium. Foaming of these agents is easily achieved with agitation. It is believed that foaming will allow more efficient sclerosis with exposure to far less sclerosing solution, as the foam can block flow into and out of the treated site.[7]

CORROSIVE AGENTS

Corrosive agents, the most diverse group of sclerosing solutions, most likely poison cell surface proteins by affecting chemical bonds within the proteins. There is some uncertainty as to which agents really belong in this category. Included are such agents as alcohols, which are not chemical poisons, but rather are solubilizing agents that affect the shape of proteins and the integrity of the cell membrane itself. With further investigation, the category probably will be narrowed to include only chemically reactive compounds that interact with cell surface proteins.

Substances now categorized as toxic or corrosive agents range from alcohols to salts to heavy metals. They act on all cell types, but are consumed in stoichiometric proportions in the process, somewhat limiting the concentration of cell injury remote from the injection site. This category includes some of the strongest solutions, such as polyiodinated iodine, but also includes one of the mildest solutions, chromated glycerin.

The strongest corrosive solutions may cause full-thickness vessel injury at the site of injection within seconds, facilitating the treatment of large varicosities. It is essential to select the proper volume and concentration so that the destructive effect does not spread beyond the targeted vessel into adjacent tissues.

Commercially Available Sclerosing Solutions

Some of the agents discussed in this chapter are not readily available in the United States, yet extensive medical literature indicates that these agents are safe and efficacious. The reasons why they are not yet approved by the FDA for labeling and distribution in the United States seem to be related more to the cost and inconvenience of the application process than to any questions about safety and efficacy. As sclerotherapy is performed more often in the United States, the economics will hopefully begin to justify application for FDA approval of these important agents.

Many sclerosing agents that are not approved by the FDA for any pharmaceutical use are nonetheless widely used both in the United States and elsewhere for sclerosis of refluxing superficial lower extremity vessels, as well as for sclerosis of esophageal varices, hemorrhoidal veins, varicoceles, vascular tumors, and other vascular and cystic structures. Paradoxically, routine use of what are widely regarded as safer, more efficacious agents has become the usual standard of care today, despite the fact that they have not been approved for this purpose by the FDA. As a reference there are numerous tables in this chapter to allow rapid comparison of a variety of issues concerning sclerosing solutions (*Table 14-3, Table 14-4, Table 14-5, Table 14-6*).

TABLE 14-3
Relative Potency of Sclerosing Solutions
(Minimal Sclerosant Concentrations)

Vein diameter	Sclerosing solution
<0.5mm	Chromated glycerin 50%
	Polidocanol 0.25%
	Sodium tetradecyl sulfate 0.1%
	Chromated glycerin 100%
	Polidocanol 0.5%
	Polyiodide iodide 0.1%
	Hypertonic saline 11.7%
	Sodium morrhuate 1%
	Ethanolamine oleate 2%
	Hypertonic dextrose and saline
0.6–1.5 mm	Hypertonic dextrose and saline
	Sodium tetradecyl sulfate 0.25%
	Polidocanol 0.75%
	Polyiodide iodide 1.0%
	Hypertonic saline 23.4%
	Ethanolamine oleate 5%
	Sodium morrhuate 2.5%
1.5–4 mm	Polidocanol 1–2%
	Sodium tetradecyl sulfate 0.5–1.0%
	Polyiodide iodide 2%
	Sodium morrhuate 5%
4–6 mm	Polidocanol 2%
	Sodium tetradecyl sulfate 1–2 %
	Polyiodide iodide 3–12%
Branch varicosities	Polidocanol 3–5%
SFJ and SPJ perforators	Sodium tetradecyl sulfate 2–3 %
	Polyiodide iodide 6–12%

Modified from Weiss MA, Weiss RA. *Sclerotherapeutic agents available in the United States and elsewhere.* In: Goldman MP, Bergan JJ, editors. Ambulatory Treatment of Venous Disease: An Illustrative Guide. St. Louis: Mosby, 1996: 37–48.

Table 14-4
Starting Doses for Sclerosing Agents (Per Point of Injection)

	Saphenofemoral or saphenopopliteal junction	Truncal varices	Non-truncal tributaries	Reticular veins	Blue spider veins	Red spider veins
Polidocanol	2 cc at 3%-4%	2 cc at 1%	1 cc at 0.5%	0.5–1 cc at 0.5%	0.2–0.5 cc at 0.5%	0.1–0.3 cc at 0.5%
Sodium tetradecyl sulfate	2 cc at 3%	1–2 cc at 1.5%–3%	1 cc at 0.5%–1.0%	0.5–1 cc at 0.2%–1.0%	0.2 cc at 0.1%–0.3%	0.1 cc at 0.1%–0.3%
Chromated Glycerin	Not used	Not used	0.5–1 cc full strength	0.5–1 cc at 80%	0.2–0.5 cc at 80%	0.1–0.3 cc at 80%
AV 15	Not used	Not used	Not used	Full strength	Full strength	Full strength
Sodium salicylate	3 cc at 30%	3 cc at 20%	1 cc at 20%	0.1–1 cc at 12%	0.1–1 cc at 12%	0.1–0.2 cc at 12%
Hypertonic saline, 23.4%	Not used	Not used	Not used	0.5–1 cc	0.1–0.2 cc	0.1 cc
Dextrose + 10% NaCl (Sclerodex™)	Not used	Not used	Not used	0.5–1 cc	0.2–0.5 cc	0.1–0.2 cc
Iodine + Sodium iodide (Variglobin®)	2–3 cc at 2%	1 cc at 2%	0.5–1 cc at 0.5–1%	Not advised	Not advised	Not advised

To avoid inflammatory hyper- or hypopigmentation, concentrations should be decreased by roughly 25% when injecting telangiectasias and reticular veins in patients with dark skin. All dilutions are made with isotonic saline.

Commonly Used Sclerosing Solutions

The solutions of hypertonic saline, hypertonic saline with dextrose, polidocanol, sodium tetradecyl sulfate, iodine, and glycerine are widely used throughout the world. For easy reference, the following panels describe each solution.

HYPERTONIC SALINE

Although approved by the FDA only for use as an abortifacient, hypertonic saline is in common daily use as a sclerosing agent by dermatologists in the United States. It is rarely used in countries where a variety of other agents are available.

Table 14-5
Maximum Doses for Sclerosing Agents per Session

Polidocanol	Approximately 4 cc at 3% (2 mg/kg)
Sodium tetradecyl sulfate	300 mg (10 cc of 3%)
Chromated glycerin	5–10 cc
AV 15	6 cc
Sodium salicylate	6 cc at 60%
Hypertonic saline, 23.4%	8 cc
25% Dextrose + 10% NaCl (Sclerodex™)	10 cc
Iodine + Sodium iodide (Variglobin®)	3 cc at 12%

Class
Hypertonic and hyperionic.

General description
Weak sclerosant with many disadvantages, quite painful for some patients.

Advantages
Total lack of allergenicity when unadulterated.
Wide availability.
Rapid response to treatment.[8]

Disadvantages
Because of dilutional effects, it is difficult to achieve adequate sclerosis of large vessels without exceeding a tolerable salt load. This can cause significant burning pain and muscle cramping for up to 5 minutes after injection.[3] If extravasated, it almost invariably causes significant necrosis and large ulcerations. Because it causes immediate red blood cell hemolysis and rapidly disrupts vascular endothelial continuity, it is prone to cause marked hemosiderin staining. It is not recommended for facial veins due to the risk of tissue necrosis with extravasation.

Principal indication
Reticular veins and telangiectasias of the lower limbs.

Accessory use
Not recommended for other sites.

Concentrations and doses in varicose veins
Not used for varicose veins.

Table 14-6
Summary of Primary Sclerosing Agents

Solution (chemical name)	Brand names	Category	Advantages	Disadvantages
Sodium tetradecyl sulfate	Sotradecol Fibro-Vein Thrombovar	Detergent: rapid dissolution of endothelium	Painless intravascular; Painful extravascular, Strong for varicose veins, Effective at low concentration, FDA approved	Skin necrosis with extravasation of concentrations > 0.25%, expensive, post-sclerosis pigmentation
Polidocanol	Aethoxysklerol Sclero-Vein	Detergent	Always painless, Cutaneous necrosis low, Effective at low concentration	Urticaria (immediate) at injection site, skin necrosis from painless arteriolar injection, not FDA approved
Hypertonic saline, 23.4%	None	Hyperosmolar: slow crenation of endothelium	Low risk of allergic reaction, readily available, rapid action, FDA use: Off-label	Painful stinging, cramping, skin necrosis
Saline and dextrose	Sclerodex	Hyperosmolar	High viscosity—remains in treated veins, low allergic risk, low risk necrosis	Too weak for larger varicosities, slight stinging, one concentration only, not FDA approved

Concentrations and doses in telangiectasias and reticular veins

20% or 23.4% solutions are used in amounts ranging from 2–8 cc per session. Each reticular injection site receives no more than 0.5 cc, and each telangiectatic injection site should receive no more than 0.1 or 0.2 cc.

Comments

Meticulous technique is necessary to obtain good results with hypertonic saline. Its use cannot be recommended to beginners, who will naturally extravasate some amount of sclerosant in the majority of their injections while developing expertise. It can be quite painful to inject and may cause a reduction in the number of patients who make return appointments. The previously widespread use of hypertonic saline in the United States caused sclerotherapy to have a reputation as a very painful procedure, which phlebologists have worked hard to overcome.

DEXTROSE AND HYPERTONIC SALINE

Produced in Canada under the trade name "Sclerodex™," this commercial solution is a mixture of 25% dextrose and 10% sodium chloride, with a small quantity of phenethyl alcohol added for stability. A primarily hypertonic agent, its effects are similar to those of pure hypertonic saline, but the reduced salt load offers certain benefits. Unlike pure hypertonic saline, it is much less painful on injection due to the hypertonicity coming more from dextrose and less from saline. It is viscous and remains where injected to allow an osmotic gradient. We have performed tens of thousands of injections with this agent and have only seen pinpoint epidermal necrosis on one occasion. We reserve this mild sclerosing solution for smaller red telangiectasias or resistant matting. It is utilized when a detergent solution in low concentration has either been ineffective or has led to marked pigmentation. This agent is not approved by the FDA for

commercial sale in the United States, but may be compounded within your own state as needed (see Chapter 27 for formula).

Class

Hypertonic and hyperionic.

General description

Weak sclerosant with some advantages, far less painful than hypertonic saline.

Advantages

Low incidence of allergies and necrosis.
Very little pain on injection.
Reportedly effective for tiny red telangiectasias and telangiectatic matting.

Disadvantages

Viscous and slightly painful upon injection, although much less so than hypertonic saline. Hyperpigmentation possible.

Principal indication

Small telangiectasias of the lower limbs or face.

Accessory use

Reticular veins and telangiectasias at other non-facial sites.

Concentrations and doses in varicose veins

Not used for larger veins. May be mixed with corrosive agents such as iodinated iodine in special situations.

Concentrations and doses in telangiectasias and reticular veins

Injected full strength. Up to 1 cc per site in reticular veins, and up to 0.2 cc per site in telangiectasia, to a total of 10 cc per treatment session.

Comments

Although this agent is better tolerated and safer than pure hypertonic saline, meticulous technique remains necessary to obtain good results.

POLIDOCANOL

Polidocanol (POL; hydroxy-polyethoxy-dodecane) is a synthetic long-chain fatty alcohol sold under many trade names (*Table 14-1*). Polidocanol is reportedly the most commonly used agent for sclerotherapy worldwide and the second most commonly used agent in the United States.

Polidocanol was first introduced in Germany in 1936 as a topical and local anesthetic agent, and was not registered as a sclerosing agent until 1967. It has been used in many foods and over-the-counter preparations, but is not approved by the FDA for commercial sale as a pharmaceutical product in the United States. Despite this fact, polidocanol has been so thoroughly studied and offers so many advantages that it is widely used as a sclerosant in the United States, and its use is taught and recommended at a number of major universities and in nearly every major medical textbook. Because of its high safety profile, many malpractice insurance carriers provide explicit waivers to cover its use.

Class

Detergent.

General description

The newest commercially available sclerosant—safe, all-purpose, moderately strong sclerosant.

Advantages

Can be used in all sizes and types of varicose, reticular, or telangiectatic veins.
Intravascular injection is painless.
Extravasation usually does not cause necrosis.
Allergic reactions are very rare.
The liquid is fluid, rather than viscous.
Easy to foam for reduced liquid volume injection.
With good technique the incidence of hyperpigmentation may be lower than most other agents.

Disadvantages

Hyperpigmentation and telangiectatic matting occur if too high a concentration or too large a volume is used.
The maximum recommended dose may be insufficient to fully treat large veins at one visit.
The FDA has not approved it for commercial distribution in the United States.
Site of action spreads furthest from site of injection; volume at higher concentration must be limited.[9,10]
Lack of pain on injection may disguise intraarteriolar injection at arteriovenous malformation sites, such as ankle.

Principal indications

Large and small varicose veins, reticular veins, telangiectasias.

Accessory use

Telangiectasias of face and trunk.

Concentrations and doses in varicose veins

The highest available concentrations may be used. In Germany the highest concentration available is 4%, but this preparation contains a significant amount of ethyl alcohol. The highest concentration available in France is 3%.

The German manufacturers of POL recommend 3% POL for varicose veins 4–8 mm in diameter, 2% POL for veins 2–4 mm in diameter, and 1% POL for reticular veins and small varicose veins 1–2 mm in diameter.

In France, polidocanol is used at its maximum available concentration for treatment directed at the saphenofemoral junction. When used for truncal varices below the saphenofemoral junction, concentrations of 1% to 3% are used depending on the size of the vein. When used for non-truncal varices, concentrations of 0.5% to 1% usually are considered sufficient.

A volume of 0.5 cc to 1.0 cc is normally used at each injection site, and the total amount per session should not exceed 120 mg (3 cc of 4% solution or 12 cc of 1% solution).

Concentrations and doses in telangiectasias and reticular veins

Reticular veins are treated with 0.5% or 1.0% solutions and up to 1 cc per site. Telangiectasias are treated with 0.25% to 0.75% solutions and 0.1 cc or 0.2 cc per site.

Comments

Because it may be injected intradermally, very rarely causing extravasation necrosis, this agent is very forgiving for beginners. The advantages of this agent can be undone if the practitioner yields to the temptation to "speed things up" by using higher concentrations and higher volumes than recommended.

SODIUM TETRADECYL SULFATE

Sodium tetradecyl sulfate (STS) (Sotradecol™, STD, Fibro-Vein™, Thromboject™) is a long-chain fatty acid salt with strong detergent properties. It is a very effective sclerosing agent that was already in commercial use before the adoption of The Federal Food, Drug and Cosmetic Act of 1938, and was therefore grandfathered by the FDA without the need to prove safety and efficacy. There is over 50 years of clinical data available, however, on file with manufacturers in the US and the UK. The safety and efficacy profile based on hundreds of thousands of treatments is extremely good.

Class

Detergent.

General description

A reasonably safe, all purpose, fairly strong sclerosant.

Advantages

Roughly twice as potent as polidocanol at the same concentration.
Can be used in all sizes and types of varicose, reticular, or telangiectatic veins.
Intravascular injection is painless.

Allergic reactions may occur, but are uncommon (minimized with latex-free syringes).
The liquid is fluid, rather than viscous.

Disadvantages
Extravasation may cause necrosis.
Hyperpigmentation and telangiectatic matting are not uncommon.
May dissolve rubber syringe plunger in higher concentrations.

Principal indication
Large and small varicose veins, reticular veins, telangiectasias.

Accessory use
Telangiectasias of face and trunk.

Concentrations and doses in varicose veins
The maximum concentration is used for treatment at the saphenofemoral junction. When used for truncal or non-truncal varices below the saphenofemoral junction, concentrations of 1.5%–3% are used for veins greater than 4 mm in diameter and concentrations of 0.5%–1.0% are used for veins 2–4 mm in diameter.

A volume of 0.5–1.0 cc is normally used at each injection site, and according to the American manufacturer, the total amount per weekly session should not exceed 300 mg (10 cc of 3% solution). The British manufacturer recommends a lower maximum dose of 120 mg per session.

Concentrations and doses in telangiectasias and reticular veins
Reticular veins are treated with 0.2%–1.0% solutions and up to 1 cc per site. Telangiectasias are treated with 0.1%–0.3% solutions and 0.1 cc or 0.2 cc per site. The recommended starting concentration for telangiectasias is 0.1%.

Comments
Aggressive or careless treatment with this agent may lead to extravasation necrosis and widespread hyperpigmentation. Use of too high a concentration for a particular vessel size may cause long-lasting hyperpigmentation, even when the injection technique is perfect.

POLYIODINATED IODINE
Polyiodinated iodine (Variglobin™) is a stabilized water solution of elemental (diatomic) iodide, sodium iodine, and benzyl alcohol that is available in concentrations from 2% to 12%. The active ingredient is the elemental iodine, which rapidly reacts with the vessel wall at the site of injection. It is a very powerful agent that causes dramatic vessel injury very rapidly. Its effects remain very localized because as it is diluted with a volume of blood, the elemental iodine is rapidly reduced to iodide, which is non-reactive. Despite the allergenicity of iodine, this solution has one of the safest and most extensive experience records worldwide. The agent is not FDA approved, and is not widely used in the United States.

Class
Chemically reactive (corrosive) agents.

General description
The strongest currently available sclerosing solution worldwide. Often used for sclerosis of widely incompetent saphenofemoral junctions.

Advantages
Highly localized reaction.
Extremely effective when properly used.
Risk of allergic reactions.

Disadvantages
Highly localized reaction.
Highly locally thrombogenic.
The liquid is brown, so blood withdrawal into the syringe is not easily seen.
Causes immediate blood coagulation in the syringe.
Very painful if extravasated.
Extravasation necrosis.
"Flulike" sensation with occasional fever after large doses.
Some patients report a metallic taste.

Principal indication
Saphenofemoral and saphenopopliteal junctions, after failure of other sclerosing solutions.

Accessory use
In the hands of highly experienced practitioners this is an all-purpose sclerosing agent for varicosities of all sizes.

Concentrations and doses in varicose veins
As a starting dose, 1 cc of a 3% solution may be used when treating at the saphenofemoral or saphenopopliteal junction. Truncal varicosities may be treated with 2 cc of 1% solution per injection point. Tributaries may be treated with 1 cc of 0.5% solution per injection point. The maximum dose per session is 5 cc of 12% Variglobin™.

Concentrations and doses in telangiectasias and reticular veins
Not used for small veins.

Comments
This is the agent of last resort when all else fails.

CHROMATED GLYCERIN
Glycerin is a tri-alcohol (1,2,3-propanetriol) that probably works by virtue of its dense hydrogen bonding capability. Glycerin is commercially available in combination with potassium chromate, but it has not been shown that the addition of the salt adds to its efficacy. Chromated glycerin (CG)(Sclérémo™, Chromex™) is a weak solution that is principally used for the tiniest of vessels, such as residual telangiectasia after an initial course of sclerotherapy. Chromated glycerin is one of the most widely used sclerosing agents in the world, but is used only rarely in the U.S. It is commercially available in a mixture of glycerin 720 mg/ml

and chrome potassium alum (a chrome salt) 8 mg/ml in an aqueous base.

Class
Uncertain (usually classed as chemically reactive).

General description
A very weak, very safe sclerosant, deserving of its appellation "the beginner's sclerosant."

Advantages
Extravasation does not cause necrosis.
Hyperpigmentation is rare.
Allergy is rare.

Disadvantages
Often too weak.
Very viscous and difficult to inject at full strength.
Painful if extravasated.
Large volumes injected into reticular veins can cause cramping.
May cause hematuria at high doses.

Principal indication
Telangiectasias.

Accessory use
Occasional use for small reticular and small varicose veins.

Concentrations and doses in varicose veins
Not used.

Concentrations and doses in telangiectasias and reticular veins
0.1–0.2 cc per site injected at full strength or diluted to 50% or 25% to reduce the viscosity. The maximum volume per session is 10 cc of full-strength solution.

Comments
Scattered reports suggest that CG may be effective for the treatment of telangiectatic matting; however, this is not proven.

SODIUM SALICYLATE (SOLUTION PRIMARILY OF HISTORIC INTEREST)
Introduced in 1919, sodium salicylate was the first reasonably safe and efficient all-purpose sclerosant. It was the beginning of modern sclerotherapy in Europe, but has been replaced by better agents today.

Class
Caustic (corrosive) agents.

General description
Obsolete, all purpose, safe, and weak, however, painful sclerosant.

Advantages
Very predictable effect.

Disadvantages
Very painful, even when injected intravascularly.
May cause tinnitus.

Principal indication
Small varicose and reticular veins.

Accessory use
None.

Concentrations and doses in varicose veins
0.5 cc–2 cc per site of a 12%–60% solution. The maximum dose is 5–6 cc of the 60% solution.

Concentrations and doses in telangiectasias and reticular veins
0.5 cc–1.0 cc of 12% solution per site in reticular veins, and 0.1 cc–0.2 cc of 7%–10% solution per site in telangiectasias.

Comments
Presented for historical purposes, but of very little clinical use today.

New and Experimental Solutions
GLYCERINE AND POLIDOCANOL
Glycerin and polidocanol (AV-15) are being combined as a new sclerosing agent now under development in France.

Class
Mixed.

General description
Brand new, weak sclerosant.

Advantages
Intended to be used without dilution.
Very few allergies.

Disadvantages
Hematuria and renal toxicity at high amounts (glycerin).

Principal indication
Telangiectasias.

Accessory use
Small reticular veins and telangiectasias of face and trunk.

Concentrations and doses in varicose veins
Not used.

Concentrations and doses in telangiectasias and reticular veins
0.1 cc–0.2 cc of full strength solution per site. Maximum dose not known.

Comments
It remains to be seen what advantages such a combination will offer.

POLIDOCANOL FOAM

Polidocanol foam is being investigated as a new sclerosing agent now under development in the United Kingdom. Polidocanol is foamed using an inert gas to the consistency of a foamy shaving cream.

Class

Detergent.

General description

Brand new, weak sclerosant.

Advantages

Same as polidocanol but includes use at lower concentrations so may have lower incidence of pigmentation and matting.
Displaces blood and remains for extended time in target vessel without being flushed.

Disadvantages

Same as polidocanol.

Principal indication

Telangiectasias and reticular veins.

Accessory use

Small reticular veins, and telangiectasias of face and trunk.

Concentrations and doses in varicose veins

Unknown.

Concentrations and doses in telangiectasias and reticular veins

Unknown.

Comments

Interesting concept to use a well-known sclerosing agent in a larger volume foam state to displace blood rather than mixing with it. Should allow more efficient use of sclerosant. Preliminary reports indicate increased efficacy. Clinical trials are ongoing world-wide.

Solutions Not Recommended

There are two FDA-approved agents available in the United States that cannot be recommended for treatment of lower extremity venous insufficiency nor for cosmetic treatment at any site. These agents are sodium morrhuate and ethanolamine oleate. Their principal use is in the sclerosis of bleeding esophageal varices, a clinical situation in which a high risk of immediate death may warrant the use of agents with a high risk of tissue necrosis and of anaphylactic reactions.

SODIUM MORRHUATE

Sodium morrhuate (Scleromate™, Palisades Pharmaceuticals, Inc., Tenafly, N.J.) is a mixture of the salts of saturated and unsaturated fatty acids in cod liver oil. Like sodium tetradecyl sulfate, this agent was "grandfathered" by the FDA, and the fact that it is approved for commercial sale does not imply that the FDA has examined it for safety and efficacy. Surprisingly, 20.8% of its fatty acid composition is unknown.[11] It is available as a 5% solution. Its use is limited by reports of fatalities secondary to anaphylaxis.[12] This agent is used for sclerosis of esophageal varices but complications (including allergic reactions) reportedly occur in up to 48% of patients.[13]

Although the FDA allows sodium morrhuate to be labeled and sold for the sclerosis of varicose veins, its frequent use for this purpose cannot be recommended. Not only has it been associated with a number of fatal reactions, it is a solution that produces dramatic and exuberant cutaneous necrosis with even minimal extravasation. One report in the literature advocates its use on leg telangiectasias.[14] The authors do not recommend its routine use in phlebology.

ETHANOLAMINE OLEATE

Ethanolamine oleate (Ethamolin™, Block Drug Co., Piscataway, N.J.) is a synthetic agent containing an organic base combined with oleic acid and supplied as a 5% solution. Its only FDA-approved indication is for the treatment of esophageal varices. Like sodium tetradecyl sulfate and sodium morrhuate, this agent was "grandfathered" by the FDA, and the fact that it is approved for commercial sale does not imply that the FDA has examined it for safety and efficacy. Ethanolamine oleate is an oily viscous solution that is thick enough to make it difficult to inject. It has been used extensively in the United Kingdom for control of acute esophageal variceal bleeding, and is reported to have a major complication rate similar to that of sodium morrhuate, but far greater than that of STS.[15] Allergic reactions have been reported with its use in leg varicosities as well.[16] Like sodium morrhuate, it produces exuberant extravasation necrosis and is not recommended for peripheral varicose veins or telangiectasias. The authors do not recommend its routine use in phlebology.

Summary

The guiding principle of modern sclerotherapy is to cause irreversible endothelial injury in the desired location while avoiding any damage to normal vessels that may be interconnected with the abnormal vessel we are treating. Our aim is to deliver the minimum volume and minimum concentration of the most appropriate sclerosant, and to inject it under conditions that will achieve the minimum effective exposure. Sclerosant concentration, volume, temperature, mixing, and patient positioning are as important in this endeavor as the choice of the actual sclerosing agent. The relative potencies of the various solutions and equivalent concentrations are important for every phlebologist to know (Table 14-3). The doses that are typically used are listed in Table 14-4 and Chapters 12, 13, and 19. Recommended maximum dosages of sclerosants are shown in Table 14-5. Typically, a phlebologist will work most often with just two to three solutions in the appropriate concentrations, but it is important to be familiar with them all *(Table 14-6)*. With attention to these details, an accomplished phlebologist can achieve good results with virtually any currently available sclerosing agent.

References

(1) Martin DE, Goldman MP. *A comparison of sclerosing agents: clinical and histologic effects of intravascular sodium tetradecyl sulfate and chromated glycerine in the dorsal rabbit ear vein.* J Dermatol Surg Onc 1990; 16:18–22.

(2) Goldman MP, Kaplan RP, Oki LN, et al. *Sclerosing agents in the treatment of telangiectasia: comparison of the clinical and histologic effects of intravascular polidocanol, sodium tetradecyl sulfate, and hypertonic saline in the dorsal rabbit ear vein model.* Arch Dermatol 1987; 123:1196–1201.

(3) Weiss RA, Goldman MP. *Advances in sclerotherapy.* Dermatologic Clinics 1995; 13(2):431–445.

(4) Imhoff E, Stemmer R. *Classification and mechanism of action of sclerosing agents.* Bull de la Soc Fran de Phlebol 1969; 22:143–148.

(5) Oscher A, Garside E. *Intravenous injection of sclerosing substances: experimental comparative studies of changes in vessels.* Ann Surg 1932; 96:691–718.

(6) De Medeiros A, Pinto Ribeiro A. *Sclerotherapy of varicose veins.* J Cardiovasc Surg (Torino) 1968; 9:268–272.

(7) Sadoun S, Benigni JP. *Bonnes pratiques cliniques et mousse de sclérosant : propositions pour une étude randomisée contrôlée, prospective, multicentrique, comparative, en aveugle, sur le traitement sclérosant par la mousse d'aetoxisclérol à 0,20 %.* Phlebol 1999;(3):291–298.

(8) Carlin MC, Ratz JL. *Treatment of telangiectasia: comparison of sclerosing agents.* J Dermatol Surg Oncol 1987; 13(11):1181–1184.

(9) Ariyoshi H, Kambayashi J, Tominaga S, Hatanaka T. *The possible risk of lower-limb sclerotherapy causing an extended hypercoagulable state.* Surgery Today 1996; 26(5):323–327.

(10) Guex JJ. *Indications for the sclerosing agent polidocanol (aetoxisclerol dexo, aethoxisklerol kreussler).* J Dermatol Surg Onc 1993; 19:959–961.

(11) Goldman MP. *Sclerotherapy treatment for varicose and telangiectatic leg veins.* In: Coleman WP, Hanke CW, Alt TH, Asken S, editors. Cosmetic Surgery of the Skin. Philadelphia: B.C. Decker, 1991: 197–211.

(12) Lewis KM. *Anaphylaxis due to sodium morrhuate.* JAMA 1936; 107:1298–1299.

(13) McClave SA, Kaiser SC, Wright RA, Edwards JL, Kranz KR. *Prospective randomized comparison of esophageal variceal sclerotherapy agents: sodium tetradecyl sulfate versus sodium morrhuate.* Gastrointest Endosc 1990; 36:567–571.

(14) Gallagher PG. *Varicose veins—primary treatment with sclerotherapy. A personal appraisal.* J Dermatol Surg Oncol 1992; 18(1):39–42.

(15) Kitano S, Wada H, Yamaga H, Hashizume M, Koyanagi N, Iwanaga T, et al. *Comparative effects of 5% ethanolamine oleate versus 5% sodium morrhuate for sclerotherapy of oesophageal varices.* J Gastroenterol Hepatol 1991; 6(5):476–480.

(16) Biegeleisen HI. *Fatty acid solutions for the injection treatment of varicose veins: an evaluation of 4 new solutions.* Ann Surg 1937; 105:610–615.

CHAPTER 15

Compression

Understanding Compression

INTRODUCTION AND HISTORY

To excel in phlebology, the physician must understand the basic concepts of compression, including physiologic effects, common terms, rationale for its use in the prevention and treatment of varicose and telangiectatic veins, and rationale and use following sclerotherapy and ambulatory phlebectomy. Although modern compression stockings are an invention of 20th century medicine, the concept of compression for varicose veins dates back to antiquity. Compression therapy for treatment of venous disease was originally mentioned in the Old Testament (Isaiah, 1:6).[1] Roman soldiers noted that the application of tight bindings to the legs could reduce leg fatigue. In the late 1700s, Theden used modified lace-up dog leather stockings originally described by Fabrizio d'Aquapendente (1537–1619), in the treatment of varicose veins of pregnancy.

Nelson Goodyear made the development of elastic medical compression bandages and stockings possible with the invention of vulcanization in 1842. Rubber harvested from the rain forests of Brazil was turned into elastic threads to weave stockings. Although uncomfortable, stockings made from rubber threads were utilized until Jonathan Sparks patented a method for winding cotton and silk around the rubber threads. This allowed more widespread use of elastic compression.[2]

As technical advances in the manufacturing process were made during the late 1800s and early 1900s, ultrafine rounded latex yarns (particularly with the later advent of circular knitting versus flat knitting techniques) became available that permitted the construction of modern compression stockings. Two-way-stretch stockings were then developed. Rubberless compression stockings became available with the development of synthetic elastomers in the 1960s, giving rise to the modern, relatively comfortable, seamless compression hose available today.

PHYSIOLOGIC EFFECTS

It is logical that the normal force generated within the venous system by muscle contraction would be additive with external applied pressure *(Table 15-1)*. This augmentation of the calf muscle pump occurs by external application of graduated compression.[3] In ambulatory patients with superficial venous insufficiency, improvement can be demonstrated with graduated compression stockings with an ankle pressure of as little as 18 mm Hg.[4] After 90 days of elastic compression with a 30–40 mm Hg graduated compression stocking, patients with cutaneous manifestations of venous stasis demonstrate noteworthy improvements in the structural pattern of dermal connective tissue.[5] Compression reduces the edema that separates the skin and dermal tissues from direct contact with the superficial capillary network, as this edema resides primarily in the papillary dermis.[6]

Graduated compression hose therefore lead to normalized nutritional exchange and waste product removal. External "graduated" compression counterbalances the lost elasticity of the tissues in order to augment lymphatic flow. This flow is also expanded through an increase in hydrostatic pressure that prevents reaccumulation of edema.[7] Compression, particularly inelastic, also decreases the size of deep muscular veins, thus increasing pressure within them and augmenting venous return.[8]

TERMINOLOGY

For the sake of understanding external compression, the process of walking is arbitrarily divided into a working phase (calf muscle contraction with plantar flexion) and a resting phase (relaxed). *Resting pressure* is the pressure arising from the compression bandage pushing against the skin without muscular action. The greater the tension and stretch of the bandage, the greater resting pressure. *Working pressure* is the compression that occurs from the bandage during muscle contraction. This pressure is the counterpressure of the stocking exerted on the calf during foot flexion phase of walking. This should not be confused with *end pressure* or *end resting pressure*, which is the additive effect of multiple compression stockings or bandages placed on top of one another to increase resting pressure. To make compliance with compression easier for an elderly individual, it is possible to place two compression stockings on top of one another. For example, two 20 mm Hg stockings can be worn to roughly equal the end pressure of a single 40 mm Hg compression stocking. Resting pressure and working pressure are important when evaluating the types of bandage or compression stocking to be employed for appropriate applications.

The terminology of the types of compression bandaging includes *non-elastic, short-stretch, and long-stretch. Non-elastic* bandages are totally rigid, unyielding to the expanding leg and capable of providing high working pressure. This pressure is transmitted directly to the deep compartment of the leg, where the deep veins are compressed and proximal flow increased. These bandages are most useful when edema of the leg is marked and muscular movement provides very little change in shape of the leg. The typical example is a zinc gel (Unna Boot [Unna-Flex: Convatec, Princeton, NJ], Gelocast [Gelocast: Beiersdorf Inc., Norwalk, CT]), which dries to an inflexible "cast" around the leg. The edema must then give way under a rigid, inflexible bandage. Application of inelastic compression must be done carefully to avoid overcompression causing arterial ischemia and/or increased compartmental pressure. Inelastic compression must be reapplied frequently as edema decreases, since working pressure rapidly drops with decreasing edema.

Table 15-1
Physiologic Effects of Compression

Mechanically externally enhances the calf muscle pump

Diverts flow into competent veins by closing incompetent superficial veins

Makes incompetent valves work by decreasing diameter between leaflets of valves in varicose veins

Reduces edema that separates skin from capillaries

Augments lymphatic flow

Short-stretch bandages are also important to treat edema and have high working pressures similar to inelastic compression. The fabric of these bandages is usually extensible, primarily because of the weave pattern; they can stretch by expanding the distance between loops without the presence of rubber, nylon, or polyurethane. They can therefore be made entirely of comfortable natural fibers, for example, Comprilan (Beiersdorf, Norwalk, CT), which is 100% cotton. Short-stretch compression is applied with fabric stretch of only 30%–50%. Short-stretch bandages exert pressure when the calf muscles are relaxed and prevent expansion in calf diameter when the muscles are contracting (working). They have a low to slight resting pressure and a very high working pressure, exerting effect mainly within the deep venous system.[9] Short-stretch bandages are comfortable when patients are recumbent (low resting pressure), and act to decrease superficial venous pressure mainly with ambulation (high working pressure). They increase deep venous flow more than they impede reflux at rest and can be worn at night. Short-stretch is recommended to clear severe edema.[10]

Long-stretch bandages can be stretched 100% to 200% in at least one direction, (usually longitudinally) and 30%–40% in the other direction (transversely). Long-stretch material is most commonly known as the graduated compression stocking. These have a high resting pressure because elastic recoil exerts high pressure on the leg as it attempts to return to the resting position.[11] Graduated compression stockings move easily during muscle contraction (the working phase), but exert significant resting pressure on the superficial venous system that minimizes reflux when the limb is at rest. Because of the ability to compress veins at muscular rest, compression stockings are useful for patients with superficial venous insufficiency who work in jobs requiring limited leg muscular contraction. When the patient is recumbent, however, these may be uncomfortable and cause arterial constriction due to the high resting pressure. Compression stockings slow the progression of disease, provide maintenance therapy, and are highly valued for postsclerotherapy compression of superficial varicosities.[12] In addition, even lightweight compression has been shown to reduce symptoms of venous hypertension.[13]

In contrast to the uniform compression available with medical stockings, the compression supplied by wrapped bandages depends greatly on the experience of the practitioner. Skilled clinicians can apply bandages with a pressure that ranges from 25–50 mm Hg, while the bandages applied by less-skilled clinicians exert pressure that ranges from 15–70 mm Hg.[14] Poor control over the amount of pressure applied can be a serious clinical problem, as compression that is too high can cause arterial occlusion and can produce trophic skin breakdown over bony prominences.

CLASSES OF COMPRESSION

Compression stockings have empirically been divided into four compression classes (*Table 15-2*) by the Compression Stocking Commission of the German Working Group on Phlebology, based on the counterpressure at complete rest

Table 15-2
Counterpressure Exerted By Various Compression Classes

Class	mm Hg	Indications
I	18.4–21.2	Leg fatigue, mild symptoms, mild varices (including pregnancy)
II	25.1–32.1	More symptoms, edema, after minor ulcerations, following sclerotherapy, moderate varicosities
III	36.4–46.5	Chronic, postthrombotic venous insufficiency, marked edema, lipodermatosclerosis, after severe ulcerations
IV	>59.0	Very severe disease unresponsive to lower compression, lymphedema

at the ankle and on the indications for that counterpressure. Class I compression is approximately 20 mm Hg at the ankle. The indications for class I compression are leg fatigue or heaviness, mild early varicose veins without associated edema, and early varices of pregnancy. Class II is roughly 30 mm Hg at the ankle. Indications for class II compression include more severe symptoms, marked varicosities, mild to moderate edema, and marked varicose veins of pregnancy. Class II compression is also indicated following sclerotherapy, ambulatory phlebectomy, or other venous surgery, and in patients with superficial thrombophlebitis or healing venous ulcers.

Class III, which provides roughly 40 mm Hg counterpressure at the ankle, is indicated for marked edema, lipodermatosclerosis, and all serious sequelae of chronic, postthrombotic venous insufficiency. Class IV, providing greater than 60 mm Hg compression, is reserved for severe disease unresponsive to the previous classes of compression and for patients with lymphedema. Class IV stockings must be specially fitted, are not routinely available without special order, and are a high risk for causing arterial occlusion.

Full-leg stockings are preferred in every patient, although with elderly patients some compromise may be necessary. Some compression is better than no compression. A patient with thigh varicosities and ankle edema who refuses to wear a thigh-high stocking will still benefit from knee-length compression, as venous return will be improved with increased efficacy of the calf muscle pump.

PRACTICAL APPLICATIONS OF LAPLACE'S LAW

Laplace's law (pressure = bandage tension/radius of surface) describes the distribution of pressure of an elastic sleeve stretched over a cylindrical surface. This principle is more clearly stated as the smaller the radius (the tighter the turn), the higher the applied pressure. Stockings that are perfectly fitted will have a constant amount of stretch at every level of the leg, thus the greatest pressure will be in the ankle, where the radius of curvature is small, and the least pressure will be in the thigh, where the curvature is most gentle.

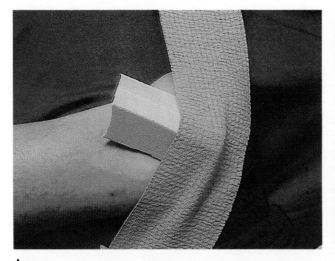
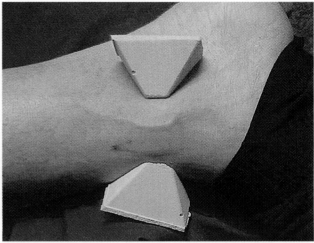

A   **B**

Figure 15-1.   Practical application of Laplace's formula. Padding is applied beneath a compression stocking to approximate the profile of a cylinder. This allows for the most even application of pressure. Pressure is most evenly distributed when approaching a cylinder. **(A)** Flat areas are rounded. **(B)** Projecting areas are made less round. LaPlace's formula (Pressure = compression divided by radius, i.e., the greater the curve or smaller radius, the greater the pressure).

Irregular contours around the knee and at the malleoli of the ankles make it difficult to maintain evenly graduated compression. To make irregular areas of the leg as cylindrical as possible, protruding surfaces (such as malleoli) must have their curve lessened with padding on each side, and flat areas must have their curve increased (with pads or cotton rolls) to produce a slight bulging, a smaller radial circle with increased pressure *(Figure 15-1)*. Laplace's law allows us to increase compression selectively over treated varicose veins: a foam pad or cotton roll over the vein will cause a smaller radius curve at the site, and will produce a greater force.

Compression Bandages and Graduated Compression Stockings

The primary differences between bandages and stockings are summarized in Table 15-3. Unlike stockings, the compression supplied by bandages is dependent on bandaging technique, as varying the amount of stretching force used during wrapping can alter pressure. The proper technique is illustrated in Figure 15-2. Principles of compression bandage application are listed in Table 15-4. A popular technique is the four-layered compression bandage.[15]

Table 15-3
Comparison of Medical Compression Bandaging with Medical Compression Stockings

Bandaging	Stockings
Textile-elastic (extensible because of weave alone without elastomeric fibers)	Elastic fibers (small percentage of elastomeric fibers to retain shape)
Short-stretch, low recoil	Long-stretch, high recoil
High working pressure—increase deep venous flow	Low working pressure—poor effect on deep venous flow
Low resting pressure—poor reflux prevention	High resting pressure—excellent reflux prevention
Risk of non-uniform application	Uniform application based on leg measurement
Must learn proper application	Easy to apply
May be worn at night—low resting pressure	May be uncomfortable at night—high resting pressure
Usage for acute problems: acute edema, dermatitis, phlebitis, acute venous ulceration	Best for maintenance, long-term treatment, prevention of recurrence of varicose leg ulcers
Initial treatment of lymphedema	Long-term treatment of lymphedema
	Additional indications of compression stockings: Pregnancy as prevention and treatment of varicose veins During exercise to minimize further dilatation of varicose veins

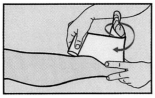

Place the beginning of the bandage plantar, guide over the outer edge of the foot over the instep up to the basal joint of the big toe. Then, coming from plantar, cross the bandage over itself on the lateral side of the basal joint of the little toe.

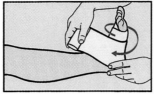

Wrap with a slightly oblique circular turn over the metatarsus medially towards the heel.

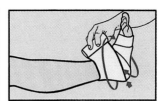

Cover the heel with one turn, then guide the bandage from lateral to medial as far as the Achilles tendon. Cover this with ⅔ of the width of the bandage, while the remaining third of the bandage runs over the heel.

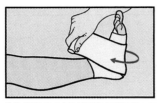

Guide the bandage from lateral to medial and cover the distal portion of the heel with about ⅓ of the bandage, then guide the the head of the bandage proximally.

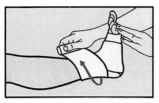

Apply the bandage in a spiral turn around the ankles, wrapping with uniform moderate compression pressure.

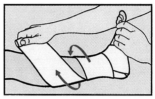

The bandage runs in a spiral turn around the calf, to the insertion of the gastrocnemius muscle below the popliteal fossa. Uncovered areas are permissible.

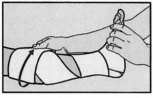

Fix the ascending spiral turn on the proximal calf with a circular turn without tension and pressure, and allow the remaining bandage to run out distally around the calf.

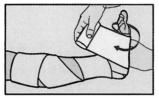

The second bandage starts plantar and leads in a circular turn around the metatarsophalangeal joints. It is also applied in the pronation direction.

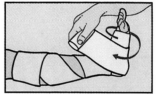

The next turn runs obliquely over the metatarsus, then over the instep medially towards the ankle.

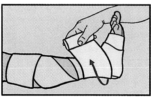

A circular turn is placed far distally around the ankles.

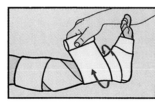

The bandage is then wrapped spirally with about 50% overlap.

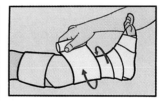

Allow the bandage to ascend proximally on the calf and take care to ensure that the turns overlap by a good 50%.

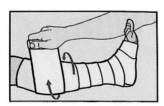

The last turn once again covers the calf muscles up to distal of the popliteal fossa.

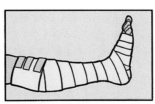

The end of the bandage is fixed with Leukoplast® strips or clips.

Figure 15-2. Proper application of compression bandage (printed with permission from Beiersdorf Medical Bibliothek, Nurnberg, Germany).

Table 15-4
Principles of Compression Bandage Application

- Usually no greater than 50% stretch applied to bandage during application.
- No gaps so that each turn overlaps 50 to 70% of the previous turn to avoid skin pinching.
- Oblique (not circular) turns of the bandage minimizes constriction of the skin.
- At the ankle and knee a two-way stretch elastic bandage better conforms to the shape of the joints and is thus more comfortable than short-stretch (one-way) elastic bandages, which are preferred on the rest of the leg.
- The ankle joint should be maximally extended dorsally when the bandage is applied.
- Some form of padding or foam should be placed on the anterior tibial and retromalleolar area to both protect thin-skinned areas and evenly distribute pressure.
- A rough textured underwrapping (such as Medirip) may be applied to minimize slippage of the compression bandage
- Local compression should be applied 5–10 cm beyond affected areas to avoid bruising, hematoma, edema, and inflammatory reactions.
- Graduated compression is achieved by applying even pressure on the bandage, which is stretched to a uniform degree while wrapping from distal to proximal direction. This occurs because Laplace's law governs that smaller diameters have increased pressures as long as tension remains constant and the leg increases in diameter from a distal to proximal direction.
- Pressure may be increased by application of multiple layers of compression bandage.

In order to minimize slipping of compression bandages, rough-textured elastic gauze can be utilized as an underbandage. When patients must apply compression bandages at home, they will require detailed instruction and supervised practice before they leave the office, as well as explicit written instructions and diagrams for use as a home reference.

Because bandages become looser over time, the principal indication for compression bandages is for temporary compression, such as in patients with marked edema or inflammatory conditions in which an improvement can be expected in a relatively short time. Bandages are useful in edema because they can be continually reapplied as the edema in the affected limb is reduced. Unlike stockings, which must be long-stretch in order to fit over the foot and ankle, limited-stretch bandages can be continually reapplied and tightened as edema is reduced. This additional pressure on the deep venous system increases its working pressure and efficiency.[8] There are few published studies comparing compression bandages with compression stockings, but one study has shown a greater success with treatment, improved patient acceptance, and reduced complications with stockings compared to bandages.[16]

Unless periodically and expertly rewrapped, compression bandages only maintain significant compression for 6–8

hours while patients are ambulatory, and lose up to 50% of their initial compression pressure in recumbent patients at 24 hours.[17] In the United States, because of insufficient training in techniques and lack of patient compliance, compression bandaging usually is reserved for patients who simply cannot be fitted with compression stockings.

Clinical Applications of Compression
PREVENTION AND THERAPY OF VENOUS INSUFFICIENCY

Veins with a high-unopposed filling pressure have a tendency to become distended, causing secondary valvular incompetence. If valves are allowed to remain incompetent for prolonged periods of time, fibrosis of the cusps may cause irreversible damage. Bandages and graduated compression stockings provide external support that can constrict dilated veins and restore competence to incompetent valves. To prevent valve fibrosis, external compression is important from the earliest stages of venous insufficiency.

COMPRESSION IN PREGNANCY

The best use of compression hose as preventive therapy is for patients with varicose veins of pregnancy.[18,19] When the factors responsible for dilation of pregnancy-induced varicose veins (excessive blood volume, hormonally induced relaxation of the vein wall, etc.) resolve, the veins often return to normal; however, after repeated pregnancies the varicose veins may become permanent. Graduated compression stockings can minimize dilatation of superficial vessels during pregnancy, and can maintain valvular competence in many patients, reducing the likelihood of permanent valvular damage. The risks of deep venous thrombosis (DVT) should also be reduced.[20]

At the first indication of pregnancy, genetically susceptible patients should initially be fitted with a 20–30 mm Hg graduated pantyhose. In multiparous women, or in those with a previous history of varicose veins, a stronger 30–40 mm Hg pantyhose should be worn. In women with large legs, or in patients who are uncomfortable with a 30–40 mm Hg pantyhose, a calf-length 20–30 mm Hg compression stocking can be worn over 20–30 mm Hg pantyhose. Even 25 mm Hg graduated compression stockings can significantly decrease subjective discomfort and ankle edema during the third trimester of pregnancy.[21]

Compression after Vein Treatment

Compression has been used as an adjunct to vein sclerotherapy since the 1940s, [22,23] and achieved widespread acceptance during the 1950s and 1960s. The addition of compression to sclerotherapy is regarded by many as the most important advance in the treatment of varicose veins since the introduction of the first relatively safe synthetic sclerosing agents in the 1940s. Postsclerotherapy compression reduces the thrombophlebitic reaction and substitutes a "sclerophlebitis" with production of a firm fibrous cord.[24] Interestingly, compression works to prevent the appearance of new varicose veins even after surgery: regular use of compression can reduce the one-year recurrence rate after surgery from 70% to just 7%.[25]

VALUE OF POSTTREATMENT COMPRESSION

When used after sclerotherapy, compression serves several important functions. Compression of the treated vessel decreases the amount and extent of thrombus formation after endothelial injury, reducing the likelihood of subsequent recanalization.[26] A decrease in thrombus formation also reduces the incidence of postsclerosis pigmentation and helps to minimize the inflammation that can lead to telangiectatic matting.[27] Compression stockings produce a marked increase in blood flow through the deep venous system, helping to prevent deep vein thrombosis, whether from direct endothelial injury or from extension of thrombus through perforating veins.[28] Immediate compression may produce direct apposition of the treated vein walls to produce more effective wall damage with a smaller concentration of sclerosing solution. A recent study demonstrates the statistical significantly improved results of 20–30 mm Hg compression hosiery after sclerotherapy. Significant clinical benefit is shown, as well as reduction in hyperpigmentation postsclerotherapy.[12]

AMOUNT OF COMPRESSION

The amount of pressure needed to fully compress a varicose vein after sclerotherapy depends on the situation. An external pressure of 30 mm Hg will produce a 96% reduction in the capacity of dorsal foot veins carrying an internal pressure of 50 mm Hg.[29] Classic compression bandaging produces an average compression of 54 mm Hg at the upper calf, sufficient to reduce the size of a vessel that is distended by an internal pressure of 90 mm Hg by 94%.[30]

DURATION OF COMPRESSION

The duration of compression needed after sclerotherapy is still a matter of controversy, although the most recommended period is 2–3 weeks. The classic descriptions of sclerosis of varicose veins described by Fegan, Hobbs, and Doran recommend compression for 6 weeks.[23,31,32] A few small randomized studies have suggested that most of the value of compression may come in the early phase, and that results may be comparable no matter whether compression is maintained for 6 weeks, 3 weeks, or only 3 days.[33,34] A recent well-controlled study concluded that 3 weeks of compression may be ideal, however, one week and 3 days of compression are sufficient to improve results.[12] In the United States, few patients can tolerate 6 weeks of uninterrupted compression, but most are able to comply with 2 weeks of compression stockings, and nearly all can tolerate a protocol that uses relatively uninterrupted compression for the first 3 days, then continues compression interrupted only for showering for the next 2 weeks.

COMPRESSION FOR SPIDER VEINS

Compression is a well-accepted part of the treatment of large varicose veins, but the use of compression when treating smaller telangiectasia is less widely accepted. A multicenter bilateral comparison study found that 3 days of compression improved the effectiveness of treatment in telangiectasia greater than 0.5 mm in diameter on the proximal leg and in telangiectasia of any size on the distal leg.[35] Compression also reduced the rate of postsclerotherapy hyperpigmentation from 40.5% to 28.5%, and reduced the incidence of posttreatment ankle edema. A recent study of flight attendants demonstrated statistically significant reduction in symptoms using only over-the-counter, ready-to-wear pantyhose compression stockings of 12–15mm Hg or 15–20 mm Hg.[13] We favor compression as adjunctive therapy for all vein sclerotherapy because the theoretical justification for compression applies equally well to small veins as to large ones, and because a significant percentage of smaller spider veins on the lateral thigh occur in direct communication with larger varicose or reticular superficial veins.[36,37]

Contraindications to Compression Modalities

Not all patients can tolerate compression stockings, and not all will benefit from them. Patients with edema may benefit more from intermittent therapy than from constant compression. Patients with arterial insufficiency may suffer more from restriction of arterial flow than benefit from enhancement of venous flow. Patients with unusual anatomy or with severe cutaneous sensitivity may be unable to tolerate placement or removal of a compression garment.

EDEMA

Marked edema, weeping stasis dermatitis, and new venous leg ulcers will benefit from bandaging or from pneumatic compression, rather than from compression stockings in the acute phase. When edema of the leg is due to cardiac failure, constant external compression may increase venous return to the detriment of the patient. It is essential to know the entire clinical situation and the cause of leg edema before instituting compression.

ARTERIAL INSUFFICIENCY

Arterial insufficiency, although not an absolute contraindication to compression, must be thoroughly evaluated before compression stockings are recommended for any concomitant venous insufficiency. When patients experience leg pain following the application of a stocking, it must be removed immediately and further examination, such as duplex ultrasound, must be performed.

It is important to check arterial pulses before and after application of compression bandages or stockings, particularly in older patients. Approximately 21% of older patients with venous disease also have decreased arterial pressure.[38] Palpable pulses of the posterior tibial and dorsal foot arteries do not exclude increased intracompartmental pressure because arterial pulsations may be normal at up to 80 mm Hg of intracompartmental pressure.[39] Sensory disturbances may be the earliest warning sign indicating excessive compression.

Even in normal limbs, arterial flow is diminished at rest, and ankle compression pressures greater than 20 mm Hg can impair calf muscle and cutaneous blood flow in bedridden patients.[40] When 30–40 mm Hg compression stockings are worn to bed, some patients may have hypoperfusion-induced discomfort in the foot, heel, and ankle that occurs during sleep and resolves with standing or walking. When double stockings are used to obtain higher compression pressures, patients must be warned to remove the outer stocking when not walking.

FITTING DIFFICULTIES

When the ankle diameter is less than 17 cm, it may be difficult to get the correct size stocking to fit over the wider portions of the foot and heel, and in this case a lower compression class may be substituted. Elderly patients with less physical strength may require assistance from a visiting nurse. A compromise solution is the use of two stockings of lower compression, one over the other, to have an additive effect. Special stockings with zippers have been developed for use in physically debilitated patients who cannot pull on an ordinary compression stocking.

How to Use Compression Stockings

MEASUREMENT

Nearly all stocking manufacturers have adopted the reference table of the GZG (Quality Seal Association for Medical Compression Stockings), which was created in 1972 by the German Association for Phlebology (Table 15-5). Measurements of circumference are taken at eight points on the leg using a non-stretchable tape measure, and patients are classified into one of six different sizes (Figure 15-3). All ready-made stockings include the ankle as one of the measuring points because a graduated stocking exerts 100% of its rated pressure here (Figure 15-3, point b). Although fitting is primarily based on ankle diameter, a custom-constructed stocking will be required if the other leg measurements are not within one size of the "best fit" as determined at the ankle. Simplified measurement methods use circumferential measurements at the ankle and at the largest diameters of the calf and upper thigh. The length of the leg is measured from the heel to the gluteal fold for pantyhose and thigh-high stockings. The length from the heel to the popliteal fossa is used for knee-high stockings. Actual gradient percentages of compression are shown in Figure 15-4.

To minimize the distorting effects of edema, fittings should be performed in the morning or immediately after the removal of a compression bandage. For lymphedema, the fit will need to be adjusted frequently once the lymph begins to be mobilized. Patients who have a wide foot do not tolerate higher classes of compression, as they often develop nocturnal foot pain if overcompressed. Up to six styles of medical compression stockings are available depending on the manufacturer; knee-length, mid-thigh, thigh, pantyhose or leotard, one-legged pantyhose, thigh with waist attachment, and maternity pantyhose. Regardless of the style, most stockings are available in three lengths: knee-length, midthigh, and thigh length. According to the standardized figure, a knee-length stocking is designated as A-D, a mid-thigh stocking as A-F, and a thigh length stocking as A-G (see Figure 15–3).

With single-leg, thigh, or calf stockings, various inexpensive methods such as adhesive tape, glue, clips, or garter belts serve to ensure proper positioning. Disadvantages of tape or glue include the pain on removal of tape from hairy legs, and irritation or allergy caused by the adhesive. For some patients, garter belts provide a desirable method for ensuring correct positioning of thigh-high stockings. A new type of silicone-beaded top-band on thigh or mid-thigh length stockings is now available from some manufacturers,

Table 15-5
Guidelines for Compression Stockings after Sclerotherapy and for Relief of Varicose Vein Symptoms

Type of vein	Suggested compression	Duration of compression
Telangiectasias	15–20 mm Hg	3 days to 2 weeks
Reticular veins (small)	20–30 mm Hg	2 weeks
Reticular veins (large)	30–40 mm Hg	3 weeks
Varicose veins	30–40 mm Hg	6 weeks
Chronic venous insufficiency	30–40 mm Hg, 40–50 mm Hg (if tolerated) (can use additive compression of lesser values)	Indefinitely or until treatment of superficial incompetence is possible
Pregnancy	20–30 mm Hg	First + second trimester
	30–40 mm Hg (or two 20–30 mm Hg)	Third trimester

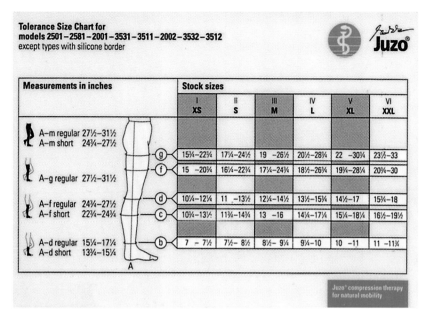

Figure 15-3. Important points of measurement for compression stockings.
(Printed with permission from Julius Zorn, Inc., Cuyahoga Falls, OH)

and in some patients this can prevent slippage without the use of glues, waist straps, or garter belts.

PROPER APPLICATION TECHNIQUE

Measures must be taken to avoid poking a hole through the stocking while pulling them onto the leg. Hand jewelry should be removed and fingernails should be smooth and

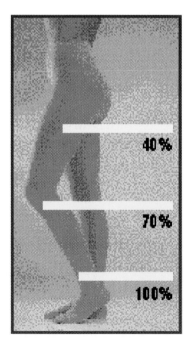

Figure 15-4. Schematic of actual gradient percentages of compression stockings.

relatively short. Rubber dishwashing gloves are recommended to prevent damage to the stockings from long fingernails and to improve the grip on the stocking. Talcum powder may be applied to the leg, or a light perlon pantyhose or stocking may be worn under the compression stocking to create a smoother leg over which to slide the stocking. Smooth fabric foot "socks" provided by some stocking manufacturers are helpful in getting an open-toe stocking over the ankle. This also helps to avoid damage from abrasive toenails and calluses.

The proper technique for putting on a compression stocking is illustrated in Figure 15-5. After taking the precautions mentioned above, the stocking is turned inside out with the foot portion tucked into the stocking. The foot opening is stretched with the fingers or thumbs of both hands and the stocking pulled up to the instep. The stocking is drawn upwards over the heel until pulling becomes difficult, and a fold that forms across the instep and heel of the stocking is pulled over the patient's heel. Finally, the stocking is pulled up in small sections, proceeding only in small steps, and taking care to avoid any creases or "bunching up" of the stocking material. It is very helpful for the physician or nurse to instruct and observe the patient applying the stocking for the first time.

Simple metal frames to aid the application of a stocking are now made by various manufacturers *(Figure 15-6)*. The compression stocking is pulled over the half-circle bracket located on the front (open) side of the device so that the heel portion of the stocking is 2–3 inches below the top on the inner circle bracket. The heel portion is positioned facing the user; the toe of the stocking is facing towards the open side of the device. The foot is then placed into the foot part of the stocking until the foot is completely on the floor or until the heel is in place. The metal grips on either side are

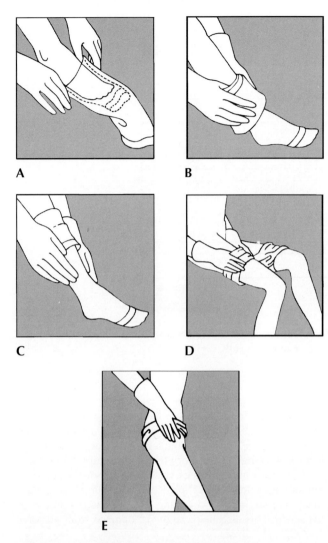

A   B

C   D

E

Figure 15-5.   Schematic diagram illustrating recommended method for application of a compression stocking. (A) Turn the stocking inside out. Tuck in the foot from the heel to the toe. **(B)** Using both hands, pull the stocking over the foot up to the instep, drawing it upwards over the heel. **(C)** Continue pulling the stocking up in small sections. **(D)** Pull the thigh section over the knee. **(E)** Gently pull stocking to waist and smooth the fit; follow by removing the foot sock, if one was used. (Courtesy Julius Zorn, Inc.)

then used to pull the rest of the stocking onto the leg. Once the stocking is above the calf, the metal frame may be pulled away and the remainder of the stocking can then be easily pulled up.

CARE OF COMPRESSION STOCKINGS

Chemical stresses from sweat, soaps, creams, and body oils, in addition to the physical stresses of near continuous stretch and relaxation with movement of the leg, result in a gradual decline in the compressive effect of the stockings. Under normal usage and proper care, compression stockings should have an effective lifespan of 4–6 months. Rub-

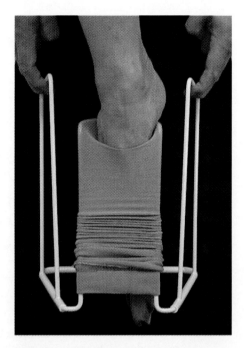

Figure 15-6.   Open frame to aid in the application of single leg compression stockings. (Medi Butler)

ber gloves should be worn when the stocking is put on to avoid tearing the threads with fingernails. Likewise, toenails should be trimmed, and hard calluses, verruca, or other rough spots on the feet should be softened or removed. The stocking (especially one composed of rubber threads) should not come into contact with ointments, creams, stain removers, or other solvents. These substances can damage the fine elastic yarns by causing them to swell, thus reducing the strength and elasticity of the fabric.

Regular and careful washing is necessary to maintain the elastic properties of the fabric, as sweat, skin oils, and environmental dirt that accumulate in the fabric while the stocking is worn have harmful effects. Compression stockings may be washed every day using a mild hand-washable soap.[22] Whenever possible, the patient should have two pairs that can be alternated between washings. Most compression stockings incorporating Spandex can be machine-washed on a fine/gentle cycle with warm (40°C) water in a mesh laundry bag. (Consult the manufacturer's guidelines for specific instructions.) Gentle detergents without bleach or alkali are best. Gentle spinning after the washing cycle expedites the drying process. Rather than being hang-dried from a line, compression stockings should be laid flat on a drying rack or towel to help maintain shape. Heat drying will cause a rapid loss of elasticity.

Summary

Compression serves many important purposes in patients with venous insufficiency syndromes. Compression is extremely valuable as adjunctive therapy when surgery or sclerotherapy is used to remove or ablate superficial veins.

POST DUPLEX-GUIDED SCLEROTHERAPY INSTRUCTIONS

1. Keep stockings on until bedtime. If your toes turn blue or feel numb, call the doctor immediately.
2. Keep the bandage on until tomorrow morning. Shower will the bandage on (it will get wet and soggy), then remove bandage when you get out of the shower and immediately put on your stockings.
3. You can resume **normal** activities today (walking is okay).
4. You can resume exercising in 3 days (no weights with the legs for 2 weeks).
5. You can take a shower in the morning but no hot baths for 1 week.
6. Wear your support hose for 2 weeks, from first thing in the morning (ideally, take a quick 5 minute shower and then put them on before doing the rest of your morning ritual), until last thing at night.
7. Schedule the next follow-up visit in 4-6 weeks.
8. Bruising, local swelling and some tenderness are normal after treatment, but please feel free to call the office if you have any questions.
9. If the vein gets hard and knotty and causes some discomfort, please call the office and schedule to have the area "nicked". This will help with the discomfort and also help the area to heal faster.

Figure 15-7. Instructions to patients for compression following duplex-guided sclerotherapy. (Instructions for compression after non-duplex-guided sclerotherapy can be found in Chapter 27)

POST AMBULATORY PHLEBECTOMY INSTRUCTIONS

1. Keep the leg elevated as much as possible until bedtime.
2. If bleeding soaks through the bandage, keep the leg elevated and call the office to reach the doctor on call. Keeping your leg elevated above the level of the heart will minimize the risk of this.
3. If your toes turn blue or feel numb, call the doctor immediately.
4. Keep the dressing dry. Do not take a shower or get the dressing wet.
5. You will see the doctor the day after surgery. At this time, the dressing will be removed and you will begin to wear the support hose.
6. Wear your support hose from first thing in the morning (ideally, keep them beside the bed and put them on before you get out of bed), until last thing at night. You may take a 5-minute shower without wearing them.
7. You must wear them in this manner for two weeks after surgery.
8. Bruising, local swelling and some tenderness are normal after treatment, but please feel free to call the office if you have any questions.
9. Walking can begin the day after surgery, but no vigorous exercise should be done for one week after surgery. Try not to bump the area treated. No weight lifting with the legs for two weeks.

Figure 15-8. Instructions to patients for compression following ambulatory phlebectomy

Table 15-6
Manufacturers of Compression Stockings

Brand	*Address*	*Special features*
Jobst	Jobst: A Beiersdorf Company P.O. Box 471048 Charlotte, NC 28247 704-554-9933	**Fast-fit** (lightweight 18-25 mm Hg or moderate 25–35mm Hg) OTC **Vairox**—available with a zipper **Ulcer care kit**—wound care + zippered stockings
Sigvaris	Sigvaris P.O. Box 570, 32 Park Dr East Branford, CT 06405 800-322-7744	Several lines available, **500** series, newest is **902**—most comprised of synthetic rubber threads covered with nylon **Delilah**—lightweight OTC
JuZo	Julius Zorn, Inc. P.O.Box 1088 Cuyahoga Falls, OH 44223 800-222-4999	**Varilastic**—increased upper portion stretch for larger thighs **Hostess**—Elastomer fibers are covered with cotton Newest thigh length have attractive **lace borders**
Medi	Medi USA, L.P. 76 W. Seegers Rd. Arlington Hts., IL 60005 800-633-6334	**Medi Plus** and **Medi 75**—**spandex** thread inlaid into every woven row **Non-slip silicone beaded band** on thigh-high Medi Plus holds stocking in place without glue or garters
Camp	Camp International, Inc, P.O. Box 89 Jackson, MI 49204	Double wrapped yarns
Venosan	Venosan North America Inc. Asheboro, NC 27204 910-672-6062	**Venosan 2000**—Combination of nylon, Lycra and cotton **Legline**—lightweight OTC graduated

OTC, over-the-counter

Table 15-7
Manufacturers of Readily Available Compression Bandages

Manufacturer	Type of bandage	Adherence / brand name
Beiersdorf Inc. Norwalk, CT 06856 (Distributed by Jobst 1-800-537-1063)	Textile elastic (low stretch)	nonhesive/**Comprilan** cohesive/**Comprihaft** adhesive/**Elastoplast**
	Elastomer (high stretch)	nonhesive/**Eloflex** cohesive/**Elohaft**
	Inelastic (no stretch)	cohesive/**Gelocast**
Se Pro Healthcare Montgomery, PA 18936	Elastomer (high stretch)	nonhesive/**Tubigrip**
3M Health Care St. Paul, MN 55144	Elastomer (high stretch)	adhesive/**Microfoam**
Convatec (division of Bristol- Myers-Sqibb) Princeton, NJ 08543	Inelastic (no stretch)	cohesive/**Unna-Flex**
Conco Medical Company Bridgeport, CT 06610	Textile elastic (low stretch)	cohesive/**Medi-Rip**

Compression alone serves as primary conservative therapy for patients with otherwise untreatable deep system insufficiency and for those with superficial insufficiency who cannot tolerate ablation of the superficial sources of reflux. Compression is an important method of prevention in pregnancy and other high-risk settings. Perhaps the most valuable role of compression is as a form of prophylaxis against deep vein thrombosis. It is a rare patient who will not benefit in some way from compression as a part of the treatment for venous insufficiency.

Sample instructions for patients are listed in Figures 15-7 and 15-8. A list of compression stocking and compression bandaging manufacturers is listed in Tables 15-6 and 15-7. (See also Chapter 27)

References

(1) Orbach EJ. *Compression therapy of vein and lymph vessel diseases of the lower extremities.* Angiology 1979; 30:95–103.

(2) Hohlbaum GG, *Zur Geschichte der Kompressions therapie.* Phlebol Proletol 1987; 16:241–255.

(3) Gronbaek K, Rasmussen AL, Struckmann J, Mathiesen FR. *The effect of the Lastosheer stocking on venous insufficiency.* Phlebol 1991; 6:199–204.

(4) Christopoulos DG, Nicolaides AN, Szendro G, Irvine AT, Bull M, Eastcott HHG. *Air-plethysmography and the effect of elastic compression on venous hemodynamics of the leg.* J Vasc Surg 1987; 5:148–157.

(5) Curri SB, Annoni F, Montorsi W. *Changes of cutaneous microcirculation from elasto-compression in chronic venous insufficiency.* In: Davy A, Stemmer R, editors. Phlebology '89. France: John Libby Eurotext, 1989.

(6) Gniadecka M. *Dermal oedema in lipodermatosclerosis: distribution, effects of posture and compressive theraphy evaluated by high-frequency ultrasonography.* Acta Derm Venereol 1995; 75(2):120–124.

(7) Partsch H. *Compression therapy of the legs. A review.* J Dermatol Surg Onc 1991; 17:799–805.

(8) Partsch H, Menzinger G, Mostbeck A. *Inelastic leg compression is more effective to reduce deep venous refluxes than elastic bandages.* Dermatol Surg 1999; 25(9):695–700.

(9) Matberry JC, Moneta GL, De Frang RD, et.al. *The influence of elastic compression stockings on deep venous hemodynamics.* J Vasc Surg 1991; 13:91–100.

(10) Spence RK, Cahall E. *Inelastic versus elastic leg compression in chronic venous insufficiency: a comparison of limb size and venous hemodynamics.* J Vasc Surg 1996; 24(5):783–787.

(11) Stoberl C, Gabler S, Partsch H. [*Indications-related use of stockings—measuring venous pump function*]. [German]. Vasa 1989; 18:35–39.

(12) Weiss RA, Sadick NS, Goldman MP, Weiss MA. *Post-sclerotherapy compression: controlled comparative study of duration of compression and its effects on clinical outcome.* Dermatol Surg 1999; 25(2):105–108.

(13) Weiss RA, Duffy D. *Clinical benefits of lightweight compression: Reduction of venous-related symptoms by ready-to-wear lightweight gradient compression hosiery.* Dermatol Surg 1999; 25(9):701–704.

(14) Yamaguchi K, Gans H, Yamaguchi Y, Hagisawa S. *External compression with elastic bandages: its effect on the peripheral blood circulation during skin traction.* Arch Phys Med Rehabil 1986; 67(5):326–331.

(15) Thomson B, Hooper P, Powell R, Warin AP. *Four-layer bandaging and healing rates of venous leg ulcers.* J Wound Care 1996; 5(5):213–216.

(16) Scurr JH, Coleridge Smith PD, Cutting P. *Varicose veins: optimum compression following sclerotherapy.* Ann R Coll Surg Engl 1985; 67:109–111.

(17) Raj TB, Goddard M, Makin GS. *How long do compression bandages maintain their pressure during ambulatory treatment of varicose veins?* Br J Surg 1980; 67(2):122–124.

(18) Zicot M. [*Venous diseases and pregnancy*]. Rev Med Liege 1999; 54(5):424–428.

(19) Sparey C, Haddad N, Sissons G, Rosser S, De Cossart L. *The effect of pregnancy on the lower-limb venous system of women with varicose veins.* Eur J Vasc Endovasc Surg 1999; 18(4):294–299.

(20) Macklon NS, Greer IA, Bowman AW. *An ultrasound study of gestational and postural changes in the deep venous system of the leg in pregnancy.* Br J Obstet Gynaecol 1997; 104(2):191–197.

(21) Austrell C, Thulin I, Norgren L. *The effects of long-term graduated compression treatment on venous function during pregnancy.* Phlebology 1995; 10(4):165–168.

(22) Orbach EJ. *A new approach to the sclerotherapy of varicose veins.* Angiology 1950; 1:302–305.

(23) Fegan WG. *Continuous compression technique of injecting varicose veins.* Lancet 1963; 2:109–112.

(24) Reid RG, Rothnie NG. *Treatment of varicose veins by compression sclerotherapy.* Br J Surg 1968; 55:889–895.

(25) Travers JP, Makin GS. *Reduction of varicose vein recurrence by use of postoperative compression stockings.* Phlebology 1994; 9(3):104–107.

(26) Fegan WG. *Continuing uninterrupted compression technique of injecting varicose veins.* Proc R Soc Med 1960; 53:837–840.

(27) Goldman MP, Bennett RG. *Treatment of telangiectasia: a review.* J Am Acad Dermatol 1987; 17:167–182.

(28) Partsch H. [*Physical prevention of thrombosis*]. [Review] [German]. Vasa Suppl 1989; 27:166–170.

(29) Somerville JJ, Brown GO, Byrne PJ, et al. *The effect of elastic stockings on superficial venous pressures in patients with venous insufficiency.* Br J Surg 1974; 61:979–981.

(30) Fentem PH, Goddard M, Gooden BA, Yeung CK. *Control of distension of varicose veins achieved by leg bandages, as used after injection sclerotherapy.* Br Med J 1976; 2:725–727.

(31) Hobbs JT. *Surgery and sclerotherapy in the treatment of varicose veins. A random trial.* Arch Surg 1974; 109:793–796.

(32) Doran FSA, White M. *A clinical trial designed to discover if the primary treatment of varicose veins should be by Fegan's method or by operation.* Br J Surg 1975; 62:72–76.

(33) Batch AJ, Wickremesinghe SS, Gannon ME, Dormandy JA. *Randomised trial of bandaging after sclerotherapy for varicose veins.* Br Med J 1980; 281:423–426.

(34) Fraser IA, Perry EP, Hatton M, Watkin DF. *Prolonged bandaging is not required following sclerotherapy of varicose veins.* Br J Surg 1985; 72:488–490.

(35) Goldman MP, Beaudoing D, Marley W, Lopez L, Butie A. *Compression in the treatment of leg telangiectasia: a preliminary report.* J Dermatol Surg Onc 1990; 16:322–325.

(36) Weiss RA, Weiss MA. *Doppler ultrasound findings in reticular veins of the thigh subdermic lateral venous system and implications for sclerotherapy.* J Dermatol Surg Onc 1993; 19(10):947–951.

(37) Somjen GM, Ziegenbein R, Johnston AH, Royle JP. *Anatomical examination of leg telangiectases with duplex scanning* [see comments]. J Dermatol Surg Onc 1993; 19(10):940–945.

(38) Callam MJ, Harper DR, Dale JJ, Ruckley CV. *Arterial disease in chronic leg ulceration: an underestimated hazard? Lothian and Forth Valley leg ulcer study.* Br Med J 1987; 294 (6577):929–931.

(39) Matsen RA, Mayo KA, Krugmire RB, et al. *A model compartment sydrome in man with particular reference to the quantification of nerve function.* J Bone Joint Surg 1977; 59:648–653.

(40) Lawrence D, Kakkar VV. *Graduated, static, external compression of the lower limb: a physiological assessment.* Br J Surg 1980; 67(2):119–121.

Veins at Other Sites

General

SPECIAL CONSENT

Because common complications such as ulceration, matting, and staining can be more distressing to the patient when they occur at sites other than the legs, patients should receive special instruction before such veins are treated. Extreme care should be taken to ensure that the patient's expectations are appropriate, and particular note should be made in the chart that the patient has been informed of the possibility of cosmetic complications. Patients should sign a special and explicit consent form acknowledging this discussion before beginning treatment; one can modify the consent forms found in Chapters 17 and 27 as needed.

LIMIT TREATMENT

Because vessels in locations other than the lower extremities do not produce significant disturbance of venous circula-

tion, treatment should be limited to the specific vessels that are symptomatic or are of immediate cosmetic concern. Only vessels that can be seen clearly in pretreatment photographs should be treated. General principles are summarized in Table 16-1.

ANTIINFLAMMATORIES

A mild local inflammatory response after sclerotherapy is common. To reduce this response when visible or sensitive body areas are treated, a nonsteroidal antiinflammatory agent can be prescribed for 3 days after each treatment session.

WATCH FOR DANGER SIGNS

Immediate investigation is indicated if the patient has any symptoms or signs that suggest more than the normal response to treatment. Patients should return immediately if they notice increasing redness or inflammation at the site of

Table 16-1
Veins Other than the Face or Legs

Site	Vein type	Treatment
Breast	Reticular veins most likely after breast implants	Sclerotherapy for reticular veins (STS 0.2–1%)
	Smaller telangiectasias on the chest from sun damage	Laser for telangiectasias
Scrotum	Varicocele	Surgical
	Angiokeratoma	Laser or intense pulsed light
Vulva	Incompetent pudendal vein origin Often painful, blue reticular varicosities	Respond well to sclerotherapy with STS 0.5%–1% or equivalent
Abdomen	Sign of serious deep venous system obstruction	Check for esophageal varices, No treatment of these shunt vessels
Foot	'Ropy' thick vein on dorsum of foot connected to dorsal venous arch	Ambulatory phlebectomy
Hand	Large blue cosmetic veins	Sclerotherapy with high strength 3% polidocanol, Ambulatory phlebectomy
Hemorrhoidal	Cause unknown, but low fiber diet suspected to contribute	Surgical removal, infrared or laser photocoagulation, injection sclerotherapy, and rubber-band ligation

treatment after the first day, any extension of redness, inflammation, or a tender palpable cord beyond the intended area of treatment, any swelling beyond the immediate area of treatment, any bleeding or drainage, or chest pain or shortness of breath of any duration.

Breast

EVALUATION

The probable cause of prominent veins on or around the breast must be ascertained before any treatment can be considered. There are a number of common problems that may cause prominent breast veins.

Some patients have familial ("essential") telangiectasia that are present on many areas of the body, including the breasts. These vessels can be treated easily, and present no special difficulty. These are usually exacerbated by sunlight exposure. Smaller telangiectasias on the chest may best be treated by lasers (Chapter 20).

Posttraumatic vessels may appear on the breast shortly after an isolated incident of trauma. These vessels can be treated easily; provided that the trauma was remote and that the vessels have not undergone any recent change.

Postoperative dilated vessels are most often noticed after breast implants (*Figure 16-1*). These may be treated, but treatment should not be undertaken for at least a year after the implant. Special care is required to avoid puncturing an

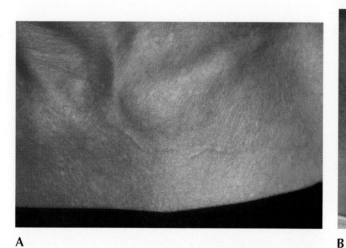

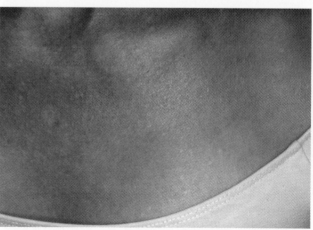

A   B

Figure 16-1.   Reticular veins prominent on the chest after breast implants. **(A)** Appearance before treatment **(B)** Appearance after one treatment with 0.2% STS, 1cc total.

implant that may have migrated or extruded into an unexpectedly superficial location.

Bypass vessels may serve to direct venous outflow around an obstruction in the axilla or the neck. These are usually identified by their location and orientation, as they extend well away from the breast towards the neck, shoulder, or axilla. These vessels should not be treated, and patients in whom this bypass syndrome is suspected should be evaluated for prior upper extremity deep venous thrombosis (DVT), for other causes of outlet obstruction such as superior vena cava syndrome, and for hypercoagulable states.

Some patients are concerned about normal vessels that are particularly prominent because of variant anatomy or because of translucent skin. Prominent normal vessels should be treated only if there is a pressing reason for doing so. Patients must be specially warned of the risks of resistance to treatment in normal vessels. Also, patients with translucent skin will always be able to see superficial veins more easily as they become more apparent with age; they must understand that maintenance treatment will be necessary.

TREATMENT

At the initial treatment session, injections should be limited to areas that are not visible in normal clothing. Treatment usually begins at the inferior outer quadrant of the breast and other areas normally covered by a brassiere. The décolletage is treated only after good results have been seen in less visible areas.

Because breast veins often drain directly into small-caliber deep vessels, the concentration and volume of sclerosant should be kept to a minimum. Typically, the starting sclerosing concentration is 0.2% STS or equivalent.

High grades of compression are not possible in the breast area, but a tight-fitting sport brassiere is recommended for the first 48 hours in order to minimize inflammation as much as possible. Patients are advised to sleep in a supine position for several days. Bruising is common.

Scrotum

EVALUATION

The scrotal veins form a complex of vessels known as the pampiniform plexus. Varicosities of this plexus present as a clump of dilated veins within the scrotum that have been described as "a bag of worms." A varicocele most often produces no symptoms, but may cause infertility, most likely because it causes an elevated scrotal temperature that reduces both the sperm count and the activity of the sperm that are produced.

Varicocele is caused by reflux into the pampiniform plexus due to malfunctioning valves in the spermatic veins. More than 90% of benign varicoceles occur on the left, and patients with a right-sided varicocele should be evaluated for the possibility of outflow obstruction caused by tumor or by thrombosis.

Angiokeratomas may occur on scrotal skin. These small round red lesions are seen commonly. Laser or intense pulsed light are best treatments *(Figure 16-2)*.

TREATMENT

The traditional treatment of varicocele requires open surgery under local or spinal anesthesia. In the traditional approach, an incision is made in the scrotum, the spermatic cord is identified, and the tortuous, dilated veins that form

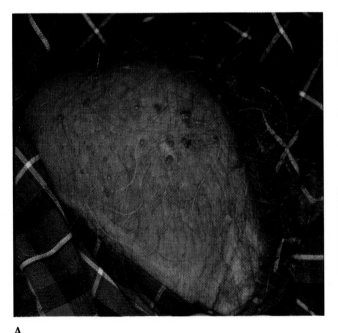

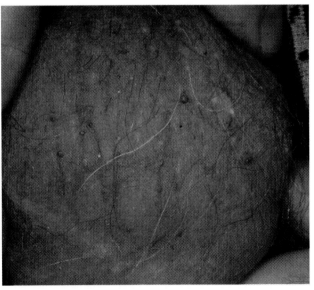

A **B**

Figure 16-2. **(A)** Scrotal angiokeratomas. **(B)** After treatment by intense pulsed light (IPL).

the varicocele are ligated and removed. Potential complications include bleeding, surgical wound infection, and inadvertent injury to the spermatic cord.

Alternative approaches include laparoscopic surgery, a retrograde approach to varicocele embolization performed via transfemoral catheter insertion or via the transjugular route, laparoscopic ligation of the internal spermatic vein, and antegrade scrotal sclerotherapy. Scrotal sclerotherapy is gaining in favor, but is not yet widely enough accepted to be considered standard treatment. If scrotal sclerotherapy is to be performed, the procedure should be carried out only after consultation with the patient's urologist. Ultrasound guidance and a catheter technique are essential to avoid inadvertent arterial injection or accidental extravascular leakage that might compromise other intrascrotal structures.

Vulva

EVALUATION

Vulvar varices may arise from incompetent pudendal veins, from tributaries of the iliac veins, from the ovarian vein, or from the greater saphenous vein *(Figure 16-3)*. They often are first noticed after pregnancy, but also are common after proximal deep vein thrombosis. In most patients, enlarged vulvar veins are more painful immediately before and during the time of menses. Interference with intercourse is a common complaint. Early treatment is preferred, because over time these vessels become progressively more painful, disfiguring, and prone to hemorrhage.[1]

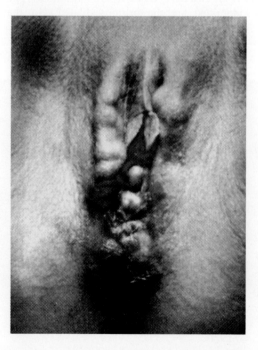

Figure 16-3. Vulvar varices as a result of pudendal vein incompetence. (Courtesy of Roberto Simkin, M.D., Buenos Aires, Argentina)

Pelvic venous congestion and pelvic varicosities can also be caused by mesoaortic renal vein compression, producing obstruction to gonadal vein outflow. Phlebography in these patients usually reveals periureteral varices as well as perirenal and ovarian varices. The demonstration of a gradient between the renal vein and the vena cava is diagnostic of this syndrome, which requires surgical intervention to protect the renal vein from compression by the superior mesenteric vein.

In some cases, vulvar varices can be a component of venous return pathways that bypass an area of deep occlusion, thus competence of the deep system should be demonstrated with ultrasound before vulvar varices are treated.

TREATMENT

Sclerotherapy of the end-branch vessels is often effective even when it is not feasible to ablate the source of reflux from the deep veins of the pelvis.

It is not necessary to shave the pubic hair in order to perform injection sclerotherapy in the vulvar region. Injections may be carried out using standard techniques, keeping the concentration and volume of sclerosant to a minimum because the varicose veins are of small volume and may have direct connections with the deep system. Typically, 0.5% STS is used to treat some of the larger vulvar veins.

Compression in this area is difficult, but may be effected with sufficient padding, tight underwear, and close-fitting Lycra bicycle shorts. A device known as the "Prenatal Cradle V2 Supporter" is made expressly for labial varicosities during pregnancy and can be used as a posttreatment compression device.[2]

Abdomen

EVALUATION

Abdominal varices (caput Medusae) are nearly always a sign of serious deep venous system obstruction. In some cases, abdominal varices are part of a bypass circuit carrying blood around an ileofemoral obstruction. More often, abdominal varices carry blood as part of a portal-systemic venous shunt caused by an obstruction to portal blood flow.

Hepatic cirrhosis is the etiology in most cases of abdominal varices. Resistance to portal flow occurs because of compression of central veins and sinusoids by hepatic fibrosis and regenerative parenchymal nodules. Anastamoses between the hepatic arteries and the portal veins also contribute to high portal venous pressures. By the time abdominal varices are visible, patients usually also have esophageal varices that may be asymptomatic until they rupture.

Rupture of esophageal varices usually results in severe bleeding, with a rebleeding incidence of 50% per year and mortality close to 50% for each episode.

TREATMENT

Acute bleeding from esophageal varices may be treated with sclerotherapy, but prophylactic sclerotherapy has not been shown to increase survival from the underlying cirrhotic disease. Abdominal varices virtually always play an important role in shunting blood around an area of obstruction, and it is rarely appropriate to treat these vessels by sclerotherapy.

Foot

EVALUATION

Foot perforators and the dorsal arch veins of the foot can contribute to serious venous problems. Indications for the treatment of foot varicosities include pain, swelling, non-healing ankle ulcers, and cosmetic concerns.

A series of perforators along the medial aspect of the foot connect the greater saphenous vein to the deep system. Valves in these veins are oriented to permit flow from the deep system to the superficial, in contrast to veins in the leg above the ankle, which direct blood inward. A high venous foot flow from the deep system of the foot toward the saphenous vein can increase venous hypertension at the ankle and can contribute to whole-leg saphenous hypertension.

TREATMENT

Although routine sclerotherapy can be performed on foot veins, the distribution of the posterior tibial artery and its branches in the lower leg is an important danger zone for sclerotherapy. Phlebectomy offers an attractive alternative for problem veins in the ankle and foot areas *(Figure 16-4)*.

If sclerotherapy is to be performed, a detailed duplex ultrasound examination is mandatory, and should include mapping of the locations of arteries (to be avoided) as well as the patterns of venous reflux to be ablated.

Hand

EVALUATION

Bulging hand veins rarely represent true venous pathology. Abnormally large hand veins that develop suddenly can be a sign of upper extremity venous outflow obstruction, but in most cases, these large veins are merely a cosmetic nuisance. They may appear as age causes a fat atrophy of the subcutaneous tissues around and below the veins *(Figure 16-5)*.

TREATMENT

Chemical ablation of these large, but otherwise normal, veins is very difficult. In many cases, attempts at sclerotherapy result in shrinkage of the vessels, but true sclerosis is uncommon. Phlebectomy may be a more effective treatment technique for these superficial veins. A recent report concludes that for hand veins, low concentrations of sclerosing agents were associated with a high incidence of failure (80%); and that use of high concentrations of 3% polidocanol produced good results in 95% of treated patients.[3] Adverse events common to sclerotherapy were observed in 90% of the treated patients. Because these vessels nearly always carry blood in an antegrade direction, ablation or removal

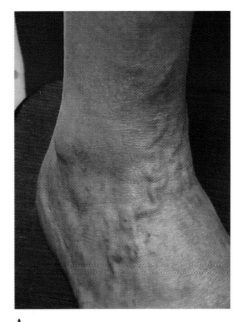

A

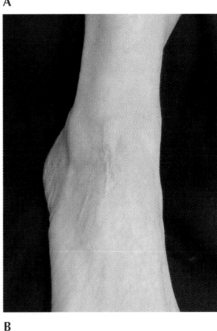

B

Figure 16-4. Foot vein. **(A)** Before treatment. **(B)** After ambulatory phlebectomy.

by any technique will cause several weeks of hand swelling while alternate pathways for venous return are developed.

Hemorrhoidal

EVALUATION

The underlying cause of most hemorrhoidal veins is not known. It is believed that a modern diet and modern lifestyle can contribute to the formation of these abnormal

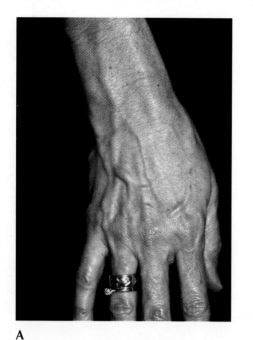
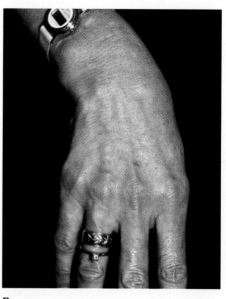

A   B

Figure 16-5. Hand veins. **(A)** Before treatment. **(B)** After sclerotherapy. (Courtesy of David Duffy, M.D., Los Angeles)

perirectal varices. Patients with portal hypertension will develop massively engorged hemorrhoidal veins along with abdominal and esophageal varices, and because these hemorrhoidal veins play an important bypass role, such patients should not be treated.

TREATMENT

Treatment alternatives for hemorrhoidal veins include surgical removal, infrared or laser photocoagulation, injection sclerotherapy, and rubber band ligation. These treatment approaches are of roughly equivalent efficacy in the reduction of symptoms.

A distinction must be made between hemorrhoids that are external and those that are internal. Internal hemorrhoids lack pain receptors, and can be ligated or banded with a rubber-banding device with very little discomfort. This technique cannot be used for external hemorrhoids, which are exquisitely sensitive to pain, and must be treated by one of the other methods described.

If sclerotherapy is to be used, the agent and dose to be used should be chosen for minimal tissue toxicity, and care should be taken to avoid extravasation that might lead to painful ulceration. The volumes injected should be sufficient to fill the varicose veins along their entire external and internal length. Sclerosis of the external component alone usually results in early recurrence.

Compression of internal hemorrhoidal varicose veins is neither necessary nor possible, but compression of external vessels will reduce the likelihood of postsclerotherapy in-

flammation and localized posttreatment thrombosis that can mimic the pain of spontaneous thrombosed hemorrhoids and can require incision and drainage for relief of the pain. A firm bulky dressing is applied and held in place with tight underwear and a leotard or bathing suit.

Summary

The pathogenesis of varicose veins is similar no matter where the veins are located, and most varicose veins can be treated following routine approaches to therapy. Ablation of proximal reflux points, when possible, will reduce the likelihood of recurrence. Just as in the legs, care must be taken to identify the cause of the abnormality, and veins that carry antegrade flow generally should not be treated.

References

(1) Ninia JG, Goldberg TL. *Treatment of vulvar varicosities by injection-compression sclerotherapy and a pelvic supporter.* Obstetrics & Gynecology 1996; 87(5:Pt 1):Pt 1):786–788.

(2) Ninia JG. *Treatment of vulvar varicosities by injection-compression sclerotherapy* [see comments]. Dermatol Surg 1997; 23(7):573–574.

(3) Duffy DM, Garcia C, Clark RE. *The role of sclerotherapy in abnormal varicose hand veins.* Plast Reconstr Surg 1999; 104(5):1474–1479.

Facial Veins

Adult Facial Vessel Disorders

Many patients who present for treatment of leg veins also are concerned about the appearance of vascular lesions on the face. We estimate that approximately 25% of patients seen for evaluation of leg veins have some form of vascular cosmetic blemish on the face. These blemishes commonly include telangiectasias that are either individual and relatively isolated, or large groups of matted telangiectasias on the cheeks. Cherry hemangioma, small round red to purple dome-shaped vascular ectasias scattered anywhere on the face or body, are also seen. In addition, patients may develop an enlargement of slightly larger venulectases that appear as purplish vessels on the cheeks, periorbital region, and vermillion. A standard terminology has been proposed which divides vascular lesions into hemangiomas, malformations, and ectasias.[1,2,3,4] The first group, childhood hemangiomas, consists of proliferative lesions with endothelial hyperplasia. The second group, vascular malformations, results from anomalies of embryologic development, and in some of them the abnormalities of the involved vessels are more functional than anatomic.

The largest category is the ectasias; this is the most common type of lesion on the face for which adults request treatment (*Table 17-1*). Ectasias have normal endothelial turnover but enlarged vascular spaces. Spider angioma, capillary aneurysm-venous lake, and telangiectasias are examples of dilations of preexisting vessels rather than vascular proliferations. Our goal in treatment is to obliterate or reduce the size of these vascular spaces so that they are no longer clinically apparent.

Special Consent for the Face

Although the face typically heals well, patients should receive special instruction as to the risks of pigmentation changes and scarring before such vessels are treated. The patient needs to understand that further sun exposure or

Table 17-1
Cosmetic Vascular Facial Lesions of Adults

Ectasias
  Cherry hemangioma
  Spider angioma
  Capillary aneurysm-venous lake
  Telangiectases
    Isolated—nasal alae
    Matting
  Reticular vessels of the periorbital region
Malformations
  Adult port-wine stains
Proliferative Lesions
  Pyogenic granuloma
  Kaposi's sarcoma
  Telangiectasias of basal cell carcinoma

---

flushing episodes may lead to recurrence. Special care should be taken to ensure that the patient's expectations are appropriate, and particular note should be made in the chart that the patient has been informed of the possibility of cosmetic complications. Small areas of posttreatment pigmentation change or even mild scarring that patients easily tolerate on their legs are typically upsetting to patients when on the face. Patients should sign a specific consent form or a note written in the chart acknowledging this discussion before beginning treatment of any form. Appendix 17-A shows a sample consent form that two of the authors use for facial treatment, modifying it for the specific laser or intense pulsed light (IPL) as needed.

Considerations: Face versus Legs

Fortunately, the treatment of facial telangiectasias is much more predictable than that of the legs. The skin heals quickly and is much less likely to scar with a similar depth of injury than on other body locations. Treatment results are often seen much more quickly, as healing is much faster on the well-oxygenated skin of the face. Facial vessels also have the advantage of a more uniform depth than the legs. The vascular walls themselves are much thinner and uniform, and hydrostatic pressure plays no major role. Occasionally, arterial pressure is a factor, as seen in spider angiomata with a small central arteriole. This is important when deciding on a method of treatment, as sclerotherapy into a bright red arteriolar-fed vessel on the cheek incurs more risks of necrosis than the use of laser or light to shut down the branches and shrink the arteriolar component.

Whereas the cause of telangiectasias on the legs is predominantly hydrostatic pressure, facial vessels appear to result from damage to the collagen of the vessel wall by sunlight. Sun exposure damages and weakens collagen with cumulative exposures, resulting in ectasia. Additionally,

there is a relatively high incidence of rosacea on the face. Rosacea consists of frequent flushing episodes associated with telangiectasias, papules, and pustules. As more individuals exercise more frequently and vigorously, the incidence of facial flushing has increased. Repeated prolonged facial flushing leads to telangiectasias. Genetic factors also play a large role, as the rosy-cheek appearance passes from one generation to the next with individuals susceptible to rosacea. Aging of the skin (accelerated by sun exposure) causes more telangiectasias with collagen breakdown.[5] Repeated trauma to the face will also induce localized erythema and ultimately vascular dilatation.

Methods of Treatment

Methods of treatment for facial telangiectasias include electrocautery (unipolar), galvanic DC current applied through fine solid needles, sclerotherapy, intense pulsed light, lasers, and ambulatory phlebectomy (Table 17-2). While all these methods of destruction carry risks of epidermal injury, electrosurgical units intentionally damage the epidermis as thermal, electrical, or radio-frequency energy is applied through it to reach underlying vessels. Fortunately, the facial skin is the most forgiving skin location, so that it is possible to "burn" right through limited areas of the epidermis and dermis but still allow healing with minimal or no scarring.

ELECTROSURGERY

Electrosurgical methods are the least specific for blood vessels. Typically operating in the 500 MHz range at 1–20 Watts, a fine metal solid needle (30 G) is applied over the region of the targeted blood vessel in a non-grounded patient. This "bounces" the energy over the skin and blood vessel, causing thermal denaturing of protein, with collagen contraction and vaporization of water. If the blood vessel receives this energy it responds with visible contraction. An uncommonly used variation of this technique include a galvanic current device in which the patient is grounded and a small DC battery generates milliamps of a 6–9 Volt current that travels through a vein that has been punctured and cannnulated by a solid metal needle.

Electrosurgery is probably the most frequently attempted since it is readily available; the units are inexpensive and widely used for other applications by many physicians.[6] Unfortunately, this form of treatment is believed to have the lowest efficacy with highest risks.[7] However, intermittent positive reinforcement keeps the physician trying this modality again and again. The patients who typically don't experience much success may reluctantly keep coming back for more. The success rate may be improved slightly by use of different frequencies and employment of very low energy (0.5–2 W) with a fine delivery tip (solid 30-gauge needle). Although sometimes effective, this treatment is not the preferred method since it incurs the highest risks of nonspecific epidermal damage and necrosis. When patients want the least expensive form of treatment, a small isolated cherry angioma may be treated, but the risk of recurrence is about 50%. Nasal alae telangiectasias are often attempted as

Table 17-2
Methods of Treatment for Facial Telangiectasias

Method	Lesion type	Success rate
Electrocautery—unipolar or Galvanic DC	Cherry angioma Isolated telangiectasia Spider angioma	Moderate—30% estimated—skill dependent
Sclerotherapy	Isolated telangiectasia Blue and purple larger veins Spider angioma	Moderate—40% estimated—skill and vessel dependent
Ambulatory phlebectomy	Larger periorbital veins	Large vessels only—90% success
Intense pulsed light	Isolated telangiectasias Rosacea Cherry angioma Venous lake Adult port-wine stains	Excellent—80% estimated

Lasers
  Argon
  Krypton
  FD Nd: YAG
  Flashlamp dye
  (PDL)
	Cherry angioma
	Spider angioma
	Isolated telangiectasia
	Telangiectatic matting (rosacea)
	Blue and purple larger veins (longer wavelengths)
	Venous lake
	Child and adult port-wine stains
		Excellent—80–90% estimated

well, but a depressed groove occurs frequently, with rapid recurrence.

SCLEROTHERAPY

Prior to the availability of vascular lasers, sclerotherapy, often in combination with electrocautery, was the preferred method. It is no longer the suggested mode of therapy for small bright red vessels of the face, as the cure rate remains low. Used in combination with electrocautery, the success rate may be improved slightly, but risks to epidermal damage are compounded when treating facial telangiectasias between 0.3 mm and 1 mm. Isolated vessels on the nose and cheeks have been rare treatment candidates, as matted groups of telangiectasia are not amenable to this technique.

For sclerotherapy, treatment is performed with the same technique as for small telangiectasias of the legs. Meticulous care is taken not to extravasate, as ulceration is highly likely even with tiny amounts of solution. A 30-gauge needle is typically used, although the thinner facial skin allows smaller gauge needles to be used if preferred. Only a few drops of sclerosing solution are injected. As the facial venous drainage drains into the cavernous venous sinuses, common sense dictates that miniscule amounts of sclerosing solutions be employed.

The typical concentration of solutions for the 0.3 mm–1 mm red vessels include sodium tetradecyl sulfate at 0.1%, polidocanol at 0.25–0.5%, saline and dextrose (Sclerodex ™) undiluted, and (rarely) hypertonic saline at 23.4%. Often these red facial vessels are at very high arterial pressures and bleed profusely once punctured. A rapidly acting detergent solution minimizes the bleeding time as damage to the vessel and swelling of the lumen occurs more quickly. The patient or assistant should hold pressure over the treated area for a minimum of 5 minutes.

For the larger (greater than 1 mm) blue reticular vessels of the cheek and periorbital region, the injection technique is the same, using only a few drops of solution. Concentrations employed are sodium tetradecyl sulfate 0.2%, polidocanol 0.5%–1%, or saline and dextrose (Sclerodex). Patients are told that edema, erythema, and bruising for a few days are the likely side effects of this form of treatment. Our experience has been an 8% incidence of pinpoint skin breakdown after sclerotherapy on the face. Fortunately, most of these patients have healed well cosmetically. Significant bruising occurs 50–75% of the time with reticular veins on the face.

INTENSE PULSED LIGHT

Intense pulsed light (IPL) consists of a non-coherent flashlamp that delivers large amounts of yellow, red, and infrared wavelengths to the skin. The advantages of this device are the large spot size and ability to control pulse duration and pulse interval times. Some selection of wavelengths is possible by use of lower-end cut-off filters. This device satisfies the criteria for selective photothermolysis, permitting blood vessels to be selectively heated over surrounding tissue. Pulses are typically separated to allow thermal relaxation time, in particular cooling of the epidermis in between pulses.

We have found this device useful for grouped telangiectasias and telangiectatic mats on the face. It allows rapid treatment of an entire cheek (*Figure 17-1*). Typical parameters employed are modified according to vessel size and are summarized in Table 17-3. The large-spot-size footprint allows large areas to be treated rapidly. Purpura is uncommon; when bruising does occur it fades very quickly in two to three days, rather than weeks as with the pulsed dye laser. The benefits and use of IPL for leg veins are discussed in Chapter 20.

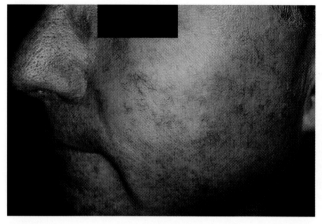

A

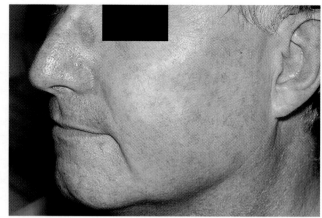

B

Figure 17-1.   Telangiectatic matting responds well to intense pulsed laser (IPL) (Photoderm™, ESC/Sharplan, Norwood, MA). The frequency of rosacea episodes is typically diminished. **(A)** Cheek of rosacea patient with widespread telangiectasia before IPL. **(B)** After IPL.

LASERS

The operation and principles of lasers are discussed in detail in Chapter 20. The success of green and yellow lasers for facial blood vessels is irrefutable. However, the side effects,

Table 17-3
Suggested Parameters for Facial Vessels for IPL[a]

Bright Red Vessels:
- For vessels < 0.2 mm diameter:
  3.0 msec
  550 nm filter[b]
  Total fluence: 22–28 J/cm2
- For vessels 0.2 mm–0.4 mm:
  2.5/2.5 msec (10 msec delay)
  550 nm filter[b]
  Total fluence: 25–32 J/cm2
- For vessels 0.4 mm–0.6 mm:
  2.4/6.0 msec (10 msec delay)
  550 nm filter[b]
  Total fluence: 30–40 J/cm2
- For vessels 0.6 mm–0.8 mm:
  2.4/7.0 msec (10 msec delay)
  570 nm filter[b]
  Total fluence: 35–45 J/cm2

Violaceous Vessels:
- For vessels 0.4 mm–0.6 mm:
  2.5/6.0 msec (10 msec delay)
  570 nm filter[b]
  Total fluence: 30–40 J/cm2
- For vessels 0.6 mm–0.8 mm:
  2.5/ 7.0 msec (10 msec delay)
  590 nm filter[b]
  Total fluence: 35–45 J/cm2

[a]Do not treat tanned patients!
[b]For patients with Fitzpatrick Types 3 and 4 skin (medium complexions who may burn but tan easily), one may need to use the 570 filter rather than the 550, or the 590 instead of the 570.
We strongly recommend doing small test areas first, before treating large areas, to assess the patient's response. Recommended fluences may vary depending on the age and number of pulses performed by the individual IPL unit.

speed of application, and pulse duration may be quite different from machine to machine. The preference for a particular laser manufacturer may also influence preference of one method over another and the rates of success reported.

There are two primary differences in lasers for the face. One group has a relatively small spot size and requires tracing out each individual vessel. The others have a large spot and use the "shotgun" approach. Pulse duration is typically in the millisecond range, although those in the microsecond range (pulsed dye) tend to have higher risks of purpura. Green and yellow light lasers are used for smaller superficial blood vessels while the longer wavelengths may be employed for larger purple vessels on the face. Table 17-4 lists the lasers commonly used on the face.

AMBULATORY PHLEBECTOMY

There is a small reticular vein plexus that courses down the temporal region to the lateral canthus, then along the lower eyelid closer to the zygomatic arch. Although barely visible in most individuals, some women with a thinner dermis develop a very prominent vein from this system. This appears immediately below the eye and may bulge above the skin surface. It is quite noticeable due to the blue to green color and is a frequent cause of cosmetic concern. Prolonged sounds of venous flow can often be heard with a 10 MHz CW Doppler, but the significance is unclear. The periorbital veins are often large enough in diameter that a significant amount of sclerosing solution is necessary to fill this large vascular space. The wall may also be thick enough that higher concentrations of sclerosing solution may be required.

Although sclerotherapy may be successful, the bruising and higher volumes and concentrations of sclerosant are worrisome for the injection into the face. Larger volumes of solution may enter the venous drainage of both the retroretinal and cavernous venous sinus in this region. For this reason, Dr. A.A. Ramelet has attempted a mini-phle-

Table 17-4

Lasers Commonly Used on the Face

Green—532nm FD Nd:YAG Diode Argon (514 nm)	Tracing vessels individually	Moderate efficacy
Yellow—PDL	Shotgun in large area	Good efficacy but results in purpura
Yellow—copper bromide	Tracing vessels individually	Good efficacy, no bruising
IPL	Shotgun for large area	Good efficacy but technique dependent
Infrared—1064 nm	Tracing	Large blue-purple (reticular) vessels only

bectomy in a series of patients using the small blue Ramelet hook. The technique involves local anesthesia without epinephrine to minimize venous spasm. A puncture is made with an 18-gauge needle over the central portion of the visible vein. The blue Ramelet hook is gently inserted and this tiny reticular vein is harpooned. The sensation of pulling at a fine string indicates that the vein has been grasped. The steps are shown in Figure 17-2. A fine glistening white loop is gently extracted. A feeling of tension along the known course of the periorbital vein should be palpable.

Only physicians well experienced with hook avulsion of leg veins should attempt this method of extraction. Compression is difficult to apply. An assistant must apply constant pressure to the region for 10 minutes after the procedure. The patient is warned to keep his or her head up for several hours after the procedure to minimize venous pressure. Bruising is surprisingly limited as long as the extraction is confined to one puncture. Patients need to be warned that other new reticular veins may occur. We have observed the formation of new veins coursing backwards from the lateral canthus or temple to the ear along with the elimination of the unsightly periorbital vein.

Specific Lesions

ECTASIAS

Ectasias are the largest group of vascular lesions on the face that are treated on adults. These increase in frequency with age. As the sun-exposed "baby boomer" generation has progressed into middle age, the demand for treatment of these lesions has markedly increased.

CHERRY HEMANGIOMA

Cherry hemangioma are small dome-shaped red papules that occur anywhere on the body but are most commonly seen on the forehead in adults. There are typically violaceous and thus respond to green, yellow, or infrared lasers. The larger lesions are best treated with infrared lasers, such as 1064 nm, with millisecond pulse durations (*Figure 17-3*). Good results may also be obtained with electrocautery. Scle-

rotherapy may result in extravasation with small punctate scarring.

SPIDER ANGIOMA

Spider angiomata are considered small A-V malformations as the central point of origin may be seen pulsating with diascopy. The yellow or infrared lasers that will achieve better penetration are best to treat these. Electrocautery can be frustrating and often causes punctate or depressed scarring. Sclerotherapy may cause ulceration as the arteriole is sclerosed. Larger lesions seen on the face after trauma may require several treatments, even when treatment is precise, accurate, and appears to completely close down flow at the time of treatment. Angiomata have a tendency to recur as the arteriolar component reanastomoses with dermal capillaries. Patients are warned about the possibility of multiple treatments (*Figure 17-4*).

CAPILLARY ANEURYSM-VENOUS LAKE

Venous lakes are most commonly seen as dark purple spots on the vermillion of the lips. These are disturbing to patients as they appear as a bruise. When raised they may bleed, and females may find it impossible to hide them with lipstick. They are usually several millimeters in depth, so that penetration with the laser is difficult. Green-light lasers typically treat only the front wall so that these must be compressed with glass or quartz during the treatment. External compression increases the success rate. Yellow lasers (PDL) typically have too short a pulse duration to thoroughly heat a vessel of this diameter. IPL is a good choice since the pulse duration and wavelengths match the requirements for photocoagulation of these lesions. Recently the use of 1064 nm (infrared) has shown surprisingly good results (*Figure 17-5*). The 1064 nm wavelength penetrates well. The larger lesions may cause extensive heat release following the laser pulse, injuring the overlying epidermis, so that external cooling before and after the laser pulse is advised.

TELANGIECTASIAS

Isolated or grouped nasal alae telangiectasias can be the most resistant area to treatment on the face. Almost all the methods and lasers have been applied with an ultimate

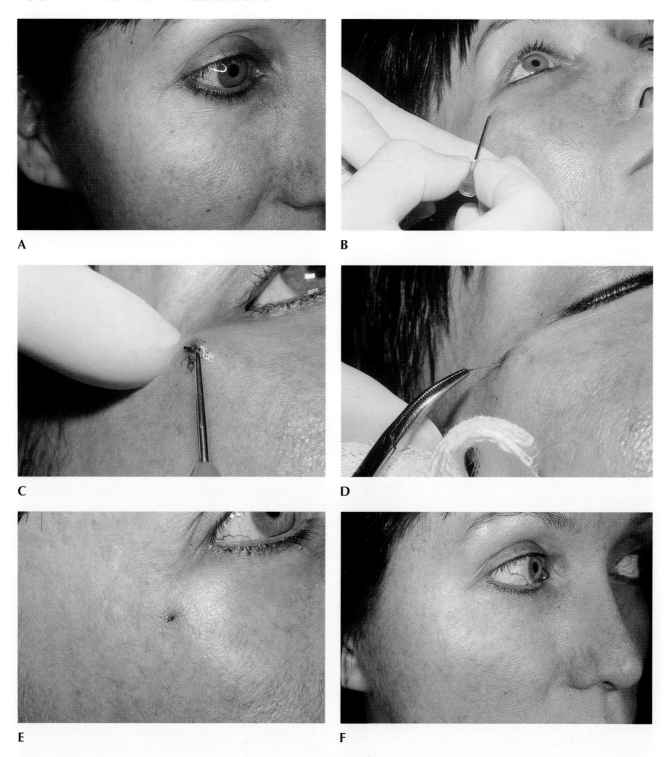

Figure 17-2.   Ambulatory phlebectomy of periorbital reticular vein: **(A)** Vein before treatment. **(B)** Puncture with 18-gauge needle. **(C)** Extraction of vein with Ramelet hook just under skin. **(D)** Vein can be pulled and stretched for about a length of 2 cm. **(E)** Results immediately after procedure. **(F)** Results after 2 years (results were excellent at 2 weeks; this is long-term follow-up).

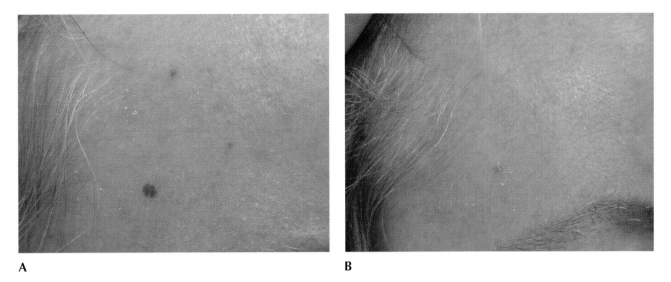

A **B**

Figure 17–3. Hemangioma on forehead. **(A)** Before. **(B)** After treatment with Cool Touch Varia™ (Cool Touch Corp, Roseville, CA). (1064-nm laser).

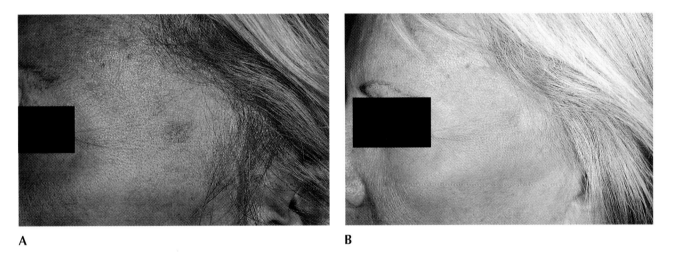

A **B**

Figure 17-4. Spider angioma on temple. **(A)** Before. **(B)** After treatment with 532-nm laser Coherent Versapulse™ (Coherent, Palo Alto, CA). Two treatments were required.

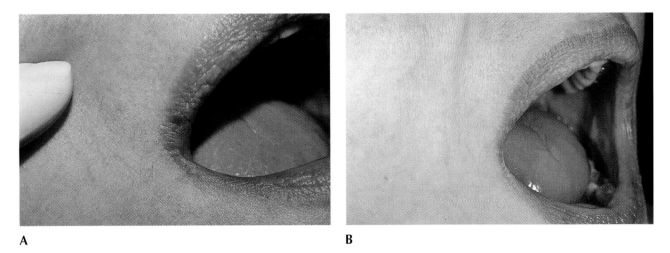

A **B**

Figure 17-5. Venous lake on the lip. **(A)** Before. **(B)** After treatment with Vasculight™ 1064-nm laser. (ESC/Sharplan, Norwood, MA).

157

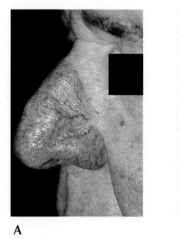 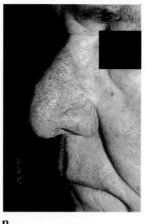

A   **B**

Figure 17-6. Nasal alae telangiectasia. **(A)** Before. **(B)** After treatment with argon laser in 1992. New vessels developed requiring additional treatment in 1996.

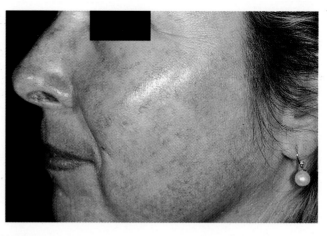

Figure 17-7. Telangiectatic matting after test pulses on the lower cheek with IPL. Notice the large spot sizes of the rectangular clearer areas. Two additional treatments cleared the entire cheek.

success rate of 65–80%. Electrosurgery and green lasers (argon and KTP) without cooling have a high risk of leaving depressed grooves at the site of telangiectasias, but the lasers can sometimes be successful (*Figure 17-6*). Yellow (PDL) leaves significant purpura that the cosmetic patients often find unacceptable. Yellow (copper bromide) allows one to trace vessels with a high success rate and low incidence of groove formation when fluence does not exceed 20 J/cm². The IPL source with both short and long pulses yields a very high success rate with minimal side effects as long as adequate gel (2 mm) is placed between the crystal and the skin.

Matting of large groups of small telangiectasias of the cheek or the bridge of the nose are best treated by large-spot-size devices. We prefer IPL since the PDL causes purpura. Recent reports indicate that larger spot sizes with the 532 nm green KTP devices may also achieve good results.[8] Typical results from IPL are shown in Figure 17-7.

RETICULAR VESSELS OF THE PERIORBITAL REGION

The methods for treatment of reticular vessels include sclerotherapy with a 30-gauge needle and small volumes of sclerosant. We typically utilize 0.2–0.5% STS with volumes of no more than 0.1–0.2 cc. Immediate swelling of the vein can be seen. This is frequently accompanied by hematoma formations lasting for 3–5 days. After injection the sclerosant is held in place by pressure from an assistant for 10 minutes to minimize bruising. Ambulatory phlebectomy may be very useful for larger vessels, as discussed above. Recent data has also shown that the infrared 1064 nm lasers may treat these veins with an immediate contraction, low incidence of bruising, and relatively few treatments. Figure 17-8 shows the immediate contraction and the results at two months after one treatment with the 1064 nm laser.

RETICULAR VESSELS OF THE TEMPLE

Many fair-skinned individuals will notice blue-green 2–3 mm veins on the temples, often in a V-shaped pattern, that begin near the periorbital rim and extend upwards onto the lateral forehead. These veins are very fragile and difficult to cannulate, but sclerotherapy can be performed very cautiously and meticulously (typically with 0.1–0.2% Sotradecol™) in small volumes (0.1–0.2 cc). The goal should be to shrink the vessels, not to make them disappear. Reports of significant necrosis of the scalp resulting from these types of injections raise concern for possible arteriovenous connections. The skin is also very thin in this area and will not tolerate extravasation. While the 1064 nm laser can be helpful also, care must be taken not to be near the temporal artery, since this laser can penetrate to its depth also. This is definitely an area that is not for the beginning phlebologist.

PORT-WINE STAINS (ADULT)

Adult port-wine stains typically have larger cavernous components and are more deep purple in color than those of childhood. Combinations of PDL for the superficial component with other laser methods to treat the deeper component are often necessary. IPL may treat the deeper portions, particularly with use of long pulse durations of around 7–8 ms.[9, 10] Recent trials using a 1064 nm laser with millisecond pulse durations show encouraging results with shrinking the violaceous cavernous component (*Figure 17-9*).

Summary

Treatment of facial venous vascular lesions in adults can be very successful. Almost all the laser devices available in the visible light range produce good results on vascular lesions of the face. Knowledge of lesion type and of differences in response by size and location can assist in selecting the procedure most likely to be successful. Wavelengths of lasers may be fined tuned for size or color of individual telangiectasias. Although electrocautery is used frequently, a more selective method is usually a better choice. Some larger facial vessels respond well to sclerotherapy or ambulatory

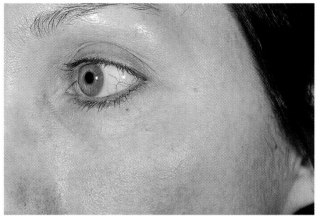

A

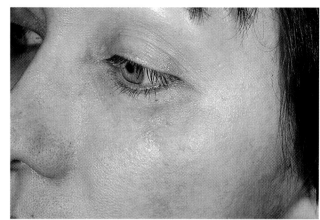

B

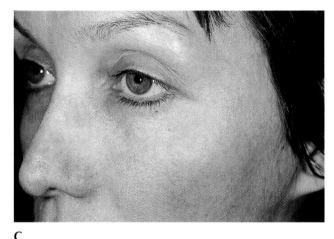

C

Figure 17-8.   Periorbital reticular veins treated with 1064-nm laser (Vasculight™) **(A)** Before. **(B)** Immediately after treatment. **(C)** Two months after a single treatment with improvement that has persisted for 2 years.

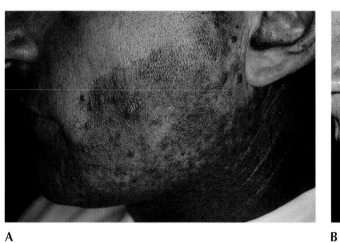

A

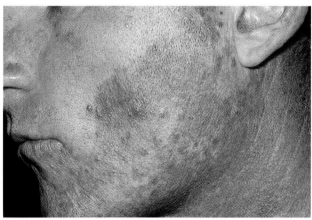

B

Figure 17-9   **(A)** Adult port wine stain (PWS) persistent after ten treatments with PDL. **(B)** After three additional treatments with IPL, the PWS is significantly lighter. The patient continued to improve with additional IPL and 1064 mm laser treatments.

phlebectomy. Larger cavernous lesions may require deeper penetration of 1064 nm (infrared) wavelengths or manipulation to reduce the total depth for laser penetration.

References

(1) Requena L, Sangueza OP. Cutaneous vascular anomalies. Part I. *Hamartomas, malformations, and dilation of preexisting vessels.* J Am Acad Dermatol 1997; 37(4):523–549.

(2) Requena L, Sangueza OP. *Cutaneous vascular proliferation. Part II. Hyperplasias and benign neoplasms.* J Am Acad Dermatol 1997; 37(6):887–919.

(3) Niechajev IA, Clodius L. *Diagnostic criteria of vascular lesions in the face.* Ann Plast Surg 1993; 31(1):32–41.

(4) Hunt SJ, Santa Cruz DJ. *Acquired benign and "borderline" vascular lesions.* Dermatol Clin 1992; 10(1):97–115.

(5) Glogau RG. *Aesthetic and anatomic analysis of the aging skin.* Semin Cutan Med Surg 1996; 15(3):134–138.

(6) Hettinger DF. *Soft tissue surgery using radiowave techniques.* J Am Podiatr Med Assoc 1997; 87(3):131–135.

(7) Goldman MP, Weiss RA, Brody HJ, Coleman WP, Fitzpatrick RE. *Treatment of facial telangiectasia with sclerotherapy, laser surgery, and/or electrodesiccation: a review.* J Dermatol Surg Onc 1993; 19:899–906; 909–910.

(8) Adrian RM, Tanghetti EA. *Long pulse 532-nm laser treatment of facial telangiectasia.* Dermatol Surg 1998; 24(1):71–74.

(9) Raulin C, Goldman MP, Weiss MA, Weiss RA. *Treatment of adult port-wine stains using intense pulsed light therapy (PhotoDerm VL): brief initial clinical report* [letter]. Dermatol Surg 1997; 23(7):594–597.

(10) Jay H, Borek C. *Treatment of a venous-lake angioma with intense pulsed light* [letter]. Lancet 1998; 351(9096):112.

Appendix 17-A

This is a sample of the consent form used for treatment with intense pulsed light and other lasers on the face by two of these authors.

ESC Photoderm VL Laser Consent

I have been fully explained this procedure by Dr._____. I realize that no promises or guarantees have been made. Intense light has been used to treat vascular lesions for several years. A vascular lesion is an abnormal collection of small blood vessels at the surface of the skin, causing a visible spot or patch. The ESC Photoderm emits a pulse of light, which penetrates the skin to a depth of about 3 mm. The light heats up and coagulates the blood vessels that are the cause of the lesion. The light beam is very effective at heating only the target blood vessels. As a result, the normal tissue surrounding the vessel is only slightly affected. The Photoderm can be used on port wine stains, leg veins, spider veins, and other vascular lesions.

I have been told of the following risks:

1. pain-feels like a "rubber band" snapping against the skin.

2. bruising-will go away in 1-3 weeks.

3. hive-like swelling-can use ice.

Very unlikely risks: less than 1%

1. crust or blister-may need to use a topical antibiotic.

2. scarring-rarely may leave a lighter area.

3. pigment changes-you must protect the area from sun exposure.

Patient   _____

Witness   _____

Date   _____

Estimated cost: test area: _____
                   per treatment: _____

Several treatments may be necessary.

CHAPTER 18

Special Situations and Problems

Failure to Respond to Sclerotherapy

Failure of sclerotherapy (defined as failure to eliminate the vessels being treated or immediate recurrence) nearly always results from an incorrect diagnosis and treatment plan, from a failure of medication delivery, or from a failure of compression compliance. Table 18-1 outlines the measures to consider when a patient doesn't respond to sclerotherapy.

DIAGNOSIS AND TREATMENT PLAN

In the majority of cases, some high-pressure source of reflux was not adequately addressed prior to sclerosis of terminal varices. After a treatment failure, Doppler examination and preferably duplex ultrasound evaluation should be performed to ensure that the pattern of reflux is fully understood. Chapter 7 includes a case study of treatment failure successfully corrected by Doppler-guided sclerotherapy. If junctional incompetence is at the root of treatment failure,

Table 18-1
When Patients Don't Respond to Sclerotherapy

- Was the Doppler exam adequate?
- Is a duplex exam required?
- Was the reticular vein adequately treated?
- Was there compliance with compression?
- Should there be a change in the solution type?
- Was the patient on hormonal therapy (hormone replacement therapy or birth control pills)?
- Is there a change in the patient's medical status?

---

surgical (Chapter 21) or endovenous occlusive (Chapter 23) elimination of the reflux is indicated before proceeding to secondary sclerotherapy or local phlebectomy. Prolonged pigmentation following sclerotherapy may also be due to continued hydrostatic pressure from a proximal source.

SCLEROSANT

In some cases, the concentration and volume of sclerosant used were insufficient to overcome dilution by blood flowing in the treated vessel. If a vessel is too large to be treated using the maximum recommended doses of available sclerosants, combinations of more than one sclerosant may be used in sequence. Some patients are resistant to one category of sclerosing solution, yet when switched to another, i.e., from detergent to hyperosmolar, they respond beautifully. Surgical removal by phlebectomy offers an excellent alternative for vessels that are resistant to chemical ablation. For those attempting to sclerose the saphenofemoral junction (SFJ) unsuccessfully, radiofrequency endovenous occlusion offers an excellent alternative.

COMPRESSION

If the amount of compression used (or patient compliance with compression) is insufficient to adequately compress a large vessel, a large thrombus will form and later recanalize. Drainage of the coagula from this thrombus followed by compression will help it sclerose (Chapter 24). Switching from a compression bandage to compression stockings may provide more dependable compression, and the use of two pairs of stockings for additive compression should be considered. The two-stocking method is particularly useful when a patient complains that he or she cannot pull a single stocking beyond the ankles. Patients who complain that they cannot be "confined" by support hose often remove compression after a few days and would be considered non-compliant as well. A vessel that cannot be adequately compressed is not a good candidate for treatment by primary sclerotherapy. Surgical removal and endovenous occlusion by means of a radiofrequency ablation catheter offer a good alternative for these cases.

Variceal Hemorrhage

Variceal hemorrhage is more common than usually realized, and rarely can result in death. These patients often complain of waking up in a "pool of blood." The bleeding varix can be

surprisingly small, as seen in Chapter 4 (*Figure 4-7*). Patients with variceal hemorrhage usually present to an emergency department, where the traditional management has been to oversew the involved vessel. In our practice, sclerotherapy has been successfully performed on an emergency basis to immediately close the bleeding site, even without eliminating reflux from above. Many of these patients have very advanced disease or are in such poor health that only palliative therapy can be offered.

OVERSEWING

Oversewing a vessel gives short-term control, but without further treatment, hemorrhage will recur. Correct treatment requires ablation or removal of the dilated superficial thin-walled vessel that has ruptured, together with correction of the major source of reflux feeding the ruptured vessel.

DEFINITIVE TREATMENT

Variceal hemorrhage can easily be treated by primary sclerotherapy or primary phlebectomy, as described in the chapters devoted to those procedures. Vessels that have dilated to the point of rupture have lost their ability to contract in spasm, and if treatment is by sclerotherapy, the solution spread must extend far enough to reach vessels proximal to the bleeding point. These vessels will then contract in spasm, reducing flow to the site. Ambulatory phlebectomy may be employed to avulse vessels leading to the bleeding site as the variceal hemorrhage point shreds with the phlebectomy hook.

Combined Deep and Superficial Reflux

When patients with superficial varices are also found to have deep system reflux, a complete normalization of venous flow will be impossible. In many cases, the superficial component of reflux may be an insignificant part of the overall disease process, no matter how impressive the superficial varices. This cannot be assumed, as recent evidence indicates that even when deep reflux exists, treatment of the superficial reflux contributes to significant clinical improvement, although in some cases the subfascial endoscopic perforator surgery (SEPS) procedure may also be necessary.[1–3] Treatment of superficial refluxing vessels may therefore be indicated not only for cosmetic reasons, but may also be indicated if there is evidence that a significant reduction in total reflux volume can be achieved.

INFORMED CONSENT

A patient with significant deep system reflux must understand and accept the possibility that symptoms may not be cured nor significantly ameliorated by sclerosis of superficial veins. It is helpful to address this issue in an informed consent document.

SUPERFICIAL VEINS AS A MAJOR REFLUX PATHWAY

If the venous refilling time (VRT) can be improved to any degree by the occlusion of superficial vessels, then ablation of superficial incompetent vessels by sclerotherapy will certainly improve overall venous function and will probably ameliorate the symptoms. If the VRT cannot be improved by occluding superficial vessels, but superficial disease is so extensive that in the clinician's judgement it is believed responsible for a significant fraction of the overall impairment of venous function, then ablation of superficial incompetent vessels by sclerotherapy may improve overall venous function, and may ameliorate the symptoms.

SUPERFICIAL VEINS AS A MINOR REFLUX PATHWAY

Varices become massively dilated in response to pressure rather than flow, thus the size of varices is not a reliable guide to the volume of reflux. No matter how large the superficial varices, if deep-system incompetence is responsible for nearly all of the total observed venous reflux, ablation of the superficial incompetent veins will not improve overall venous function and will not ameliorate any symptoms. Treatment in this special case should be performed only for cosmetic purposes.

Sclerotherapy in Patients at Special Risk for Venous Thromboembolism

Patients at high risk for new or recurrent deep venous thrombosis (DVT) and pulmonary embolism are poor candidates for any surgical procedure, and probably are poor candidates for sclerotherapy as well. Although sclerotherapy is an extremely safe procedure, the risk is not zero: there are rare reported cases of pulmonary embolism (PE) in patients undergoing sclerotherapy, and some of these have resulted in death. Even patients who survive DVT and PE often suffer severe morbidity, with lifelong post-phlebitic syndrome and cor pulmonale.

If sclerotherapy is contemplated in a patient at high risk, every effort should be made to mitigate the risks through prophylaxis. Treatment is only justified if the benefits can be said to outweigh the risks, and the patient and clinician both must be prepared to shoulder those risks knowingly.

RISK CRITERIA

Many of the hematologic risk factors for DVT and PE are not clinically apparent, but there are a number of clinical situations that should serve as "red flags" to the clinician.

- Prior history of deep or superficial blood clots or of pulmonary embolism
- Family history of blood clots
- Duplex scan evidence of prior deep vein thrombosis
- Known hypercoagulable state
- Limited ability to ambulate

After sclerotherapy, patients may develop new risk factors within 4 weeks from:

- Lower extremity cast
- Forced bedrest
- Long-distance travel

STRONGER CONTRAINDICATIONS TO SCLEROTHERAPY

Except under rare circumstances, sclerotherapy should not be performed in patients with a confirmed deficiency of antithrombin III. This is because a deficiency of antithrombin III can cause thrombus to propagate into the deep veins after even minor endothelial injury, causing deep vein thrombosis. To make matters worse, heparin is ineffective in the absence of antithrombin III, so there is no immediately safe and effective therapy for deep vein thrombosis in these patients.

A combined history of deep vein thrombosis and heparin-induced thrombocytopenia is a strong contraindication to venous sclerotherapy for the same reason: should deep vein thrombosis occur, there would be no safe and effective therapy.

REQUIRED WORKUP

A bilateral color-flow duplex ultrasound exam is required before starting sclerotherapy for a patient at high risk for DVT and PE. Most cases of DVT do not produce symptoms, thus the ultrasound examination should be repeated approximately 1 week after each treatment session and again several weeks after the last treatment.

SPECIAL PROTECTIVE MEASURES

There is no regimen that can entirely eliminate the risks of DVT and PE, but the risks can be reduced dramatically through routine prophylactic measures.

Antiinflammatories

Antiinflammatory and antiplatelet drugs should be taken during the entire at-risk period.

Compression garment

Strict adherence to a compression-stocking regimen is required. High-grade (30–40 mm Hg gradient or higher) compression stockings must be worn at all times except when showering and changing. Compression should be continued for 6 weeks after completion of sclerotherapy.

Ambulation

Increased ambulation is an absolute necessity when a high-risk patient is being treated.

Anticoagulation

Fractionated low-molecular-weight heparin (LMWH) should be used prophylactically throughout the period of treatment in patients with a history of recurrent DVT, in those with a deficiency of protein C or protein S, or those with resistance to activated protein C. A 5-day course of LMWH following each treatment session is probably sufficient, but a color-flow duplex examination to rule out occult deep vein thrombosis should be performed on the fifth day (prior to the discontinuation of LMWH) and again 3–4 days later.

SPECIAL INFORMED CONSENT

Patients with a prior history of DVT or PE, those with a known hypercoagulable state, and those with a strong family history of DVT or PE must sign a special consent form indicating that they understand the following concepts:

- Hypercoagulability causes a lifelong increased risk of spontaneous and recurrent DVT and PE.
- Varicose veins are believed to increase the risk of DVT and PE, although this is not well proven.
- Surgical treatment of varicose veins, like almost all surgery, is associated with a high postoperative rate of recurrent DVT. This is a proven risk that can be reduced with proper preventative measures.
- Nonsurgical treatment of varicose veins probably presents an increased risk of recurrent DVT during and for several weeks after treatment. This risk has never been proven to exist, but the possibility cannot be ignored. The theoretical risk can be reduced with preventative measures.

TREATMENT

Treatment begins only after duplex ultrasound has confirmed the absence of preexisting fresh thrombus in the iliac veins, the femoral veins, and the calf veins of both legs. Routine treatment techniques are used, with careful attention to the minimal effective concentration for each vein being treated.

FOLLOW-UP

Immediate repeat duplex scan is indicated if the patient develops any new leg pain, swelling (even if minimal), or redness anywhere other than at an injection site. Immediate repeat duplex scan and pulmonary ventilation-perfusion (V/Q) scan are indicated if the patient develops chest pain of any type or duration whatsoever, shortness of breath of any duration, palpitations, or syncope.

Pregnancy and Sclerotherapy

Many thousands of patients have been safely treated by sclerotherapy during pregnancy, and many physicians around the world continue to treat varicose veins in pregnant patients by injection sclerotherapy. There is no evidence that this is unsafe or harmful in any way. If a patient discovers that she is pregnant while she is in the midst of treatment, she may be reassured that the treatments she has had will almost certainly have no impact on her pregnancy.

However, since pregnancy is well recognized as a hypercoagulable state that places a patient at high risk for deep vein thrombosis and pulmonary embolism, it is best to avoid the possibility of increasing that risk further by performing sclerotherapy during pregnancy, except for unavoidably urgent cases. In the untoward event that a pregnant patient treated with sclerotherapy developed a

DVT or PE, the medicolegal uncertainty as to whether that condition was caused by pregnancy or sclerotherapy would place the treating physician in a difficult position, at least in the United States. A recent study demonstrated that maximum changes of venous enlargement are seen in the superficial venous system in the thigh; however, changes in reflux returned to pre-pregnancy levels in the puerperium.[4]

We recommend avoiding sclerotherapy in any patient who is known to be pregnant, who has indicated that she is actively attempting to become pregnant, or who has been pregnant in the last three months. Should sclerotherapy be absolutely necessary, the informed consent discussion must be well documented.

NEW OR WORSENING VARICOSE VEINS IN PREGNANCY

Development or worsening of varicose veins is a recognized complication of pregnancy. The benign causes of this phenomenon include hormonally induced changes in vein wall and vein valve elasticity, expanded intravascular volume, and increased hydrostatic pressure in the lower extremities due to outflow obstruction caused by the gravid uterus. Unfortunately, the sudden onset of varicose veins may also be an indicator of deep vein thrombosis, for which pregnancy is a major risk factor. Any pregnant patient who reports acutely changing varicosities, or varicosities in association with leg pain or swelling, should receive a duplex evaluation for possible deep vein thrombosis.

COMPRESSION

To reduce the likelihood and severity of varicose veins, all pregnant patients should be placed in gradient compression hose as tolerated. The ideal regimen is 30–40 mm Hg gradient hose in maternity waist-height (pantyhose) style. Lighter grades of compression are acceptable if they will result in higher compliance. If thigh-high hose are preferred, they should always be used with a waist strap or other mechanism to keep the stockings up and prevent rolling.

SCLEROTHERAPY AFTER PREGNANCY

Sclerotherapy may be commenced or recommenced three months after pregnancy, as long as patients understand that early treatment may be premature, as spontaneous remission of varicosities may occur up to a year after pregnancy.

Many changes in venous flow dynamics occur in pregnancy, and previously competent junctions and perforators may become incompetent without producing overt clinical signs. A proper diagnosis and treatment plan is essential, thus a detailed examination must be performed or repeated, including venous refilling time, maximum venous outflow, and continuous wave Doppler examination. Duplex ultrasound evaluation is also strongly advised prior to early treatment after pregnancy.

Because there have been reports of a hypercoagulability of pregnancy that may persist beyond three months, patients must be hypervigilant for any of the warning signs of DVT and PE.

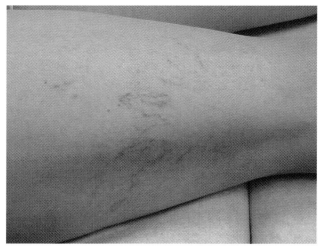
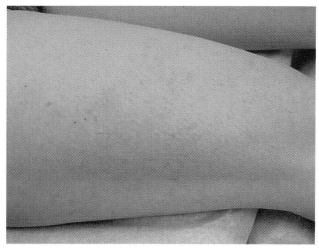

A   B

Figure 18-1.   **(A)** Lateral venous system developed during pregnancy. Patient desires treatment 6 months postpartum; however, the patient is still breastfeeding. Concern for products in breast milk led to a trial of hypertonic saline-dextrose sclerosant mixture. **(B)** Results at 6 weeks show excellent results with this solution, which is safe to use while breastfeeding.

BREASTFEEDING

Hypertonic saline is safe during breastfeeding, but other sclerosants are of unknown safety. Detergent sclerosants are small lipid-soluble molecules that will pass into breast milk. The substances used are simply dilute soapy alcohols solutions in extremely small quantities, but there is no factual evidence as to their safety during breastfeeding. A theoretically acceptable plan is to have patients use a breast pump and store milk before a treatment session, and then wait 4–6 hours after treatment before breast feeding. Figure 18-1 shows the successful treatment of telangiectasias with a solution of hypertonic saline and dextrose (the equivalent of Sclerodex™) in a breastfeeding patient.

Summary

A variety of unforeseen circumstances may arise in patients contemplating or undergoing treatment for superficial venous insufficiency. More contraindications to varicose vein

sclerotherapy are discussed in Chapter 12 *(Table 12-6)*. In most cases, problems and potential problems can be easily managed though common-sense approaches and careful attention to the basic tenets of diagnostic evaluation, treatment planning, and monitoring of progress.

References

(1) Sakurai T, Gupta PC, Matsushita M, Nishikimi N, Nimura Y. *Correlation of the anatomical distribution of venous reflux with clinical symptoms and venous haemodynamics in primary varicose veins.* Br J Surg 1998; 85(2):213–216.
(2) Scriven JM, Hartshorne T, Thrush AJ, Bell PR, Naylor AR, London NJ. *Role of saphenous vein surgery in the treatment of venous ulceration.* Br J Surg 1998; 85(6):781–784.
(3) Stuart WP, Adam DJ, Allan PL, Ruckley CV, Bradbury AW. *Saphenous surgery does not correct perforator incompetence in the presence of deep venous reflux.* J Vasc Surg 1998; 28(5):834–838.
(4) Sparey C, Haddad N, Sissons G, Rosser S, De Cossart L. *The effect of pregnancy on the lower-limb venous system of women with varicose veins.* Eur J Vasc Endovasc Surg 1999; 18(4):294–299.

CHAPTER 19

Duplex Ultrasound Guided Sclerotherapy

Background

Color-flow duplex ultrasound has proven its value for anatomic imaging and mapping venous reflux in patients with venous insufficiency. When used for preoperative mapping and postoperative assessment of results, ultrasound can dramatically improve outcomes by directing the intent of therapy precisely to where it is needed.

In experienced hands, ultrasound can also be used intra-operatively to guide the delivery of sclerosant to areas of reflux. This procedure is often referred to as ultrasound-guided sclerotherapy, but is more properly specified as "injection of sclerosant with direct ultrasound visualization." Some of the literature terms this technique echo-guided sclerotherapy (EGS) or duplex ultrasound guided sclerotherapy (DUS). Some describe the use of a long catheter within the saphenous veins as the ELLE (extended long line echo-sclerotherapy) technique. Some physicians or clinics have tried to trademark various names as proprietary, but the technique is the same. A simpler technique for veins palpable on standing but not supine has been described with CW Doppler.[1] The complete duplex ultrasound procedure involves five essential steps:

1. Preoperative localization and external marking of reflux areas to be treated.

2. Ultrasound visualization of the correct placement of a needle or catheter into a vessel, with or without

threading of a catheter up to the level at which sclerosant will be delivered.

3. Injection of the sclerosing agent under direct visualization, and control of the direction of flow of the injected sclerosant.
4. Observation of vasospasm as a predictive marker of successful treatment.
5. Postoperative assessment of results in vessels and areas that are not visible on the surface of the skin.

Although injection with direct ultrasound visualization is an important advance in sclerotherapy, this procedure is not without risks. When ultrasound is used to guide injections through needles placed directly into anatomic danger zones, the risk of injury to nerves and arteries exists.[2-5]

Indications

In expert hands nearly any vessel can be treated with traditional sclerotherapeutic techniques, but it is more difficult to treat larger vessels, vessels with a high-grade source of reflux, vessels with a complex pattern of reflux, and vessels that lie deeper beneath the surface of the skin. Failures can be due to incorrect assumptions about the patterns of flow, incomplete understanding of the anatomy, or incorrect placement of the delivery catheter or needle.

Direct ultrasound visualization offers an alternative to "blind" sclerotherapy with one very important advantage: after a treatment under direct visualization, there can be no doubt that sclerosant has been delivered where it was intended, and that all areas of reflux have been exposed to the sclerosing solution. An important secondary benefit is that observable spasm is a predictor of vessel closure.[6] Table 19-1 lists common indications for injection of sclerosant with direct ultrasound visualization. The best application for this technique is to treat saphenous tributaries not visible from the surface; an illustrative case is shown in Chapter 7.

Table 19-1
Indications for Injection with Ultrasound Visualization

Greater saphenous vein without junctional incompetence
Lesser saphenous vein without junctional incompetence
Truncal or tributary vessels with large failed perforating veins
Non-truncal varicosities larger than 5 mm diameter
Extensive networks of varicosities
Varicosities eroding into soft tissues
Vulvar or scrotal varices
Varicosities of any type in the obese patient
Varicosities with saphenofemoral incompetence
Varicosities with saphenopopliteal incompetence
Varicosities with large open connections to the deep venous system
Resistance to other techniques of sclerotherapy
Early recurrence after other forms of treatment (e.g., surgery)

Equipment

Injection with direct ultrasound visualization requires high-quality images of the vascular system and surrounding tissues. For most patients, an ultrasound machine with a linear array transducer in the 7.5–10 Mhz range is optimal (*Figure 19-1*). Obese patients and those with variant anatomy may occasionally require a lower frequency transducer to allow clear imaging at depths below 3 cm. Color-flow duplex ultrasound equipment improves and speeds up the pretreatment diagnostic evaluation and mapping procedure, but injection with ultrasound visualization can be carried out very effectively with a grayscale machine only.

Technique

Preoperatively, the ultrasound examination begins with a careful scan of the deep system to rule out deep vein thrombosis and deep system incompetence (see Chapter 10). The superficial system is then examined, and every identifiable area of superficial reflux is mapped and recorded in the chart. This is the most important part of the ultrasound-guided approach to sclerotherapy: if the underlying diagnosis and reflux mapping are not correct, subsequent treatment often will be unsuccessful.

At each treatment session, the deep system is again scanned quickly to make sure there is no occult deep vein thrombus, and a focused superficial reflux examination is restricted to areas to be treated at that session.

CATHETER INFUSION TECHNIQUE

In this approach, an intravenous catheter is placed into the vessel to be treated and is attached to an open extension tub-

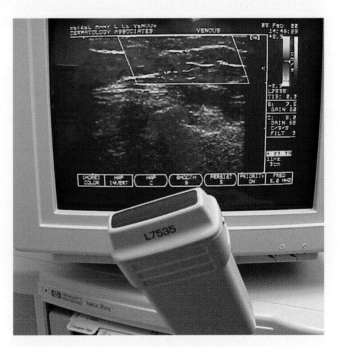

Figure 19-1. Duplex ultrasound with linear array transducer rather than mechanical rotating head.

ing. If a short catheter is used, the sclerosant will be delivered as a large-volume infusion; the direction and extent of flow will be observed and directed under ultrasound visualization. If a long catheter is used (*Figure 19-2*), the catheter tip is threaded intravenously (either proximally or distally) to reach the desired point of treatment, and small aliquots of sclerosant may be injected at selected points as the catheter is withdrawn. Compared to the direct needle injection technique, the catheter infusion approach is more technically difficult, more time consuming, and more expensive, but is equally effective and offers a wider margin of safety.

A syringe is prepared containing the sclerosant of choice. The size of the syringe is chosen to be convenient for the entire volume of sclerosant that will be infused. No needle is used on the sclerosant syringe, but a second syringe containing normal saline will be used with a needle for placement of an intravenous catheter. This second syringe is fitted either with a 2-inch, 27-gauge over-the-needle catheter, such as are commonly used for routine peripheral intravenous lines, or with a needle from an over-the-wire catheter placement kit, such as are commonly used for placement of small arterial lines and peripheral intravenous lines via the Seldinger technique.

The areas to be treated and the site at which the catheter will be placed are identified and localized, and the ultrasound transducer is positioned over the introduction site along the vessel in the longitudinal direction. Initial catheter placement is chosen to be at a site where there are no important arteries or nerves, well away from the anatomic danger zones. If necessary, a long catheter can be placed at a safe entry point and then threaded inside the vessel to reach any desired point of treatment.

A small amount of local lidocaine is infiltrated into the skin, and a catheter-insertion or wire-insertion needle is passed into the subcutaneous tissues as close to the transducer as possible. As the needle descends obliquely under the transducer towards the vessel, it becomes visible on the ultrasound display. When the needle appears to enter the

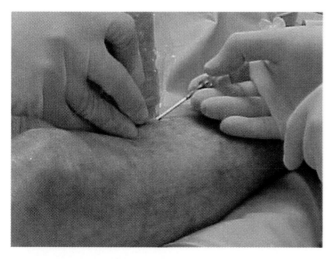

Figure 19-2. Long catheter placed into vein under duplex guidance.

vessel lumen, a small amount of blood is withdrawn to verify placement. The correct placement of the needle tip is inferred when venous blood can be easily withdrawn, when the ultrasound image shows the bevel appearing to be within the vein, and when there is no pain at the needle site.

If the catheter to be used is an over-the-needle type, it is now advanced into the lumen of the vessel exactly as though a peripheral intravenous line were being started. Direct visualization permits verification that the catheter remains within the vessel lumen. If a wire guide (Seldinger technique) is being used, the wire is now threaded into the vessel under direct visualization, the needle is withdrawn, and the long catheter is advanced over the wire and passed into the vessel. A long catheter is now threaded within the vessel to the point at which the first injection is to be given.

With the catheter in place, extension tubing is attached and opened to air in order to detect any arterial pulsations that might suggest arteriovenous malformation or inadvertent arterial cannulation.

The leg is elevated and the catheter position and flow dynamics are verified using an initial infusion of agitated normal saline under direct ultrasound observation. The area of flow of the agitated saline is compared to the mapped areas to be treated. If saline does not flow into all areas where treatment is desired, the catheter may be repositioned as needed for multiple small infusion aliquots, or another catheter may be placed in order to extend the area of coverage. If saline flows directly into the deep venous system, the catheter is repositioned to prevent this.

Sclerosant is infused in concentrations and volumes appropriate to the size and location of vessels being sclerosed. If leg elevation and vessel compression permit the vessel to be maintained in a collapsed and low-flow state, then dilution will be minimal. In this case, low volumes and low concentrations of sclerosant may be used. A rule of thumb for the popular detergent sclerosants (sodium tetradecyl sulfate and polidocanol) is that the concentration after dilution with blood must be approximately 0.5% if large-vessel treatment is to be effective. For a vessel with a 1 cm inside diameter, the static volume of dilution is a little less than 1 cc per centimeter of length. If the concentration of sclerosant is 3%, then approximately 1 cc of sclerosant is needed for every 5 cm (2 inches) of vessel to be sclerosed. Dynamic blood flow through the vessel will increase the amount needed, whereas any maneuver that can prolong contact between the sclerosant and the vessel wall will increase the efficacy and the range of the sclerosant.

DIRECT NEEDLE INJECTION TECHNIQUE

In this approach (*Figure 19-3*), the needle tip is placed in the vessel under direct visualization at multiple points of injection, and a small amount of sclerosant is injected at each site. Compared to the catheter infusion approach, the direct injection approach is equally effective, more rapid, less technically difficult, and less expensive, but offers a more narrow margin of safety.

A 3-cc syringe is prepared containing the sclerosant to be used. Needles should be 21 gauge to 27 gauge, and 1 inch or 1.5 inch long, as smaller and longer needles are too flexible to permit reliable control of tip placement.

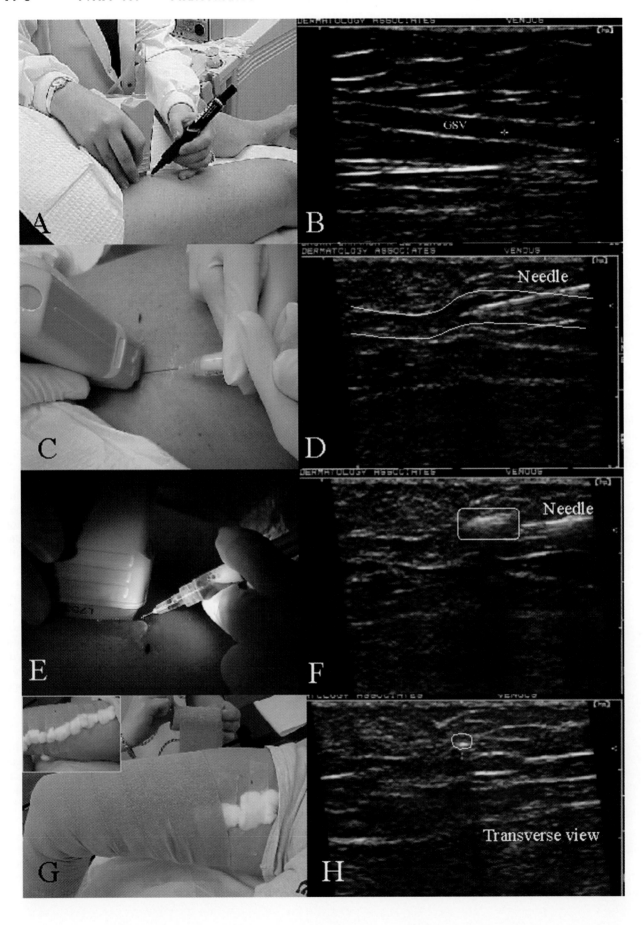

The area to be treated is identified and localized, and the ultrasound transducer positioned over the vessel in the longitudinal direction. The needle is inserted with the bevel facing up as close to the transducer as possible. As the needle descends obliquely under the transducer towards the vessel, it becomes visible on the ultrasound display. When the needle appears to enter the vessel lumen, a small amount of blood is withdrawn to verify placement. The correct placement of the needle tip is confirmed when venous blood can be easily withdrawn, when the ultrasound image shows the bevel appearing to be within the vein, and when there is no pain at the needle site.

The injection is initiated with only a few drops of medication. There should be no resistance to injection and no pain upon injection. The ultrasound screen should show the solution flowing in the vessel; in color mode there would be a burst of color as the solution flows out of the needle, and in grayscale mode there is a "snowstorm" of echogenicity moving with the injection flow. The patient is told to immediately report any pain occurring at any time during the injection.

External pressure with the hand is used to reduce the speed and volume of flow through the area to be treated, and the sclerosant is injected in an amount and concentration appropriate to the size of the vessel. The patient is placed in Trendelenburg when possible to reduce the vein size. Because this technique usually is reserved for large vessels that are dilated with blood, a high concentration of sclerosant is used. Sodium tetradecyl sulfate may be used at 3%, polidocanol at 3% or 4%, or iodinated iodine at 2%. In most cases, the volume per injection site is limited to no more than 1 or 2 cc. Immediately after injection is complete, the needle is removed and continuous pressure is applied for one minute. This increases contact with the vessel wall and reduces flow dilution in the area.

Although there are those who attempt to place the needle directly within an incompetent junction, this approach is fraught with danger. For those phlebologists who choose to treat junctional incompetence with sclerotherapy, it usually is sufficient to make the initial injection 3–4 cm distal to the saphenofemoral or saphenopopliteal junction. When spasm of the treated segment is seen, subsequent injections are made approximately 5 cm apart at progressively more distal sites along the course of the vessel to be treated. Persistent vasospasm of the entire treated portion of the vessel often is observed after four to six injections of 1 cc each, or alternatively, one or two injections of 3 cc each.

FOAM TECHNIQUE

Some clinicians prefer to use a "foam technique," in which the syringe contains a small amount of foam developed by vigorously shaking the syringe of detergent sclerosant prior to injection, or by pulling back so hard on the plunger that air is drawn past the glass plunger into a glass syringe of sclerosant. Some claim that the total amount of sclerosant used by foaming is greatly reduced and that flow away from the site of injection is minimized. When this foam is injected, typically at the end of the infusion of sclerosant, it becomes immediately and dramatically visible under ultrasound (Figure 19-4), and the size, volume, and movement of the foam aliquot allow a clear assessment of the volume of the treated vessel and the rate of flow within that vessel. It also allows assessment of tributaries or branches into which sclerosant has settled. The foam remains visible even after vein contraction has occurred.

After the injections are complete, ultrasound visualization permits documentation of surrogate endpoints of treatment, including contraction of the vein and reduction or absence of flow through the treated vessel. If these endpoints are not observed, injections may be repeated if necessary, provided the maximum dose of sclerosant has not been reached.

Relative Risks of Injection Techniques

There are several reasons why the risk of injury to nerves or arteries can be higher with a direct needle approach than with the more cumbersome catheter-infusion approach.

- Wherever a needle is inserted, misplacement remains a possibility, as two-dimensional imaging is not a reliable way to guarantee the 3-dimensional location of a needle tip (Figure 19-5). Needle placement is especially critical when inserted in close proximity to critical structures.

- With a needle directly attached to a syringe there is no opportunity to detect the pulsations that could alert the clinician to inadvertent arterial cannulation or to unsuspected arteriovenous malformation, whereas with an open catheter infusion set, these pulsations can be seen.

Figure 19-3. Sequence for injection using duplex ultrasound. **(A)** Marking the intended site for injection by duplex. **(B)** Site visualized on simultaneous duplex. **(C)** Lining up needle with center of transducer prior to insertion. **(D)** Needle insertion seen by duplex. Vein tip in saphenous tributary (outlined in *white*). **(E)** Easy flashback of venous blood prior to injection. Note foamed solution in syringe. **(F)** Initial squirt of sclerosant seen as reflective "puff" without distortion of vein outline. Sclerosant outlined by *white rectangle*. **(G)** Following injection cotton balls are placed along the treated vein (inset). Short stretch or inelastic wrap placed over cotton balls. Elastic compression stocking will then be placed over this wrap. **(H)** Transverse view (since vein can no longer be visualized in longitudinal view) of totally contracted vein. Small amount of foamed sclerosant is seen in the center of the treated vein, now 1 mm in diameter (*white circle*).

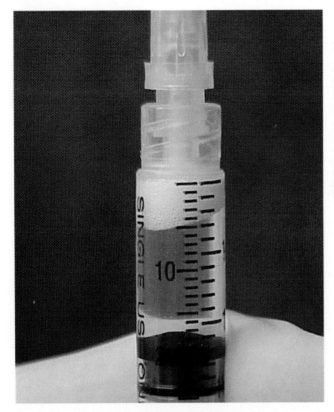

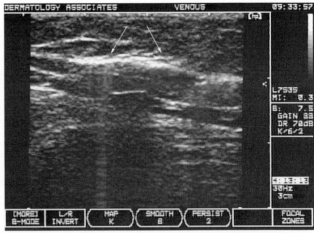

A

Figure 19-4. **(A)** Foam in syringe. **(B)** Foam as seen on duplex as a highly echogenic snowstorm (*arrows*).

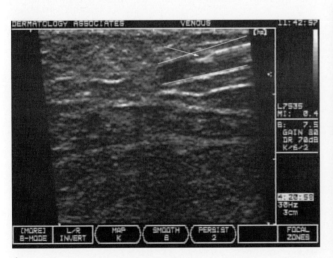

A

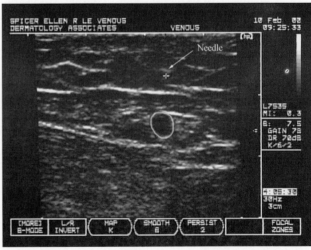

B

Figure 19-5. Transverse and longitudinal views of needle placement. **(A)** In the longitudinal view, the needle tip (*arrow*) appears to be in the vein, but is actually lateral to it. No blood can be drawn back into the syringe. This is the reason that overconfidence in this technique and failure to confirm with aspiration of blood prior to injection can lead to extravascular injection and severely deleterious consequences. **(B)** Checking the position of the needle in transverse view allows one to note whether the needle is centered over the vein. The saphenous vein is *circled*, and the needle is indicated by *arrow*. Note that the needle is slightly off center in this view, but on the longitudinal view would misleadingly look exactly centered.

- During injection, patient movement or movement of the clinician's hand can permit the sharp needle tip to migrate out of the vessel.
- Even when the patient's and clinician's movements are perfectly controlled, vessel spasm can cause the needle to pass through the vessel or can make the vessel pull away from the needle, leading to perivascular deposition of sclerosant with a risk of arterial and nerve injury.

These risks are low, but they are very real: numerous case reports have been published describing catastrophic outcomes after ultrasound-directed needle placement for sclerotherapy.[2,7] Chapter 24 (Figure 24-10) documents such a case, in which inadvertent intraarterial injection occurred during duplex-guided sclerotherapy, leading to severe tissue necrosis. Infrequent cases have resulted in loss of a limb or of life. Besides the published literature, the authors are aware of a number of other similar cases that have proceeded to litigation, but have not been published in the medical literature. Recent analysis of several cases has allowed a few safety principles to be suggested (*Table 19-2*).[8]

Injection of sclerosing agents through a needle placed directly into an anatomically high-risk site (such as the saphenofemoral junction or the popliteal fossa) is not a safe technique for beginners. Although the approach seems easy enough, overconfidence in this technique can lead to disaster. Should any solution extravasate or inadvertently enter an artery, severe tissue necrosis and nerve injury can occur. This technique is best reserved for those with extensive experience, solid credentials, and a practice that is stable enough to withstand a catastrophic outcome should one occur.

Posttreatment Care

A wide range of management alternatives has been recommended following injection sclerotherapy with ultrasound visualization. Some clinicians advise keeping the leg elevated as high as possible for 15 minutes after the injections,

Table 19-2
Principles for Increasing Safety of Direct Injection Duplex-Guided Sclerotherapy

---

A small bolus of air or foam precedes the injection of sclerosant when possible

Draw venous blood (low pressure and darker) freely back into syringe before injection

Visualize initial injection of several drops of foam or sclerosant

Stop if distension around the vein or vein wall is seen on the duplex image

Stop if the patient complains of discomfort at the first moment of injection

Avoid injection directly at the SPJ or SFJ, inject 3–4 centimeters below

---

and send patients home with instructions to elevate the legs for many hours. Others advise immediate walking on a treadmill for 20 minutes to clear sclerosant from the local circulation. Some use no compression, others use compression stockings or compression bandages, and some use both bandages and stockings together. Some restrict activity, and others do not. A conservative approach errs on the side of safety in all of these areas. Two of the authors' posttreatment instructions are detailed in Chapter 15 (Figure 15-7).

COMPRESSION

Whether compression is needed for effective treatment remains controversial, but compression stockings are highly recommended, if only for their proven role in prophylaxis against deep vein thrombosis.[9]

Elastic stockings strong enough for ambulatory compression of large proximal vessels usually are too tight to be tolerated at night. An alternative is to apply two pairs of compression stockings during the day, and to remove one pair at night. The optimal approach may be to apply an inelastic short-stretch postoperative bandage, which has a low resting pressure but a high working pressure, followed by an overdressing of elastic compression stockings to be worn during the day but removed at night.

If compression is to be effective at holding these large vessels closed, it should be maintained as completely as possible for several weeks. Patients vary in their ability to tolerate uninterrupted compression, and the compression may be removed for showering when the patient can no longer tolerate it. Many practices find that patients can tolerate 3 to 7 days of continuous compression. After showering, another pair of compression stockings should be applied at home, but short-stretch bandages can rarely be safely or correctly reapplied by the patient. Patients may use a plastic sleeve expressly made for this purpose (STD Pharmaceutical, Hereford, England) over the compression stocking while showering. Patients must then be warned of the slippery surface underfoot and the need for assistance into and out of the shower. Chapter 15 further discusses the details of compression.

ACTIVITY

Many factors have been said to affect the likelihood of successful fibrosis after sclerotherapy of large varicose veins. Because the Valsalva maneuver can be shown to cause a large temporary increase in the filling size of incompetent vessels, activities that induce Valsalva (such as heavy weightlifting and resistance training) should be avoided until the vessel is completely closed. The most important advice regarding activity is that the patient should remain active. Prolonged bedrest or any type of prolonged immobility is ill advised after the deliberate induction of endothelial injury.[9]

TRAVEL

Because of the thrombogenic effects of travel,[10] patients should avoid long trips for up to 6 weeks after sclerotherapy of large varicose veins. This may be more important when proximal vessels have been treated, because thrombus in the proximal greater saphenous vein may progress through the saphenofemoral junction.

Intravascular Coagulum

As for all forms of sclerotherapy, pain and inflammation related to intravascular coagulum should be treated by syringe aspiration and manual coagulum expression. This will relieve pain and also reduce the likelihood of recanalization and of persistent hyperpigmentation. Visible hyperpigmentation occurs with decreased incidence in veins 5 mm or more below the skin surface.

Summary

Injection of sclerosant under direct ultrasound visualization is a non-patented, relatively new technique that offers great promise for the experienced practitioner. It is clear that the efficacy of this approach must be greater than the efficacy of "blind" sclerotherapy, if only because direct visualization removes any ambiguity about which reflux pathways remain open after a partial course of treatment. What is not clear is whether the long-term efficacy of this approach will prove to be any higher than that of other sclerosing procedures when applied to high-grade junctional reflux that could reasonably be considered an indication for surgery or RF endovenous occlusion. Standardized techniques and outcome studies of 7–10 years from multiple independent sites will be needed to answer that question. In the meantime, it can be said that the technique does have a high rate of immediate success, and has been reported to have a 2-year success rate of roughly 65–75% when used to treat junctional incompetence.[11,12]

References

(1) Cornu-Thenard A, de Cottreau H, Weiss RA. *Sclerotherapy. continuous wave Doppler-guided injections.* Dermatol Surg 1995; 21(10):867–870.

(2) Biegeleisen K, Neilsen RD, O'Shaughnessy A. *Inadvertent intra-arterial injection complicating ordinary and ultrasound-guided sclerotherapy.* J Dermatol Surg Onc 1993; 19:953–958.

(3) Goldman MP, Sadick NS, Weiss RA. *Cutaneous necrosis, telangiectatic matting, and hyperpigmentation following sclerotherapy. etiology, prevention, and treatment.* [review]. Dermatol Surg 1995; 21(1):19–29.

(4) Baccaglini U, Pavei P, Spreafico G, Sorrentino P, Fontebasso V, Castoro C, et al. [*Echo-sclerotherapy in the management of varices of the lower extremities*]. [Italian]. Minerva Cardioangiol 1995; 43(5):191–197.

(5) Baccaglini U. Consensus Conference on Sclerotherapy—Padua, 24 September 1994. International Angiology 1995; 14(3):239–240.

(6) Kanter A. *Clinical determinants of ultrasound-guided sclerotherapy outcome. Part I: The effects of age, gender, and vein size.* Dermatol Surg 1998; 24(1):131–135.

(7) Benhamou AC, Natali J. [*Complications of sclerosing and surgical treatment of leg varices. Apropos of 90 cases*]. Phlebologie 1981; 34(1):41–51.

(8) Bergan JJ, Weiss RA, Goldman MP. *Extensive tissue necrosis following high-concentration sclerotherapy for varicose veins.* Dermatol Surg. 2000; 26(6):535–541.

(9) Feied CF. *Deep vein thrombosis: the risks of sclerotherapy in hypercoagulable states.* Semin Dermatol 1993; 12:135–149.

(10) Eklof B, Kistner RL, Masuda EM, Sonntag BV, Wong HP. *Venous thromboembolism in association with prolonged air travel* [see comments]. Dermatol Surg 1996; 22(7):637–641.

(11) Zummo M, Forrestal M. *Sclerotherapy of the long saphenous vein—a prospective duplex-controlled comparative study.* Phlebology 1995;Suppl.1: 571-573. Phlebology 1995; 1(Suppl):571–573.

(12) Kanter A, Thibault P. *Saphenofemoral incompetence treated by ultrasound-guided sclerotherapy.* Dermatol Surg 1996; 22(7):648–652.

CHAPTER 20

Lasers and High Intensity Pulsed Light

Introduction

The success and "Star Wars" mystique of lasers and intense pulsed light for facial veins has helped spark recent patient interest in lasers or light for leg vein treatment. Those seek-ing cosmetic treatment for their legs often request laser, as they believe it is more effective, less painful, and less inva-sive than sclerotherapy. While sclerotherapy causes an inflammatory reaction capable of inducing postsclerosis pig-mentation[1] and/or telangiectatic matting, lasers cause destruction by heat and release of denatured protein, which can also lead to an inflammatory reaction with unwanted side effects. One of the responsibilities of the treating physician is to explain the differences between thermal and chemical destruction in terms of efficacy, risks, and side effects. Some recent advances have permitted lasers and intense pulsed light (IPL) devices to become methods for treating telangiectatic vessels of the leg with reduced risks of adverse effects and greater efficacy. The debate over which is the best laser to treat leg veins is frequently approached with "religious" fervor. Only analysis of the principles involved can allow the physician to choose a laser or light source suitable to the size, location, and oxygenation state of a targeted vessel.

Laser versus Sclerotherapy

A complicating factor for laser treatment of leg veins is that most telangiectases are associated with high reverse pressure from associated reticular veins. Most lasers or IPL (except possibly 1064 nm lasers) will not treat associated high-pressure reticular veins. The success rate is therefore greatly diminished not only for lasers, but also for any treatment of telangiectasias when proximal hydrostatic pressure remains. Additional problems with treating leg veins, as opposed to facial veins, are the deeper location of leg veins, their thicker and larger walls, the overall larger vessel diameter through which the laser must penetrate, and the reduced oxygenation state leading to a violaceous (rather than red) color. Red telangiectasia have been found to have an oxygen saturation of 76%, compared to blue telangiectasia, which have an oxygen concentration of 69%.[2] Thus, each type of telangiectasia may have a slightly different optimal wavelength absorption based on its color, in addition to basis on its relative size and depth. With all of these hurdles, it is inherently more difficult to get photons safely and in sufficient number through melanin into the target chromophore in leg veins as compared to facial vessels. One must employ specific measures to decrease the risk of burning the epidermis when treating leg veins.

It must be understood that for leg telangiectasias, sclerotherapy remains the gold standard of treatment. Lasers are adjunctive and not replacement therapy. The newest technological improvements of lasers, however, have improved the rate of success and are slowly beginning to challenge these perceptions. These modifications include:

- Longer wavelengths that penetrate more deeply and interact less with melanin
- Use of epidermal cooling devices, including dynamic (spray cooling) versus contact cooling to protect the epidermis
- Longer pulse durations that allow more thorough heating of larger vessels
- Larger spot sizes that allow more photons to reach the target

One must explain to patients that injection directly into the target vessel with subsequent spread of solution into connecting telangiectasias is a more efficient method than laser, treating larger areas more quickly. Particularly when patients have large reticular networks, they are informed that failure to eliminate hydrostatic pressure sources will render the laser treatment less effective, and more short term, and will require many more repeated treatments. In spite of these explanations, patients may be irrationally fearful of an invasive needle puncture, have excessive fears of allergy to sclerosant, or may question the skill of a novice practitioner of sclerotherapy. For these patients, laser is often the treatment of choice.

When possible, consider performing tests of both methods (laser and sclerotherapy) on the initial visit, thus allowing the patient to choose the modality at the subsequent treatment session. Often a combination of treatments will allow efficient elimination of associated reticular veins, with treatment of the smaller, more difficult to cannulate telangiectasias done with the laser or light source. A very simplified comparison of sclerotherapy versus laser therapy can help guide patient decision making (Table 20-1).

Table 20-1
Simplified Comparison of Laser Therapy and Sclerotherapy

	Laser	Sclerotherapy
How it works	Heats blood to the boiling point of water	Chemical irritation
Pain	Intense heat for fraction of a second	Small pinprick. Only painful with hypertonic saline
Area treated per session	Small	Large
Risks of epidermal injury	1–10%	Less than 1%
Treatment of tanned legs	No (except 1064 nm)	Yes
Risks of pigmentation changes	Up to 50% with lower wavelengths, greatly reduced with epidermal cooling	Hyperpigmentation in 8–25%
Cost	Up to 100% more per treatment than sclerotherapy	Variable depending on total time of treatment
Number of treatments	2–10	1–5
Need for repeat treatments	Frequent	Less frequent

Table 20-2
Primary Indications for Lasers/IPL for Leg Veins

A-V malformations—bright red, central source
Ankle telangiectasias
Resistance to sclerotherapy
Fine matting postsclerotherapy
Hemangiomas (ectasias)—cherry, venous lake
Needle phobia
Patients prone to pigmentation from sclerotherapy (choose wavelength wisely)

Indications for Primary Laser Treatment of Leg Veins

Although sclerotherapy is the treatment of choice for most small telangiectasias, there are several clinical states in which lasers or IPL are primarily indicated (*Table 20-2*). When no apparent connection exists between deep collecting and reticular vessels and the superficial telangiectasia, this telangiectasia may arise from a terminal arteriole or arteriovenous anastomosis.[3] These telangiectasias may be treated without consideration of underlying forces of hydrostatic pressure. They occur far more commonly near the ankle and appear as bright red telangiectasias with a central point of origin. Use of sclerotherapy incurs the risk of injection into the arteriolar component with subsequent risk of delayed skin necrosis.

In patients prone to hyperpigmentation from sclerotherapy, the destruction of endothelial cells through thermal damage caused by lasers and IPL is theoretically believed to produce less inflammation and subsequent hyperpigmentation as compared to the chemical irritation of the vessel wall caused by sclerotherapy. This assumes that the patient's natural pigmentation is taken into account when choosing and utilizing the laser or IPL.

When patients have been repeatedly treated by sclerotherapy without good results, and all the measures outlined in Chapter 18 have been followed, then lasers should be strongly considered as an alternative treatment. The needle-phobic patient who becomes vasovagal at the sight or thought of a needle penetrating the skin is also an excellent candidate. Laser best treats some superficial vascular ectasias, such as cherry angiomas and deeply purple venous lakes. Sclerotherapy has no advantage in these cases, incurs a greater risk of necrosis, and is technically very difficult. Lasers may also treat resistant matting following sclerotherapy; in particular, those devices that treat bright red superficial blood vessels, such as the yellow light lasers and IPL, have the best results.

Principles of Lasers for Vascular Lesions

In 1981, Anderson and Parrish introduced the theory of selective photothermolysis, which is the basis of most of the lasers and light sources in use today.[4] This principle re-

quires that selective destruction of the target take place with minimal damage to surrounding structures. Selective light-induced thermal damage occurs by selecting a wavelength that is maximally absorbed by the targeted structure combined with a pulse duration that is less than the thermal relaxation time of the target, or the time required for the target to dissipate 50% of the heat acquired following laser irradiation. The most widely understood example of selective photothermolysis is that of pulsed dye lasers in the treatment of port wine stains.[5]

To understand the best wavelength to treat superficial red vessels, one must know that oxyhemoglobin's primary absorption peaks are in the blue-green-yellow portion of the visible range (418, 542, and 577 nm), but that the lowest wavelength peak of 418 nm is strongly absorbed by melanin and cannot be utilized (*Figure 20-1*). Even light with wavelengths at the peak of 542 nm, unless cooling is used to protect the epidermis, will have too much absorption by melanin and therefore fail to be photoselective, with probable epidermal damage. There is a fourth broad-band hemoglobin absorption peak from 800 nm to 1000 nm, which becomes more significant for more deeply situated vessels, as these wavelengths may penetrate over 3 mm into the dermis to actually reach these deeper vessels. In general, longer wavelengths penetrate more deeply into skin, with less scattering of the photons and their energy.

We now understand that telangiectasias and venulectases of the leg are, at certain points, deeper vessels (over 1 mm), thus requiring a longer wavelength to allow penetration. However, even at a penetrating wavelength, pulse duration must be matched to vessel size. The pulse duration is determined by the thermal relaxation time, which can be up to 160 ms for a 0.4 mm vessel. As depth and size of vessel changes, so do the absorption characteristics (*Figure 20-2A*).[6] Large diameter vessels require a longer pulse duration to allow sufficient time for diffusion of heat evenly throughout the cylindrical vessel lumen.[7]

Various lasers have been utilized in an effort to enhance clinical efficacy and minimize the adverse sequelae of telangiectasia treatment. The optimal light source would have a wavelength specific for the vessel treated and have

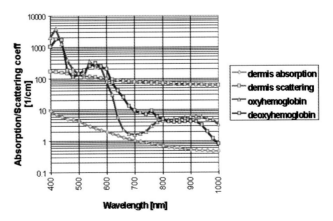

Figure 20-1. Absorption spectrum of hemoglobin. (Courtesy of ESC/Sharplan, Norwood, MA.)

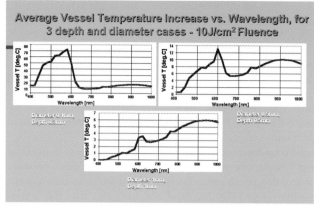

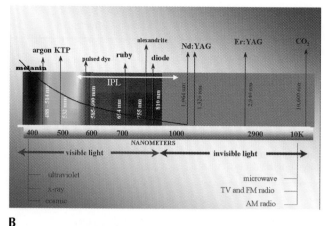

A   **B**

Figure 20-2. **(A)** Vessel heating as a function of size and depth. (Courtesy of ESC/Sharplan, Norwood, MA) **(B)** Color spectrum guide for lasers with melanin absorption shown in brown. Melanin absorbs very little at 1064 nm.

the ability to penetrate to the depth and diameter of the vessel through its entire course. Unfortunately for the treating physician with a laser, leg telangiectasias course along at different depths in the skin and subcutaneous tissue,[8] unlike facial vessels, which are more uniform in distance from the epidermis. For leg veins, wavelengths of 600–900 nm have been predicted to be most useful for vessel depth.[9] Ideally, a light source should have a pulse duration that would allow the light energy to build up in the target vessel so that its entire diameter is thermocoagulated.

During the process of delivering a sufficient quantity of energy to thermocoagulate the target vessel, the overlying epidermis and perivascular tissue should be unharmed. This requires minimal interaction with melanin and/or some form of protective epidermal cooling. A number of different laser and IPL systems have been developed with this goal in mind.

The principles of laser treatment of leg veins are outlined in Table 20-3. Lasers should be analyzed in terms of the color of light they produce, starting with green, then yellow, red, and infrared. Table 20-4 shows the current lasers available, manufacturers, and their associated color output. A color spectrum diagram to assist in understanding the laser wavelengths relative to melanin absorption is shown in Figure 20-2B.

Laser Sources for Phototherapy of Telangiectasia

ARGON (488 AND 511 NM, BLUE-GREEN)

The argon laser (488 nm and 511 nm) produces wavelengths absorbed by hemoglobin and to a lesser, although significant, extent, by melanin. Its relatively short wavelength, combined with a spot size of 1 mm or less, prevents its penetration much beyond 0.5 mm. When the patient is pigmented or tanned, epidermal melanin will selectively absorb the laser energy, preventing penetration below the

epidermis. This absorption of heat by the epidermis typically results in thermal injury. Thus, the argon laser is not recommended for leg veins due to its relative nonspecificity and associated unacceptably high risk of adverse sequelae in treating leg telangiectasia. Hypopigmented scarring is a frequent occurrence, as is treatment failure (*Figure 20-3*). For these reasons, the use of this laser for the legs has been all but abandoned.[10–12]

KTP AND FREQUENCY-DOUBLED ND-YAG (532 NM, GREEN)

Modulated krypton triphosphate (KTP) lasers have been reported to be effective at removing leg telangiectasia using pulse durations between 1–50 ms. The 532-nm wavelength is one of several hemoglobin absorption peaks. Although

Table 20-3
Principles of Laser Treatment for Leg Veins

Smaller superficial bright red vessels need shorter wavelengths of green or yellow:

Green—532 nm, KTP, krypton, 511 nm argon

Yellow—585 nm PDL, 578 nm copper bromide

Yellow, red and infrared—Intense pulsed light (epidermal cooling required on shorter wavelengths to protect epidermis from thermal injury)

Deeper blood vessels require longer wavelengths of infrared light:

Alexandrite—755 nm

Diode—800 nm, 980 nm

Nd:YAG—1064 nm

Other points:

Larger blood vessels need pulse durations of 10–50 millisec

Spot size diameter should be double the size of targeted vessel

Pigmented skin will be damaged by shorter wavelengths (minimize risk by cooling)

Table 20-4
Manufacturers of Lasers for Vascular Lesions

Manufacturer	Product Name	Laser Type	Wavelength	Energy Output	Pulse Duration	Accessories
Aesculap-Meditec	Pro-Yellow	Diode/copper	511/578 nm	8.5 w	Continuous	Handpieces: .6mm / 1.5 mm Contact skin cooling
Altus Medical	CoolGlide	Long pulse Nd: Yag	1064 nm	10–100 J	10–100 ms	ClearView handpiece: 9 mm ×9 mm square spot Contact cooling
Candela	GentleLase	Alexandrite	755 nm	100 J	3 ms	Dynamic Cooling Device (cryogen)
	ScleroPLUS SkinPLUS (KTP alone)	Pulsed Dye YAG (KTP)	up to 600 nm 532 nm	up to 20 J 10–15 mJ	1500 ms Quasi-CW	Dynamic Cooling Device SkinScan no scanner
Coherent	VersaPulse C	Multiple	1064 nm 755 nm 532 nm/long	400 mJ 450 mJ 200 mJ/4000 mJ	5 ns 45 ns 4 ns/2–50ms	VersaSpot QS handpiece / VersaSpot Chill Tip
	VersaPulse V	Green	532 nm	4000 mJ	2–50 ms	VersaSpot Chill Tip
Cynosure	V-star	Dye	585–600 nm	12 J	3–12 ms	With SmartCool
	VLS	Dye	585–600 nm	20 J	450–1500 ms	With SmartCool
	Erasure	Dye	532–595 nm	20 J	450 ms	With SmartCool
	Illustra	DPSS	532 nm	3 J	10–200 ms	
Diomed	LaserLite	Diode	810 nm	up to 350 J	50–250 ms	Scanning handpiece
	A100	Diode	810 nm	up to 90 J	50–250 ms	
ESC	MultiLight VascuLight	Pulsed light YAG and pulsed light	515–1200 nm 1064 nm 515–1200 nm	up to 90 J up to 150 J	up to 25 ms up to 14 ms	Handpiece: 8 mm × 35 mm PhotoDerm upgrade available
IRIDERM	Diolite 532	DPSS green	532 nm	up to 3W up to 950 J	1–100 ms	Comes with 5 spot size handpieces, polarized light head set, carry-all case, safety glasses, patient goggles, Scanlite, optional/marketing materials
Cool Touch Corporation	CoolTouch Varia	Nd:Yag	1064	up to 150 J	up to 200 ms	Pulsed cooling handpiece
Laserscope	Aura	KTP	532 nm	1–999 J	1–50 ms	Scanner (up to 13 mm)/handpieces 250 mm, 1-, 2-, 4 mm
	Lyra	YAG	1064 nm	100 J	10–50 ms	Scanner (up to 25mm) handpieces 3-mm, 5 mm
Nidek	Prima KTP 532	YAG	532 nm	up to 990 J	3 to 700 ms and CW	PrimaScan pattern generator/ optional

(Courtesy of Medical Laser Insight, Medical Insight, Inc., Mission Viejo, CA, Michael Moretti, Editor)

this wavelength does not penetrate deeply into the dermis (about 0.75 mm), damage can occur in the vascular target by selecting a more vessel specific pulse duration (10–50 ms, compared to the argon laser's 100 ms), although absorption by melanin is still significant. KTP lasers that utilize a 1- or 2-mm-diameter beam focus too much heat in one spot in the target vessel with less than optimal results (*Figure 20-4*).[13]

A redesigned long-pulse 532 nm laser (frequency-doubled Nd:YAG) (Versapulse, Coherent, Inc., Palo Alto, CA) is more effective in treating leg veins due to its larger spot sizes and the use of epidermal cooling. Utilizing fluences between 12–20 J/cm² delivered with a 3–5 mm diameter spot size, a train of pulses is delivered over the vessel until spasm or thrombosis occurs. For leg vessels less than 1 mm in diameter that are not directly connected to a feeding reticular vein, and with use of a 4°C chilled tip to protect the epidermis, this method can be effective. There is considerable variation in results reported by individual physicians, with more than one treatment typically necessary for maximal vessel improvement.[14] This laser is best used for vessels recalcitrant to other lasers, intense pulsed light and sclerotherapy treatment, or postsclerotherapy matting. Recent enhancements with a longer pulse duration of 20–50 ms and an increase in spot size to 5 mm, for the highest fluence of 20 J/cm², have improved the performance of the 532 nm frequency-doubled Nd:YAG. It has shown increased efficacy with reduction in non-specific pigmentary changes seen with the shorter pulse duration (*Figure 20-5*).

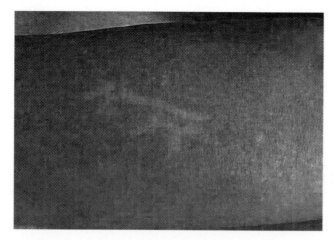

Figure 20-3. Hypopigmentation after argon laser on the legs. Similar hypopigmentation can occur after 532 nm treatment.

FLASHLAMP-PULSED DYE LASER (PDL) (585 NM, YELLOW)

The PDL has been demonstrated to be highly efficacious in treating cutaneous vascular lesions consisting of very small superficial vessels, including port wine stains (PWS), hemangiomas, and facial telangiectasia.[15] The depth of vascular damage is estimated to be 1.5 mm at 585 nm. The pulse duration of the first generation of PDL was 450 μs, optimal for the 50–100 μm diameters of PWS vessels. This pulse duration has also been shown to be effective for treating leg telangiectasia less than 1 mm in diameter.[16–18] Vessels that should optimally respond to PDL treatment are predicted to be red telangiectasia less than 0.2 mm in diameter, particularly those vessels arising as a function of telangiectatic matting postsclerotherapy. The primary problem for treatment

of cosmetic telangiectasias on the leg is the purpura that becomes long-standing hyperpigmentation. Patients thoroughly detest the long-lasting pigmentation that commonly replaces the fine telangiectasias for months before fading *(Figure 20-5B).*

The PDL produces vascular injury in a histologic pattern that is different than that produced by sclerotherapy.[19] The PDL alters intravascular fibrin, which is believed to occur through thermal alteration of fibrin complexes or proteolytic cleavage of fibrinogen.[16,19,20] A relative decrease in perivascular inflammation is seen with PDL therapy as compared to vessels treated with sclerotherapy alone.[19,21] These two factors may minimize the induction of angiogenesis that can be seen with sclerotherapy. Long-lasting hypopigmentation may occur in some patients with tanned skin.

LONG PULSE PDL (585–600 NM, YELLOW)

In an effort to thermocoagulate larger diameter blood vessels, the pulse duration of PDL has been lengthened to 1.5 ms and the wavelength increased to 600 nm.[22] This theoretically permits more thorough heating of a larger vessel. Studies utilizing a 595-nm PDL at 1.5 ms found 50–75% clearance of leg veins.[23–25] Vessels ranging in diameter from 0.6–1 mm were treated with an elliptical spot size of 2x7 mm through a transparent hydrogel-based wound dressing.

Adding cooled gel or epidermal ice cube cooling has reportedly improved the efficacy of this long-pulse PDL laser system.[24] In these studies cooled Vigilon gel decreased fluence by 35%, in addition to decreasing skin temperature 5°C for one minute. Ice cube cooling produced a 15°C decrease in skin temperature for 1 minute. With ice cube cooling, clearance of greater than 95% occurred in 20% of patients with veins of less than 0.5 mm in diameter and no veins between 0.5–1 mm in diameter treated at 600 nm with 18 J/cm². Clearance of 50–95% occurred in 82% of veins of less than 0.5 mm in diameter and 50% of veins between 0.5–1 mm in diameter at a fluence of 20 J/cm².

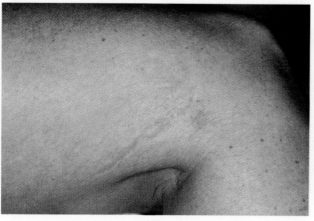 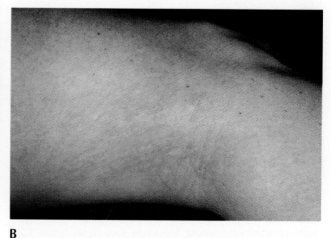

A B

Figure 20-4. Frequency doubled Nd:YAG with 10 ms pulse duration and epidermal cooling. **(A)** Immediate (10 min) linear urticarial reaction is seen along the treated vessels, a desired visual endpoint. **(B)** Hypopigmented streaks are seen along with vessel clearance at one month. Most of the hypopigmentation cleared after 6 months.

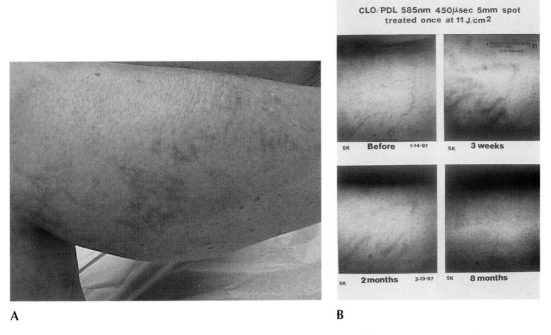

A   B

Figure 20-5. Postlaser hyperpigmentation. **(A)** Hyperpigmentation after KTP. **(B)** Pigmentation following PDL treatment of telangiectasias lasting as long as 8 months. (Courtesy of Cyrus Chess, M.D., Norwalk, CT.)

An even longer pulse PDL has also been developed with a pulse width of 4 ms and a wavelength of 595 nm. The longer pulse duration was added to better achieve the requirements for thermal relaxation times of larger vessels *(Table 20-5)*. This laser has been used to treat leg veins of less than 1 mm in diameter with a 2x7 mm, 5 mm or 3x5 mm spot size. No difference in vessel response between a 4 ms 16J pulse, a 4 ms 20J pulse, and a 1.5 ms 14 or 16J pulse can be observed.[26] Overall, approximately 60% improvement was seen in these groups. Purpura occurred with treatment, but with decreased incidence over shorter pulse PDL.

COPPER BROMIDE (578 NM, YELLOW)

The copper bromide laser, while at the theoretical peak of specific hemoglobin absorption, has not gained wide accep-

tance due to the large physical size of the machine, complex operation with necessity of heating the copper bromide for 15 minutes, and small spot size. Newer, more compact units, are presently entering the marketplace (Aesculap Meditec, Germany) with spot sizes of 1.5 mm. Pulse durations of 10–50 ms should permit treatment of small bright-red superficial telangiectasias on the leg, especially combined with epidermal cooling *(Figure 20-6)*. Unlike the PDL, the longer pulse durations of this yellow laser do not lead to

Table 20-5
Thermal Relaxation Times of Blood Vessels

Diameter (mm)	Seconds
0.1	0.01
0.2	0.04
0.4	0.16
0.8	0.6
1.0	1.0
2.0	4.0

Presented by RR Anderson at the Annual Meeting of the North American Society of Phlebology, Washington, DC, November 1996.

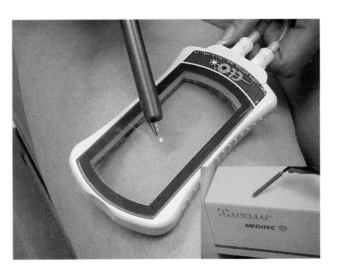

Figure 20-6. Use of copper bromide yellow laser with cooling device placed directly on the skin. (Aesculap Meditec, Germany; Cool Laser Optics, Norwalk, CT)

purpura. Rapid clearing of bright red vessels is predicted to occur. Risks of pigmentation changes should be reduced with cooling and the absence of purpura.

LONG-PULSE INFRARED ALEXANDRITE (755 NM, LONG PULSE INFRARED)

In order to penetrate more deeply to treat larger vessels and to allow for greater thermal diffusion time, the alexandrite laser has been modified to allow pulse durations of up to 20 ms. This wavelength theoretically penetrates to 2–3 mm in depth. In its early clinical trials, this wavelength has been effective in clinical and biopsy studies. Using 10–20 ms pulse durations and fluences of 20 J/cm^2 with three treatments at 4-week intervals, subjective grading indicated a 63% reduction in leg telangiectasias.[27] Biopsies revealed vessel wall endothelial cell necrosis at 5 days with fibrosis occurring at 3 weeks. Some treatments also included sclerotherapy with 23.4% hypertonic saline. Alexandrite laser was concluded to be most effective for leg telangiectasias 0.4–3.0 mm in diameter, and was significantly improved with the addition of sclerotherapy. Newer higher fluences devices of 60–80 J/cm^2, combined with dynamic spray cooling (of up to 60 ms), show some promise for greater efficacy of small red telangiectasias with fewer treatments (Kauvar–personal communication) *(Figure 20-7)*.

DIODE LASERS (800 NM, INFRARED)

Three new diode pumped lasers have recently entered the U.S. market including a 532 nm and 810-nm (gallium-arsenide) laser (LaserLite, Boston, MA), and an 800-nm diode array with a fixed spot size of 9x9mm (Star Medical, Inc., a division of Coherent). Diode lasers generate coherent monochromatic light through excitation of small diodes. These devices are therefore lightweight, reliable, and portable, with a relatively small desktop footprint. Dierickx and coworkers evaluated an 800-nm diode array laser (Star Medical, Inc, a division of Coherent) on eight areas of leg veins.[28] The laser was utilized at 15–40 J/cm^2 given in 5–30 ms pulses as double or triple pulses separated by a 2 s delay time. Veins were treated every 4 weeks for three sessions and evaluated 2 months after the last treatment. Clearing of 100% occurred in 22%, 75% clearing in 42%, and 50% clearing in 32%. Garden et al.[29] utilized an 810-nm diode laser with a 750 μm spot size at 40 w, and 50 ms pulses for a total of 453J/cm^2 of fluence delivered. There was a mean clearance of 60% after 2.2 treatments.

Diode lasers show promise in the treatment of larger telangiectasias of the leg. Some interaction with pigmentation still occurs and tanned legs must not be treated. Epidermal cooling is also advisable. Large-scale studies for leg veins have not yet been conducted for these lasers.

ND:YAG (1064 NM, INFRARED)

The Nd:YAG (1064 nm) laser with long pulse durations (seconds) was first used to treat leg telangiectasia with intravascular fiberoptics.[30] The average depth of penetration in human skin is 0.75 mm, and reduction to 10% of the incident power occurs at a depth of 3.7 mm.[31] This wavelength should theoretically be well suited to treat blood vessels within the mid-dermis. The 1064 nm wavelength is absorbed by both hemoglobin and water, but to a much lesser degree by melanin. Paradoxically, the primary benefit for treatment of larger vessels is complete penetration since hemoglobin does not effectively stop 1064 nm absorption (compared to 578 nm for example). However, high energies must be utilized for adequate penetration and vessel heating. Only with sufficient fluence and facilitation of heat dissipation can the posterior wall of a larger diameter (1–2 mm) vessel filled with deoxygenated hemoglobin be reached and heated to a target temperature of 100°C.

Newer 1064-nm lasers with pulse durations between 1–50 ms have recently been developed and tested on leg telangiectasia by various manufacturers (Veinlase™, HGM Medical Laser, Salt Lake City, UT; Vasculight™, ESC Sharplan Medical Systems, Needham, MA; CoolTouchVaria™, Cool Touch Corp, Roseville, CA; and Lyra™, Laserscope, Boston, MA). The effectiveness of these systems is presently being evaluated in a large number of patients.

Our initial studies with a prototype device in 1998, have found the wavelength used by the Vasculight™ to be effec-

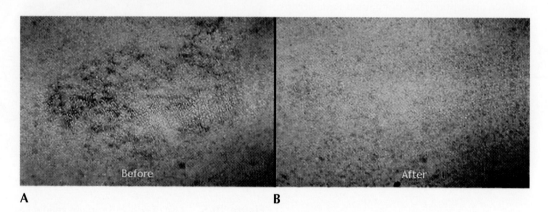

Figure 20-7.   Alexandrite 755-nm laser **A)** before and **B)** after on the lateral thigh. (Courtesy Cynosure, Chelmsford, MA)

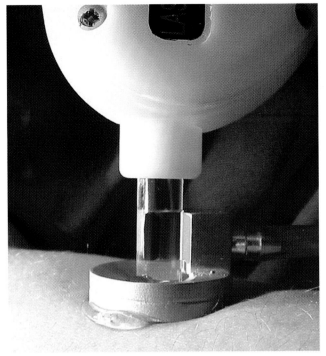

Figure 20-8. A water-cooling device clips onto the Vasculight (1064-nm) crystal. (Zel Technologies, Dallas, TX).

tive with fluences of 80–150 J/cm² and pulse durations of 10-30 ms. The first published report on this type of laser indicated that this 1064 nm laser with single pulses of up to 16 ms was a valuable modality for immediate closure and subsequent elimination of ectatic leg veins in about 75% of cases. Epidermal injury was unlikely, as the near infrared wavelength has minimal interaction with melanin. At 3 months follow-up, 75% improvement was noted at treatment sites.[32]

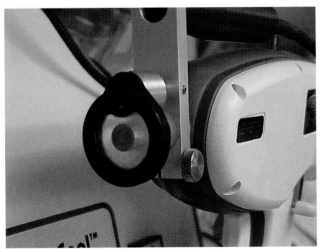

Figure 20-9. A sapphire crystal is chilled with cryogen and clamped onto the 1064 nm crystal. (Derma Cool, Boston, MA).

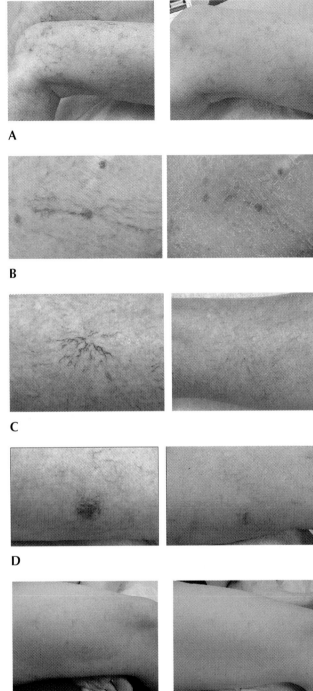

A

B

C

D

E

Figure 20-10. Clinical results of 1064 nm laser for leg veins. **(A)** Before and after on lateral thigh (Vasculight™, ESC/Sharplan, Needham, MA); **(B)** Before and after on medial thigh–a keratosis is unharmed and does not block penetration of 1064 nm (Vasculight™ ESC/Sharplan, Needham, MA); **(C)** Before and after of an ankle AV malformation, a primary indication for laser therapy. (Vasculight™ ESC/Sharplan, Needham, MA); **(D)** Before and after of more cavernous lesion resulting in hyperpigmentation posttreatment. (Vasculight™ ESC/Sharplan, Needham, MA). **(E)** Before and after on lateral thigh (Cool Touch Varia™, Cool Touch Corporation, Auburn, CA).

Epidermal cooling may be provided through cold gel, cryogen spray, or a skin-chilling device at 1–4°C, primarily for patient comfort *(Figure 20-8, Figure 20-9, and Figure 20-16C)*. As interaction with melanin is extremely small, the use of the 1064 nm wavelength allows treatment of skin types up to Fitzpatrick V that is not possible with the other lasers. Results utilizing the 1064 nm Vasculight™, which allows pulses of up to 16 ms to be synchronized with specific thermal relaxation intervals (10–30 ms), and the CoolTouch-

Varia are shown in Figure 20-10. Vessels of up to 3 mm can be treated with this wavelength and pulse duration.

HIGH-INTENSITY PULSED LIGHT (IPL) (YELLOW, RED, AND INFRARED)

The high-intensity pulsed light (IPL) source was developed as an alternative to lasers in an attempt to improve efficacy for treating leg veins (PhotoDerm® VL, ESC Sharplan, Nor-

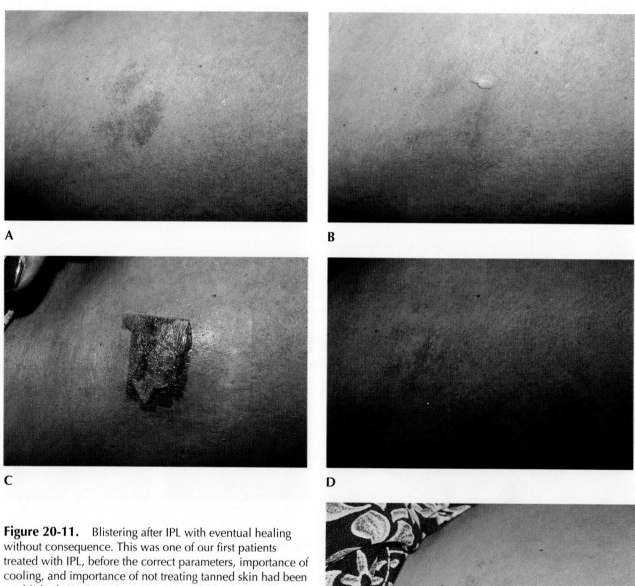

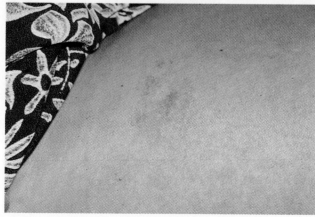

Figure 20-11.   Blistering after IPL with eventual healing without consequence. This was one of our first patients treated with IPL, before the correct parameters, importance of cooling, and importance of not treating tanned skin had been established. **(A)** Port wine stain on tanned leg before IPL with 515 filter, no cooling. **(B)** Immediately after treatment: gray skin and blistering. **(C)** One week after treatment (patient noncompliant with wound care). Patient was reinstructed regarding wound care and need for sun protection. **(D)** Two months after treatment, well healed with hypopigmentation. **(E)** Three months after treatment, with resolved hypopigmentation and significant improvement of port wine stain. The patient was satisfied with this result.

wood, MA). This device permits sequential pulsing of 1–12 ms duration separated and synchronized with 1–100 ms rest intervals utilizing a filtered flashlamp to produce non-coherent wavelengths of 515–1000 nm. This encompasses primarily the yellow and red wavelengths, as well as some infrared. Pulsing is microprocessor controlled.

A device that produces a non-coherent light as a continuous spectrum longer than 550 nm should theoretically have multiple advantages over a single-wavelength laser system. First, both oxygenated and deoxygenated hemoglobin will absorb at these wavelengths. Second, larger blood vessels located deeper in the dermis can be affected. Third, thermal absorption by the exposed blood vessels should occur with less overlying epidermal absorption since the longer wavelengths will penetrate more deeply.

Utilizing these theoretical considerations, IPL emitting in the 515–1000 nm range was used at varying energy flu-ences (5–90 J/cm^2) and various pulse durations (2–12 ms) to treat venulectasia 0.4–2.0 mm in diameter. Although clinical trials using various parameters with IPL demonstrated an efficacy ranging up to 90% clearance in leg vessels less than 0.2 mm in diameter, 80% in vessels from 0.2–0.5 mm and 80% in vessels 0.5–1 mm in diameter,[33-35] we now observe after hundreds of treatments that the actual clearance rate of leg telangiectasias in day-to-day clinical use is lower.

Our experience is 30–40% clearance with two to three treatments of the legs. In the technical method described, the incidence of adverse sequelae is minimal, with hypopigmentation occurring in 1–3% of patients resolving within 4–6 months. Tanned or darkly pigmented Fitzpatrick Type III patients were likely to develop hypo- and hyperpigmentation in addition to blistering and superficial erosions *(Figure 20-11)*. These all cleared over a few months. Treatment parameters that were found to be most successful ranged

Table 20-6
Treatment Parameters for IPL and Vasculight™ (1064 nm)

Parameters for IPL of Leg Veins:

For vessels 0.1 mm–0.4 mm (red):
2.5/ 7.0 ms (10–20 ms delay)
570-nm filter (590 nm filter for purple vessels)
Total fluence: 40–44 J/cm^2
With cooling: 45–55 J/cm^2

For purple or larger vessels 0.5–1 mm:
8.0/ 8.0 ms (20–30 ms delay)
590-nm filter
Total fluence: 45–55 J/cm^2
With cooling: 55–70 J/cm^2

Parameters for Vasculight™ (1064 nm):

Size	Pulses	Delay	Fluence
General purpose, starting leg veins	16-ms single pulse		120–135 J/cm^2
Prominent, concentrated, purple leg veins	10ms/10ms	40 ms	125 J/cm^2
< 0.1 mm legs	2 ms/2 ms/2 ms	10 ms/10 ms	120 J/cm^2
< 0.5 mm legs	10 ms		100 J/cm^2
0.5–0.7 mm	10 ms/10 ms	20 ms	120 J/cm^2
1–2 mm	10 ms/ 10 ms	30–50 ms	130–140 J/cm^2
Face (eye reticulars)	12 ms		80 J/cm^2

Important technical features with Vasculight:

- For smallest vessels need to increase distance from skin by holding crystal 1–2 cm away from skin, using thin layer of gel, and decreasing fluence to 80–100 J
- Angling crystal will allow photocoagulation over greater distances with each pulse (1–2 mm) vessels
- Some form of epidermal cooling required for patient tolerance on reticular veins
- May compress larger reticular veins to decrease depth of target.
- Do not overlap pulses as more hemosiderin deposition with subsequent hyperpigmentation will occur
- Using too high a fluence causes prolonged telangiectatic matting—start off with minimal fluence to cause visual photocoagulation

from a single pulse of 22 J/cm^2 in 3 ms for vessels less than 0.2 mm or a double pulse of 35–40 J/cm^2 given in 2.4 and 4.0 ms with a 10 ms delay. Vessels between 0.2–0.5 mm were treated with the same double pulse parameters or with 3.0 and 6.0 ms pulses at 35–45 J/cm^2 with a 20 ms delay time. Vessels above 0.5 mm were treated with triple pulses of 3.5, 3.1, and 2.6 ms with pulse delays of 20 ms at a fluence of 50 J/cm^2 or with triple pulse of 3, 4, and 6 ms with a pulse delay of 30 ms at a fluence of 55–60 J/cm^2. The choice of a cut-off filter was based on skin color, with light-skinned patients using a 550-nm filter and darker-skinned patients using a 570- or 590-nm filter.

More recently, increased efficacy was achieved by increasing the pulse durations to a maximum of 12 ms in two consecutive pulses separated by a 20–30 ms delay with a 570–590 nm cut-off filter and fluences of 70 J/cm^2. A response rate of 74% in two treatments with an 8% incidence of temporary hypo- or hyperpigmentation has been reported.[36] By combining a shorter pulse (2.4–3 ms) with a longer pulse (7–10 ms), it is theoretically possible to ablate smaller and larger vessels adjacent to each other in the dermis. Smaller more superficial vessels theoretically absorb the shorter pulses more selectively, while the larger diameter vessels absorb the longer pulses. Table 20-6 outlines IPL parameters for various lesions.

Technique for IPL

When a group of spider veins on the leg is to be treated, parameters are set based on vessel color and size. Light-red small vessels are treated with the 570-nm filter parameter *(Table 20-6)*. Medium-sized violaceous vessels are treated with the 590-nm filter, but the largest violaceous vessels are treated with the longest pulse durations.

If a contact-cooling device is utilized, a small layer of water-based gel is placed on the cooling collar of the treatment crystal. This remains in contact for at least 10 seconds to chill down to the temperature of the circulating water set at 1–4°C. With absolutely minimal pressure, the cooling device with the crystal is placed directly onto the skin overlying the targeted area *(Figure 20-12A)*. No pressure is applied as the target vessels shut with compression. No EMLA® cream is used before treatment as there is a high incidence of vasoconstriction produced by the prilocaine component of EMLA. ELA-MAX® is a better choice but is usually not necessary with cooling.

When a cooling device is not utilized (but we do not recommend this), then a thick layer of gel must be placed onto the crystal and absolutely no pressure applied as the crystal is placed over the target area *(Figure 20-12B)*. Compressing the 2–3 mm layer of gel will result in crystal placement too close to the skin, thus greatly increasing the risk of epidermal injury. Spacers have now been developed to increase the uniformity of distance of crystal and thickness of gel *(Figure 20-12C)*. Cooling with IPL has been shown to produce better results *(Figure 20-13, and Figure 20-14)*. For light-colored legs with very fine telangiectasia, excellent results can usually be obtained; when large areas are involved, the large spot size of the IPL allows rapid treatment *(Figure 20-15)*.

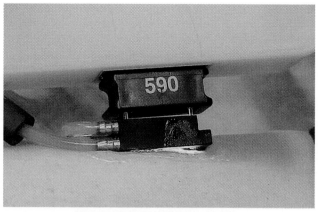

A

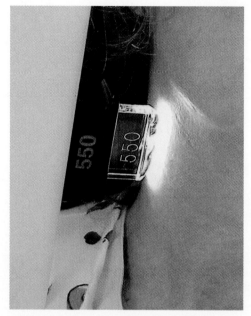

B

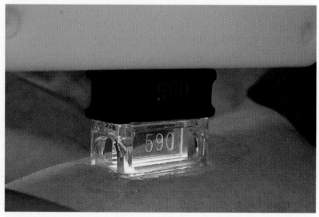

C

Figure 20-12. Placement of IPL crystal. **(A)** Proper placement of the IPL crystal with use of a cooling device. **(B)** Proper placement of the IPL crystal with a thick layer of gel. **(C)** Spacer to aid in proper IPL crystal and gel spacing.

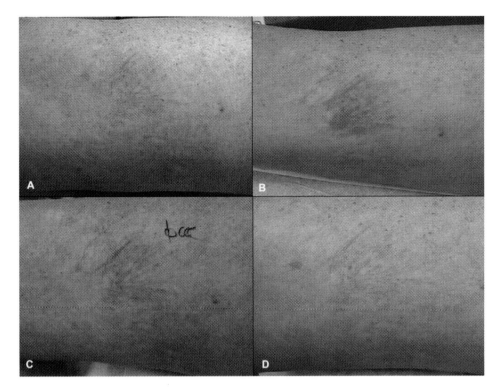

Figure 20-13. IPL treatment sequence without initial cooling. **(A)** Leg telangiectasia before IPL. **(B)** 10 minutes after IPL without cooling, with marked urtication and inflammation. **(C)** One month later, with slightly increased matting. **(D)** After retreatment using cooling device, with marked improvement.

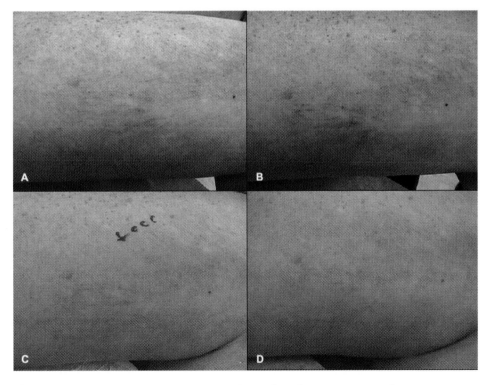

Figure 20-14. IPL treatment sequence with initial cooling. **(A)** Opposite leg, same patient, before IPL using cooling device. **(B)** 10 minutes after IPL with cooling, with less immediate inflammation. **(C)** One month later, with markedly better results than opposite leg treated without cooling. **(D)** After second treatment with cooling, with excellent results.

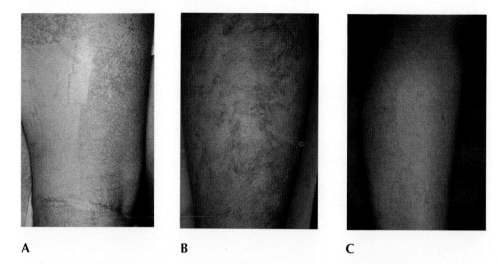

A   B   C

Figure 20-15. Treatment of large areas of fine telangiectasias using IPL with cooling. **(A)** Only one side of this thigh with severe actinically induced telangiectasias was treated initially (for demonstration purposes). **(B)** Leg with sclerotherapy-resistant telangiectasia before IPL. **(C)** Good response after three sessions with IPL.

Technique for Laser (1064 nm)

DIRECT CONTACT

It is critical to wear protective glasses when using the 1064-nm wavelength, as it is one of the most penetrating and damaging to the eyes. Most of the 1064-nm devices available are based on a fiber delivery system with a contact or dynamic cooling device. The Vasculight may be used without a cooling device, and its crystal can be placed directly on the skin *(Figure 20-16, A and B)*. For the contact cooling devices, water-based gel is placed directly on the skin and the crystal or spacing device is held directly against the skin. For dynamic cooling devices no gel is necessary *(Figure 20-16C)*. Minimal pressure is placed against the skin since the target may be compressed with excessive hand pressure. In cases in which a larger reticular vein is targeted for a 1064-nm laser, slight pressure may be used to minimize the total diameter of the vein, allowing greater penetration and less total heat accumulation by virtue of less hemoglobin heated. This may make the treatment slightly less painful *(Table 20-6)*.

OFF-SKIN TECHNIQUE

Some of the devices allow a defocused beam or divergent collimated beam to be used. A small layer of gel is placed on the skin and the crystal or fiber delivering the laser energy is held 1–3 cm from the skin. This causes a sudden change in interface from air to water, permits a larger spot size, causes more lateral spread of thermal energy, and causes some of the smaller vessels (0.3–0.5 mm) to visibly contract. Increased visualization of the treatment area is the primary advantage; greater heat accumulation towards the skin surface is the main disadvantage.

DYNAMIC COOLING TECHNIQUE

Some devices allow an integrated cryogen spray to be timed and synchronized with the laser pulse. For smaller vessels, the cryogen is typically sprayed before the laser pulse; however, for larger leg veins, Cool Touch Corp., (Roseville, CA) introduced the concept of Thermal Quenching™. By synchronizing the cryogen spray immediately after the laser pulse, damage from dissipated heat from larger vessels is reduced. It is thus possible to have a dynamic cooling spray both before and after the laser pulse for increased patient comfort and increased safety of the epidermis. Higher fluences can thus be delivered. The main advantage of the dynamic cooling lasers for leg veins is excellent visibility during treatment; the main disadvantage is accumulated cold injury should too many pulses be delivered in the identical spot. The key to safety and increased patient comfort is to allow each pulse to be separated by at least 2–3 mm and to keep the cumulative cryogen time to less than 60 ms.

Clinical Endpoints and Pitfalls of Laser Treatment

Regardless of the laser equipment utilized, there are some features and pitfalls common to all devices. For effective treatment, the treating physician should observe the immediate visual endpoint darkening of the targeted vessel, followed by urtication within 10 minutes and loss of the visual vessel margins *(Figure 20-17)*. With some of the infrared lasers it is possible to see immediate vessel contraction, but for the vast majority of lasers urtication continues to evolve up to 30 minutes after the laser treatment.

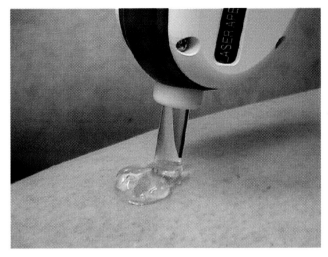

A

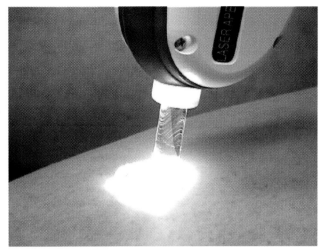

B

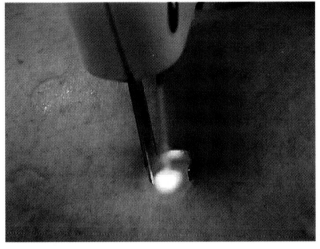

C

Figure 20-16. Delivery methods for 1064 nm short pulsed. **(A)** Vasculight™ crystal placed directly onto the skin with gel. **(B)** With the Vasculight™, the gel provides a continuous interface during the laser pulse. **(C)** Dynamic cooling with the Cool Touch Varia™—no gel is necessary as the cryogen spray cools the skin.

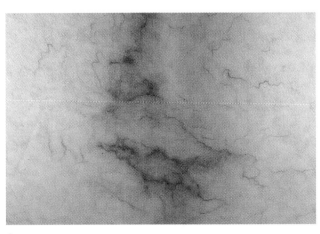

A

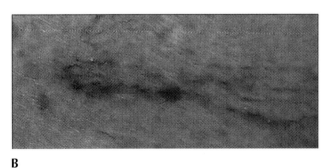

B

Figure 20-17. Visual endpoints of treatment are seen: darkening of the targeted vessel, followed by urtication within 10 minutes and loss of the visual vessel margins. Clinical results are usually good when this correct end point is achieved. **(A)** After IPL. **(B)** After 1064 nm.

Blanching of the skin is to be avoided with all the devices. With the 1064-nm lasers, lateral spread of thermal effects within the vessel beyond the point of treatment is frequently noted so that overlap is not necessary; pulses should be spaced at least 1 mm apart. For the other lasers or light sources, up to three passes may be performed over the treated areas. For intense pulsed light, a 2-mm layer of gel must always be present between the crystal and the skin when no epidermal cooling device is used. One does not want to see an immediate gray tone to the skin in the shape of the crystal; erythema and urtication in the shape of the crystal are not unexpected.

One of the greatest pitfalls for the novice laser user is the temptation to re-treat an area when no instantaneous changes are apparent. One should wait at least 5 minutes after providing a treatment with the correct parameters of fluence, pulse duration, and so on, for the recognized signs of thermocoagulation to occur. Often the treating physician will turn up the fluence in an attempt to get a better response; however, this increases risks to the epidermis. Often just waiting will reveal the changes of vessel blurring and slight urtication, and no further treatment at that session will be required. Minimal treatment with the lowest effective fluence is the course we recommend. Excessive thermal injury of the epidermis will often lead to long-term pigmentation changes causing long-term patient dissatisfaction. Patients must understand that multiple conservative treatments are often necessary to minimize the risk of pigmentation change.

Summary

Laser treatment of leg veins continues to evolve into a more useful modality. Optimal efficacy in treating common leg telangiectasia may often be achieved with a combination of sclerotherapy followed by laser or intense pulsed light. Combination treatment allows sclerotherapy to treat the feeding venous system, while laser or IPL effectively seals superficial vessels to prevent extravasation, thereby theoretically minimizing pigmentation, recanalization, and telangiectatic matting. Longer wavelengths, such as 1064 nm, used at pulse durations of 10–50 ms, improve the capability of lasers to treat larger deeper deoxygenated blood vessels of the leg, thus addressing the origins of hydrostatic pressure. It minimizes the risks to the skin even when patients are tanned. Other wavelengths have been made safer with the addition of epidermal cooling devices.

The ethical way to offer laser treatment is to consider a test of both sclerotherapy and lasers, thereby permitting the patient to decide. Explanations of cost and time differences are essential. Failure to address sources of backpressure or reflux will render any treatment ineffective, including laser. Vessels below the ankle are particularly suitable for lasers or IPL since, for a variety of reasons, sclerotherapy in this area is associated with a relatively high incidence of complications. Patients who have vessels that are resistant to sclerotherapy or experience matting from sclerotherapy are excellent laser candidates.

References

(1) Goldman MP, Kaplan RP, Duffy DM. *Postsclerotherapy hyperpigmentation: a histologic evaluation.* J Dermatol Surg Onc 1987; 13:547–550.

(2) Sommer A, Van MP, Neumann HA, Kessels AG. *Red and blue telangiectasias. Differences in oxygenation?* Dermatol Surg 1997; 23(1):55–59.

(3) deFaria JL, Moraes IN. *Histopathology of telangiectasias associated with varicose veins.* Dermatologica 1963; 127:321–329.

(4) Anderson RR, Parrish JA. *Microvasculature can be selectively damaged using dye lasers: a basic theory and experimental evidence in human skin.* Lasers Surg Med 1981; 1(3):263–276.

(5) Tan OT, Murray S, Kurban AK. *Action spectrum of vascular specific injury using pulsed irradiation.* J Invest Dermatol 1989; 92(6):868–871.

(6) Smithies DJ, Butler PH. *Modelling the distribution of laser light in port-wine stains with the Monte Carlo method.* Phys Med Biol 1995; 40(5):701–731.

(7) Dierickx CC, Casparian JM, Venugopalan V, Farinelli WA, Anderson RR. *Thermal relaxation of port-wine stain vessels probed in vivo: the need for 1-10 millisecond laser pulse treatment.* J Invest Dermatol 1995; 105:709–714.

(8) Braverman IM. *Ultrastructure and organization of the cutaneous microvasculature in normal and pathologic states.* J Invest Dermatol 1989; 93:28.

(9) Kienle A, Hibst R. *Optimal parameters for laser treatment of leg telangiectasia.* Lasers Surg Med 1997; 20(3):346–353.

(10) Landthaler M, Haina D, Brunner R, Waidelich W, Braun-Falco O. *Effects of argon, dye, and Nd:YAG lasers on epidermis, dermis, and venous vessels.* Lasers Surg Med 1986; 6(1):87–93.

(11) Van GM, de KW, Henning JP. *Temperature behaviour of a model port-wine stain during argon laser coagulation.* Phys Med Biol 1982; 27(9):1089–1104.

(12) Dixon JA, Rotering RH, Huether SE. *Patient's evaluation of argon laser therapy of port-wine stain, decorative tattoos, and essential telangiectasia.* Lasers Surg Med 1984; 4:181–184.

(13) West TB, Alster TS. *Comparison of the long-pulse dye (590–595 nm) and KTP (532 nm) lasers in the treatment of facial and leg telangiectasias.* Dermatol Surg 1998; 24(2):221–226.

(14) Adrian RM. *Treatment of leg telangiectasias using a long-pulse frequency-doubled neodymium:YAG laser at 532 nm.* Dermatol Surg 1998; 24(1):19–23.

(15) Garden JM, Bakus AD. *Clinical efficacy of the pulsed dye laser in the treatment of vascular lesions.* J Dermatol Surg Oncol 1993; 19(4):321–326.

(16) Polla LL, Tan OT, Garden JM, Parrish JA. *Tunable pulsed dye laser for the treatment of benign cutaneous vascular ectasia.* Dermatologica 1987; 174(1):11–17.

(17) Goldman MP, Martin DE, Fitzpatrick RE, Ruiz-Esparza J. *Pulsed dye laser treatment of telangiectases with and without subtherapeutic sclerotherapy. Clinical and histologic examination in the rabbit ear vein model.* J Am Acad Dermatol 1990; 23(1): 23–30.

(18) Goldman L, Kerr JH, Larkin M, Binder S. *600-nm flash-pumped dye laser for fragile telangiectasia of the elderly* [published erratum appears in Lasers Surg Med 1993;13(4):485]. Lasers Surg Med 1993; 13(2):227–233.

(19) Goldman MP, Martin DE, Fitzpatrick RE, Ruiz-Esparza J. *Pulsed dye laser treatment of telangiectases with and without subtherapeutic sclerotherapy. Clinical and histologic examination in the rabbit ear vein model.* J Am Acad Dermatol 1990; 23(1):23–30.

(20) Nakagawa H, Tan OT, Parrish JA. : *Ultrastructural changes in human skin after exposure to a pulsed laser.* J Invest Dermatol 1985; 84:396–399.

(21) Goldman MP, Fitzpatrick RE. *Pulsed-dye laser treatment of leg telangiectasia: with and without simultaneous sclerotherapy.* J Dermatol Surg Oncol 1990; 16(4):338–344.

(22) Edstrom DW, Ros AM. *The treatment of port-wine stains with the pulsed dye laser at 600 nm.* Br J Dermatol 1997; 136(3):360–363.

(23) Hsia J, Lowery JA, Zelickson B. *Treatment of leg telangiectasia using a long-pulse dye laser at 595 nm.* Lasers Surg Med 1997; 20(1):1–5.

(24) Hohenleutner U, Walther T, Wenig M, Baumler W, Landthaler M. *Leg telangiectasia treatment with a 1.5 ms pulsed dye laser, ice cube cooling of the skin and 595 vs 600 nm: preliminary results.* Lasers Surg Med 1998; 23(2):72–78.

(25) Perez B, Nunez M, Boixeda P, Harto A, Ledo A. *Progressive ascending telangiectasia treated with the 585 nm flashlamp-pumped pulsed dye laser.* Lasers Surg Med 1997; 21(5):413–416.

(26) Alora MB, Herd RH, Szabo E. *Comparison of the 595 nm long pulse (1.5 ms) and the 595 nm ultra-long pulse (4 ms) laser in the treatment of leg veins.* Lasers Surg Med 1998;10[Supplement], 38.

(27) McDaniel DH, Ash K, Lord J, Newman J, Adrian RM, Zukowski M. *Laser therapy of spider leg veins: clinical evaluation of a new long pulsed alexandrite laser.* Dermatol Surg 1999; 25(1):52–58.

(28) Dierickx CC, Duque V, Anderson RR. *Treatment of leg telangiectasia by a pulsed, infrared laser system.* Lasers Surg Med 1998; 10[Supplement], 40.

(29) Garden JM, Bakus AD, Miller ID. *Diode laser treatment of leg veins.* Lasers Surg Med 1998;10[Supplement], 38.

(30) Apfelberg DB, Smith T, Maser MR, et al. *Study of three laser systems for treatment of superficial varicosities of the lower extremity.* Lasers Surg Med 1987; 7:219–219.

(31) Glassberg E, et al. *The flashlamp-pumped 577-nm pulsed tunable dye laser: clonical efficacy and in vitro studies.* J Dermatol Surg Onc 1988; 14:1200

(32) Weiss RA, Weiss MA. *Early clinical results with a multiple synchronized pulse 1064 nm laser for leg telangiectasias and reticular veins.* Dermatol Surg 1999; 25(5):399–402.

(33) Goldman MP, Eckhouse S. *Photothermal sclerosis of leg veins. ESC Medical Systems, LTD Photoderm VL Cooperative Study Group* [see comments]. Dermatol Surg 1996; 22(4):323–330.

(34) Schroeter C, Wilder D, Reineke T, et al. *Clinical significance of an intense, pulsed light source on leg telangiectasias of up to 1 mm diameter.* Eur J Dermatol 1997; 7:38–42.

(35) Raulin C, Weiss RA, Schonermark MP. *Treatment of essential telangiectasias with an intense pulsed light source (PhotoDerm VL).* Dermatol Surg 1997; 23(10):941–945.

(36) Weiss RA, Weiss MA, Marwaha S, Harrington AC. *Non-coherent filtered flashlamp intense pulsed light source for leg telangiectasias: Long pulse durations for improved results.* Lasers Surg Med 1998; 10[Supplement], 40.

Surgery for Truncal Varicose Veins

A great controversy has arisen over the question of whether surgery alone, sclerotherapy alone, or some combination of the two may be the better approach to one or another type of venous insufficiency. Each author invariably cites numerous studies supporting his or her preference, and argues the case with sometimes near-religious fervor. As in most medical matters, continuous improvements in technology have made direct comparisons to historical experience difficult, as improved equipment and new understanding lead to lower complication rates and increased diagnostic accuracy. What is clear is that every treatment approach has its own treatment failures, major and minor complications, risks, and benefits. A good procedure loses efficacy in the hands of an unskilled practitioner, and a highly skilled practitioner can obtain good results with a poor procedure. Yet when all is said and done, in certain settings a surgical approach can offer unique benefits that will be apparent to any qualified practitioner.

Older surgical approaches were unpalatable to the patient because of poor cosmetic outcomes, prolonged hospitalizations, and a high rate of complications (*Figure 21-1*). Even with modern surgical approaches, incorrect or incomplete diagnosis in the preultrasound era often led to incomplete treatment, or even to stripping of the wrong vein, with a high rate of early recurrences. Modern approaches allow complete treatment with a good cosmetic outcome, do not require hospitalization, and have acceptable rates of complications.

Objectives of Surgical Treatment

FUNCTIONAL IMPROVEMENT
The primary goal of surgical therapy is to improve venous circulation by correcting venous insufficiency through the removal of major reflux pathways.

COSMETIC OUTCOME
A good cosmetic outcome requires appropriate placement and orientation of incisions of minimum length. It also requires careful attention to learn what aspect of venous disease is most bothersome to the patient. If small telangiectasias are the primary concern, correction of axial reflux may be necessary, but it will not be sufficient for patient satisfaction.

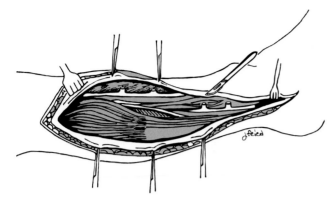

Figure 21-1.   Many historical surgical approaches were unpalatable to patients. The Linton procedure used an open approach for removal of incompetent vessels and subfascial interruption of perforating veins.

MINIMIZE COMPLICATIONS

The most serious potential complication after venous surgery is deep vein thrombosis and pulmonary embolism, which can be fatal. Strict enforcement of postoperative compression and ambulation are essential, and chemical prophylaxis is indicated for any patient with a prior history of venous thrombosis or with an unmodifiable risk factor. The most annoying of complications are dysesthesias from injury to the sural nerve or the saphenous nerve. Subcutaneous hematoma is a common complication that is readily managed. Other complications, such as postoperative infection and arterial injury, are less common, and may be kept to a minimum by strict attention to good technique. Table 21-1 lists the common complications that may be seen with superficial venous surgery.

Saphenectomy for Axial Reflux

High ligation without saphenectomy has a high rate of early recurrent reflux through the same incompetent vein. A recent study shows that high ligation can be combined with sclerotherapy with good results, at least in the short term,[1] but complete saphenectomy guarantees the elimination of axial reflux through the segment of vein that has been re-

Table 21-1
Potential Complications after Vein Surgery

Hyper or hypopigmentation
Neuritis and neuropathy
Postoperative wound infection
Pulmonary embolism
Recurrence of reflux
Scarring
Superficial or deep thrombophlebitis
Telangiectatic matting

moved. A recent study has shown that stripping in addition to flush ligation reduced the risk of reoperation by two thirds after 5 years.[2] Saphenous veins once removed will not regrow, but accessory veins, collateral veins, and tributary veins can dilate rapidly under the influence of high pressure, and can appear in the same distribution as the vein that has been removed. Patterns of recurrent varicose veins reveal that limbs that had previously undergone saphenofemoral ligation in the groin had an open recurrent saphenofemoral junction 65% of the time.[3]

PREOPERATIVE EVALUATION

A careful history and physical examination, including continuous-wave Doppler, is essential to developing an appropriate diagnosis and treatment plan. Preoperative mapping of all major reflux pathways is essential. Venography has largely been replaced by color-flow duplex mapping in the evaluation of venous insufficiency. For a good outcome, all surface vessels to be removed should be marked with a skin marker prior to treatment.

A correct diagnosis is essential. Veins should be surgically treated only if incompetent. Removal of a saphenous vein with a competent termination will not aid in management of non-truncal tributary varices.

TECHNIQUE

Before removing the greater saphenous vein (GSV), the saphenofemoral junction and its tributaries must be flush ligated through a 2–3 cm incision placed in a skin line slightly above the groin crease (*Figure 21-2*). The incision is begun over the femoral artery and is extended medially, and the saphenofemoral junction is exposed by blunt dissection.

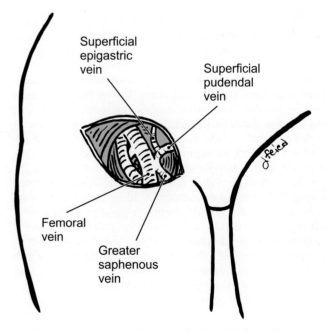

Figure 21-2.   Before stripping the greater saphenous vein, all tributaries of the saphenofemoral junction must be identified and flush ligated to minimize the incidence of early recurrence.

After ligation and division of the junction and all of its tributaries, the GSV is pulled from the leg with the aid of a stripping tool. Most surgeons use an endovascular stripper rather than an external stripping device for removal of truncal varices. With this approach, the stripping instrument (usually a stiff, but flexible, length of wire or plastic) is passed into the GSV at the groin and is threaded through the incompetent vein distally to the level of the upper calf, where it is brought out through a small incision (5 mm or less) approximately 1 cm from the tibial tuberosity at the knee. An acorn-shaped stripping head is then attached to the stripper and pulled through the leg, tearing the vessel loose as it proceeds. An older technique of stripping all the way to the ankle has fallen into some disfavor because of a high incidence of complications, including damage to the saphenous nerve, which is closely associated with the vein below the knee.

The most popular technique for saphenectomy today is the perforate-invagination (PIN) method, which uses an internal stripping tool and a special small-caliber inverting

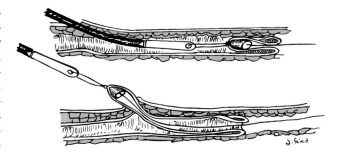

Figure 21-4. The PIN stripper is used to invert the vessel and pull it through itself using endovenous traction, reducing the likelihood of injury to adjacent structures.

head that is attached to the stripper at the groin and is secured to the proximal end of the vein. The vessel is then inverted into itself *(Figure 21-3)* and pulled through itself all the way from groin to knee. Each tributary and perforator is stretched and torn loose as the vein and the stripper are pulled downward through the leg and out through the incision in the upper calf *(Figure 21-4)*. If desired, a long gauze or ligature may be secured to the stripper before invagination, allowing a hemostatic packing to be left in place for a period of time after stripping is complete. A recent prospective randomized trial of PIN versus conventional stripping in varicose vein surgery demonstrated no statistically significant differences between the two techniques in terms of time taken to strip the vein, percentage of vein stripped, or the area of bruising after 1 week. The size of the exit site, however, was significantly smaller with the PIN device.[4] Another recent comparison, however, showed a slight reduction in the incidence of saphenous nerve injury and pain with PIN stripping as compared to traditional stripping.[5]

Removal of the lesser saphenous vein (LSV) proceeds by the same method, but is complicated by a highly variable local anatomy at the saphenopopliteal junction and by a risk of injury to the adjacent popliteal vein and peroneal nerve. The saphenopopliteal junction must be located by duplex examination before beginning the dissection, and adequate direct visualization of the junction is essential. After ligation and division of the junction, the stripping instrument (often a more rigid stripper that facilitates navigation) is passed downward into the distal calf, where it is brought out through a small incision (2–4 mm). The stripper is secured to the proximal end of the vein, which is invaginated into itself as it is pulled downward from knee to ankle and withdrawn from below.

Ligation of Varicosities Alone

Traditionally taught in vascular surgery programs in the 1970s and 1980s, the concept of ligating visible varicosities is an antiquated one doomed to failure. In this older approach, multiple incisions are made overlying visible varicosities, and ligatures are placed every 2–3 cm. Modern understanding of venous reflux and its origin in the saphenous trunk has made it clear why this method is ineffective: Only after

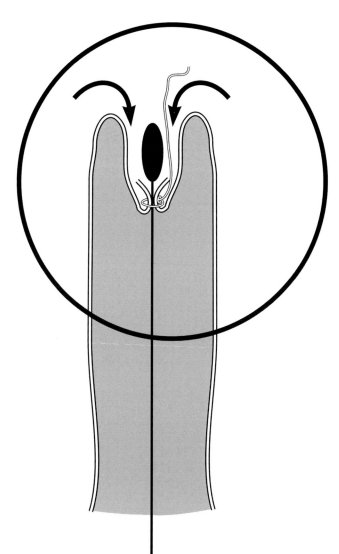

Figure 21-3. Close-up of an invagination stripper being used to turn a vein inside out.

reflux has been properly addressed at its origins can the removal of secondary visible varicosities be effective. Simple ligation of visible varicosities not only fails to correct the origin of venous reflux, but also fails to extirpate the varicosities themselves. Patients treated in this way usually return after a few months with recurrent varicosities immediately adjacent to the site of the incisions.

Ambulatory Phlebectomy

The stab-avulsion technique allows removal of short segments of varicose and reticular veins through tiny incisions, using special hooks developed for the purpose. This procedure, discussed in Chapter 22, is extremely useful for treatment of residual clusters after saphenectomy and for removal of non-truncal tributaries when the saphenous vein is competent. There is a growing enthusiasm for the use of this external technique for removal of the entire greater saphenous trunk as an alternative to stripping. The LSV is not as amenable to this approach because the likelihood of sural nerve injuries is very high.

Summary

Surgical removal of varicose veins is an effective mode of treatment that can provide cosmetic results in an outpatient treatment setting, with an acceptable success rate and a good safety profile. Advances in diagnostic capability help to improve outcomes by providing therapy that correctly addresses the underlying problem in each case. Surgery plays an especially effective role in the treatment of junctional incompetence, where high-pressure reflux makes all forms of treatment difficult and where recurrences are common.

References

(1) Ishikawa M, Morimoto N, Sasajima T, Kubo Y, Nozaka T. *Treatment of primary varicose veins: an assessment of the combination of high saphenous ligation and sclerotherapy.* Surg Today 1998; 28(7):732–735.

(2) Dwerryhouse S, Davies B, Harradine K, Earnshaw J J. *Stripping the long saphenous vein reduces the rate of reoperation for recurrent varicose veins: five-year results of a randomized trial.* J Vasc Surg 1999; 29(4):589–592.

(3) Jiang P, van Rij AM, Christie R, Hill G, Solomon C, Thomson I. *Recurrent varicose veins: patterns of reflux and clinical severity.* Cardiovasc Surg 1999; 7(3):332–339.

(4) Durkin MT, Turton EP, Scott DJ, Berridge DC. *A prospective randomised trial of PIN versus conventional stripping in varicose vein surgery.* Ann R Coll Surg Engl 1999; 81(3):171–174.

(5) Lacroix H, Nevelsteen A, Suy R. *Invaginating versus classic stripping of the long saphenous vein. A randomized prospective study.* Acta Chir Belg 1999; 99(1):22–25.

Phlebectomy

Introduction and History

This safe, aesthetic, effective, and economical operative technique enables the physician to remove nearly any incompetent vein below the saphenofemoral and saphenopopliteal junctions, although the junctions themselves cannot be treated by simple phlebectomy. Large truncal veins can be removed by this method, together with their major tributaries, perforators, and reticular veins, including small reticular veins that supply annoying telangiectasias. A sharp phlebectomy hook enables the extraction of veins through skin incisions or needle punctures as small as 1 mm. A vein that has been removed by this method is gone forever, and the small size of the skin punctures usually results in mini-

197

mal or no scar. In comparison with sclerotherapy, surgical extraction avoids the risks of intraarterial injection, extravasation skin necrosis, and residual hyperpigmentation.

Phlebectomy, first described by Cornelius Celsus (25 BC–45 AD), has been performed since ancient times. Phlebectomy hooks were in regular use as early as 1545, as illustrated in the *Textbook of Surgery* of W.H. Ryff, published in that year.[1] Phlebectomy was forgotten during the Middle Ages, but the technique was later reinvented and (with later research) rediscovered in 1956 by Dr. Robert Muller, a Swiss dermatologist in private practice in Neuchâtel, Switzerland. Dr. Muller developed his method following modern techniques[2,3] and taught it to a great number of disciples.[4–6] A modest man, Muller always attributed the technique to his historic predecessor, calling his operation Celsus' phlebectomy. Several societies devoted to phlebectomy have since been created in Europe and the United States.

Indications

The goals of ambulatory phlebectomy depend on the patient's particular medical situation. Sometimes phlebectomy is a definitive treatment that addresses both the root source of reflux and its visible expression. In other cases local phlebectomy is purely palliative, as when a painful varicose vein is removed in a patient unwilling or unable to consider a more extensive treatment. Sometimes phlebectomy may be used to eradicate a short varicose segment or feeding vein that is responsible for a leg ulcer.[4–8]

All types of primary and secondary varicose veins (truncal, reticular, telangiectatic, and perforating) may be removed by Muller's phlebectomy. The technique may be used in isolation, or in conjunction with other surgical procedures, such as flush ligation of the saphenofemoral junction and stripping of incompetent saphenous veins.

Veins most readily treated by phlebectomy include accessory saphenous veins of the thigh, pudendal veins, reticular varices in the popliteal fold or on the lateral thigh or leg, veins of the ankles, and the dorsal venous network of the foot. Phlebectomy can also be used in the immediate treatment of superficial phlebitis: a typical needle-puncture or incision is made, intravascular coagulum is expressed, and the vein segment is then extracted through the same incision, assuring definitive treatment and immediate relief of pain. The indications for phlebectomy are listed in Table 22-1.

Although any varicosity may be removed by hook extraction, inexperienced phlebologists should avoid the popliteal fold, the dorsum of the foot, and the prepatellar and pretibial areas because they often present significant surgical difficulties. Recurrent varicose veins after phlebitis or sclerotherapy also may be particularly difficult to extract because prior inflammation produces adhesions and local scar tissue.

Preoperative Evaluation of the Patient

A detailed general and phlebological examination is mandatory before any phlebological treatment.[4] Careful attention must be paid to the patient's medical history and to the gen-

Table 22-1
Comparative Indications of Phlebectomy and Sclerotherapy

	Phlebectomy	Sclerotherapy
Groin		
Pudendal veins	+++	++
Thigh		
Greater saphenous (without junctional insufficiency)	+++	+
Saphenous accessory	+++	+
Perforators (Dodd, etc.)	+++	++
Reticular	+++	++
Albanese veins	+++	++
Knee		
Prepatellar	+++	+
Popliteal perforator	+++	+
Albanese perforators	+++	++
Popliteal fold veins	+++	+
Calf		
Greater and lesser saphenous	+++	++
Saphenous accessory	+++	++
Perforators (Boyd, Cockett, etc.)	+++	+
Reticular	+++	++
Albanese (lateral)	+++	++
Foot		
Perforators	+++	+
Dorsal venous network of the foot	+++	-
All Locations		
Feeding veins of leg ulcers	++	+++
Feeding veins of telangiectasias	++	+++
Thick telangiectasias	+	+++
Postsurgical residual varicosities	++	+++
Postsurgical recidivism	+++	++
Other Body Areas		
Eyelids, arms, hands	+++	+
Superficial Thrombophlebitis	+++	-

Key: + = low; ++ = good; +++ = highly recommended; - = none.

eral state of the patient, including any contraindications to local anesthesia or to the surgical procedure itself. The integrity of the deep venous system and the proper function of the calf muscle pump should be assured, and it is also essential to perform preoperative clinical and ultrasonographic detection and mapping of all types of varicosities and of their origin. Important sources of reflux (such as the saphenofemoral or saphenopopliteal junctions) should be corrected before any effort is made to address end-branch disease.

Operating Environment and Operative Materials

This ambulatory procedure requires an operating table allowing the Trendelenberg position and good lighting. Direct intraoperative support is seldom necessary, but the presence

Table 22-2
Materials for Phlebectomy

Permanent or skin marking pen or KMnO₄ (7,5%)
Antiseptic solution
Disposable facemask
Sterile gloves
Local anesthetic
Saline or Ringer solution
Syringes and needles
Resuscitation material
Clamps
Sterile gauzes
18 gauge needle
11 scalpel
Mosquito forceps
Hydrogen peroxide (for postoperative washing of the leg)
Absorbant dressings
Tubular dressings
Elastic bandages

---

of a nurse or an assistant in the office is mandatory. Emergency equipment and supplies should be at close hand. Only a small number of surgical instruments are required to perform Muller's phlebectomy (see Table 22-2). A number

11 scalpel or an 18-gauge needle is used to perform microincisions. Tiny ophthalmological scalpels are available, but offer few advantages to offset their expense. Phlebectomy hooks are used to pick up the vein and bring it through the incision, and mosquito forceps are used to grasp the veins as they are extracted.

PHLEBECTOMY HOOKS

The ideal hook should have a comfortable grip to prevent fatigue, and a sharp harpoon to catch the adventitia of the vein. Blunt hooks (boot-hook type) have been used by some surgeons, but require a larger incision (*Figure 22-1*) and a more aggressive venous dissection.

Two sizes of hook are enough to perform all types of phlebectomies. A large hook with a thicker stem is indicated in extraction of larger truncal varicosities and perforators. A thinner device is necessary to remove smaller reticular venous networks. Several types of hooks are listed in Table 22-3 and shown in Figure 22–2. The choice of hook type is personal, although we often have all sets of hooks available on the surgical tray.

Muller

Muller's hook, available in four sizes, was the first modern hook device to be developed. The grip is not very comfortable, the stem and its angulation are suitable, but the harpoon is not sharp enough. Any physician inclined to tinker may modify this barb portion.

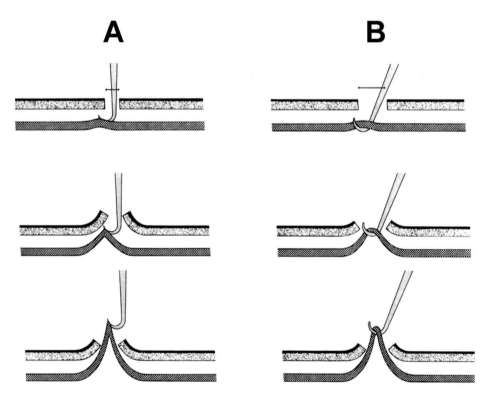

Figure. 22-1. **(A)** The ideal hook should have a sharp harpoon to grip the adventitia of the vein, allowing its removal through a minimal incision. **(B)** A larger incision is needed if using blunt hooks (boot-hook type). (Adapted from Ramelet A.A., Monti M.: Phlébologie, 4ᵗʰ ed. Paris, Masson, 1999, with permission.)

Table 22-3
Phlebectomy Hooks: Sets, Manufacturers, and Distributors

Muller's hooks (four sizes, also available for the left-handed)
Etablissements L. Padulli, Pont-Astier, F-6390 Lezoux, France
Salzmann AG, Unterstrasse 52, CH-9001 St-Gallen, Switzerland
Tel: (+41) 71 228 43 13 Fax: (+41) 71 228 43 10
Venosan North America Inc., 718 Industrial Park Ave., P.O. Box 4068, Asheboro, N.C. 27204-4068, Fax: (888)639-7642
Voice Mail: (800) 619-3705

Oesch's hooks (three sizes, also available for the left-handed)
Theodor Tüscher, Ziegelackerstrasse 11, CH-3027 Bern, Switzerland
Salzmann AG, Unterstrasse 52, CH-9001 St-Gallen, Switzerland
Tel (+41) 71 228 43 13   Fax (+41) 71 228 43 10
www.salzmann-group.ch
Venosan North America Inc., 718 Industrial Park Ave., P.O. Box 4068, Asheboro, N.C. 27204-4068, Fax: (888)639-7642
Voice Mail: (800) 619-3705

Ramelet's hooks (two sizes, also available for the left-handed)
Maillefer SA, CH-1338 Ballaigues, Switzerland
Salzmann AG, Unterstrasse 52, CH-9001 St-Gallen, Switzerland
Tel (+41) 71 228 43 13   Fax (+41) 71 228 43 10
Venosan North America Inc., 718 Industrial Park Ave., P.O. Box 4068, Asheboro, N.C. 27204-4068, Fax: (888)639-7642
Voice Mail: (800) 619-3705

Varady's hooks (four sizes, two phlebodissectors; may be used by both right- and left-handed)
Aesculap AG, D-7200 Tuttlingen, Germany
Tel (+49) 74 61 95 0   Fax (+49) 74 61 95 2600
www.aesculap.com

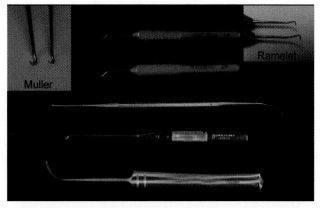

A

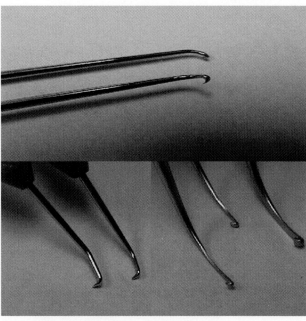

B

Figure. 22-2 **(A)** Phlebectomy hooks. Top to bottom: Ramelet (*blue* and *green*), Varady, Muller-Padulli, Oesch. **(B)** Detail of stems and hooks, (from top to bottom,) Muller, Ramelet, Oesch.

Oesch

Oesch's hook, available in three sizes, is characterized by a massive grip, although one cannot roll it between the fingers. The "barb" or spike end is of relative help for "harpooning" the vein and cannot be modified. This sensible device, highly valued by many surgeons, is very effective for removing larger veins, but less efficacious for reticular veins.

Varady

Varady's phlebextractor combines two devices on one stem. The vein is first dissected with the spatula end, and then grasped with the hook end of the phlebextractor. The device must be frequently reversed in the operator's hand. Because the hook end is blunt, harpooning is not possible. The spatula-dissector portion has no advantage in our opinion. Some believe that it injures the surrounding tissues and does not expedite the procedure nor improve the result.

Ramelet

Ramelet's hook[9] was developed by this author (AAR) to address perceived shortcomings of other existing instruments. The instrument is very economically priced com-

pared with other hooks, yet offers several advantages. Ramelet hooks are produced in two sizes that are easily distinguishable by the different color of each handle. A smaller, fine hook is designed to remove reticular or medium-sized truncal varicose veins, while a larger hook with a thicker stem is useful for extracting large truncal and perforating veins. The hook includes a plastic-coated aluminum handle and a stainless-steel stem, ensuring strength and durability. The grip is easy to grasp, well-adapted to the operator's hand, and does not slip or risk tearing the surgeon's gloves. The cylindrical shape of the grip permits a gentle rolling of the hook between the fingers, diminishing the amount of rotation of the wrists and minimizing wrist and hand stress during the procedure. The shape of the handle also does not

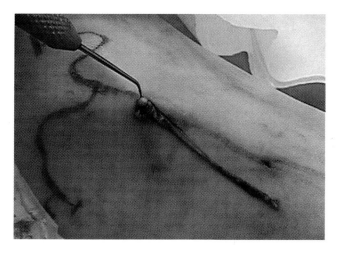

Figure 22-3. Ramelet hook with the sharp harpoon grips the vein by the perivenous collagen bundles and tunica externa, limiting the damage to the surrounding tissues and lymphatics.

cause fatigue during long operations. The hook stem is short, allowing precise and close work as well as vigorous traction. The hook angulation facilitates vein dissection and anchoring. The sharp harpoon grips the vein by the perivenous collagen bundles and tunica externa *(Figure 22-3)*, limiting the damage to the surrounding tissues and lymphatics. It has an additional advantage in that it may be modified by the user.

Patient Preparation and Anesthesia

Premedication is rarely required and should be avoided as much as possible, as it may hinder immediate postoperative walking, which is the best means of prevention of potential vascular complications. The varicose veins are carefully drawn with KMnO4 or with an indelible marking pen on the standing patient. The patient is then placed supine for further marking. Cutaneous transillumination may be helpful in locating reticular veins (see Chapter 27).[10] Local anesthesia is injected after routine skin disinfection *(Figure 22-4A)*.

The most common anesthetic used for phlebectomy is perivenous infiltration with lidocaine (0.25%–1% with or without epinephrine). Regional nerve blocks are occasionally used when the area to be treated is extensive. To minimize the pain that accompanies injection of a normally acid anaesthetic solution, commercial lidocaine–epinephrine solutions can be buffered to a near neutral pH by adding 1 cc of an 8.4% sodium bicarbonate solution for every 10 cc of lidocaine solution used. This preparation may be stored up to 2 weeks when properly refrigerated. [11]

When lidocaine is used without epinephrine, the recommended dose is up to 4.5 mg/kg, to a maximum of 300 mg. The addition of epinephrine slows the absorption of lidocaine and permits the use of up to 7.0 mg/kg to a maximum of 500 mg in a single session. Phlebectomy itself reduces ab-

sorption, and higher doses may be tolerated in phlebectomized patients. [12,13]

Tumescent anesthesia is a popular technique in which a normal dose of lidocaine is highly diluted in saline or Ringer's solution, and then injected in very large volumes until the perivenous tissues are engorged and distended. The advantages of this technique include painless injection, low toxicity, easy dissection of the vein, a local perioperative compression effect, a postoperative rinsing effect, and longer-lasting anesthesia. The traditional tumescent anesthetic solution consists of normal saline containing lidocaine at a concentration of 0.05%–0.1% and epinephrine at 1:1 million dilution. As for any use of acidic lidocaine preparations, burning and stinging on injection can be minimized if the solution is buffered to a near neutral pH by adding 1 cc of an 8.4% sodium bicarbonate solution for every 10 cc of lidocaine solution used.

A typical tumescent preparation for phlebectomy would consist of 200 mg lidocaine (20 cc of 1% lidocaine) diluted with normal saline to a volume of 200 cc, with the addition of 2 cc of 8.4% bicarbonate solution, the entire volume to be injected along the course of the veins to be removed. Tumescent anesthesia is regarded by many as a major advance in ambulatory phlebectomy.[14,15]

Allergic and toxic reactions are very rare, but the operator must always be prepared with IV perfusion solutions, resuscitation equipment, epinephrine, injectable steroids, and IV diazepam.

Technique

Cutaneous incisions with the number 11 scalpel or the 18-gauge needle *(Figure 22-4B)* should be vertically oriented along the thigh and lower leg and should follow the skin lines at the knee or the ankle. The distance between the incisions varies from 2 to 15 cm, according to the experience of the surgeon, the size of the vein, presence of perforators, previous episodes of phlebitis, or previous sclerotherapy.

The varicose vein is gently dissected by undermining with the stem of the phlebectomy hook. Undermining is largely carried out along the course of the vein, but is extended slightly in a perpendicular direction *(Figure 22-4C)*. When freed of its fibroadipose attachments, the liberated vein can then be grasped by the harpoon of the hook *(Figure 22-4D)* and easily removed with the help of a mosquito forceps held in the other hand *(Figure 22-4E,F)*. The left hand also grips a sterile gauze strip and assures hemostasis by local compression of the already removed venous network.

The whole varicose vein is then extracted progressively from one incision to the next *(Figure 22-5)*. Incompetent perforators are carefully dissected and eliminated by gentle traction or torsion. Venous ligation is not necessary: hemostasis is achieved with intra- and postoperative local compression. Areas in which postoperative compression is most difficult (popliteal folds, thighs, groin, deeper and larger perforators) are surgically removed first, to permit the maximum time for hemostasis while the patient remains supine. No skin closure is needed if the operator respects the basic principle of minimal incisions (1–3 mm) and good postoper-

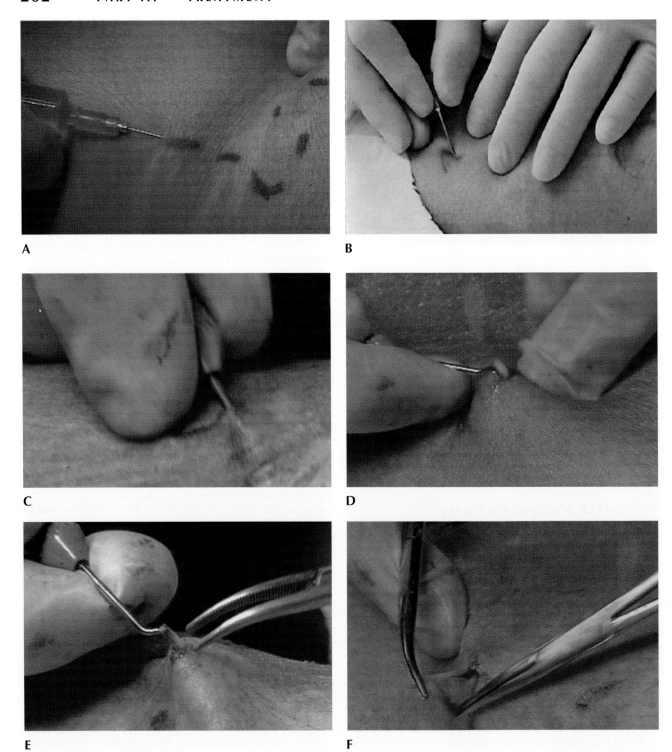

Figure. 22-4 Ambulatory phlebectomy, step by step: **(A)** Tumescent anesthesia after marking and sterile preparation of site. **(B)** Cutaneous puncture with 18 gauge needle (for reticular and telangiectatic varicosities) or minimal cutaneous incision with the edge of # 11 blade. **(C)** Introduction of Ramelet's phlebectomy hook through the incision and gentle dissection by undermining with the stem of the hook. **(D)** Adventitia of the liberated vein is grasped by the harpoon of the hook. **(E)** Varicose vein is removed with the help of a mosquito forceps. **(F)** Further extraction of the vein with two mosquito forceps.

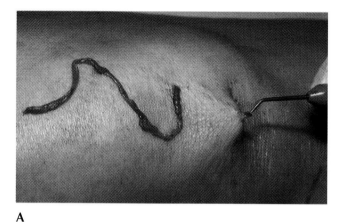

A

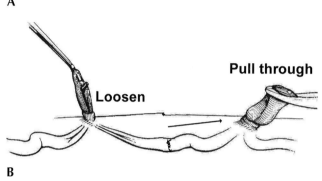

Pull through

Loosen

B

Figure. 22-5 **(A)** The whole varicose vein is then extracted from one incision to the other, after loosening vein loops at several sites as shown in **(B)** the schematic diagram.

ative compression. With experience, it usually is possible to remove extensive venous networks on both legs in a single session of 60 to 120 minutes.

Complementary fine-needle sclerotherapy of telangiectasias can be performed immediately before or after the eradication of their nourishing venules.[16,17] Larger telangiectasias may also be destroyed by gentle subcutaneous curettage with the harpoon of the hook, debris of venectasias being removed through tiny incisions.

At the end of the operation, the leg is carefully cleansed with hydrogen peroxide (H_2O_2). If there is persistent oozing at any site, it is easily controlled by additional local compression. Application of antiseptic powder is useless and must be avoided, as it may induce silicotic granuloma several years later. [18]

Drugs and Prophylactic Anticoagulation

Postoperative pain seldom occurs. A mild agent such as acetaminophen may be used if necessary. Aspirin and non-steroidal antiinflammatory agents may be used, but can lead to increased bruising. Except in patients with a prior history of deep vein thrombosis and pulmonary embolism, prophylactic anticoagulation need not be considered, as the patient

continues to move the legs during the operation and walks immediately after the phlebectomy with a compression bandage.

Postoperative Care and Bandaging

Adequate dressing is an essential step in the procedure and should be carefully applied by the operator or a well-trained assistant. The incisions are covered with a protective film, over which sterile gauze or absorbent pads *(Figure 22-6A,B)* are affixed with tape. In applying tape, it is important to avoid skin tension, which will produce large "shearing" skin blisters.

If the phlebologist is experienced with bandaging, a second dressing with a high elasticity (long-stretch) bandage is applied to the leg *(Figure 22-6C)*. This compression dressing prevents postoperative hemorrhage and reduces the likelihood of pain, bruising, seroma formation, and other complications. The long-stretch bandage is applied from the foot up, beginning at the toe joints, including the heel, and extending proximally to cover all incisions. To avoid a tourniquet effect, an elastic dressing must never be applied over the proximal leg without beginning at the feet.

If the phlebologist is not experienced with bandaging, compression stockings may provide an alternative means of compression. A single pair of 40–50 mm Hg compression hose may be used, or two layers of 20–30 mm Hg stockings may be applied for additive effects. If two layers of stockings are used, the topmost pair may be removed at night and replaced in the morning.

Daily ambulation should be increased as much as possible in the immediate postoperative period. Under no circumstances should a patient be placed at bedrest after venous surgery. Patients may return to work immediately after the operation, but should not drive an automobile until the next day, as distal motor function may be subtly impaired due to prolonged anesthesia, particularly after local anesthesia in the popliteal region.

Dressings are removed after 24 or 48 hours, and the wounds are cleansed with antiseptic and sprayed with a protective film (opsite). If the incisions are of minimal size, further wound dressings are not necessary, but ongoing compression therapy (elastic bandages or compression stockings) is mandatory for 7 to 21 more days, depending on the size of the removed veins and the degree of reflux that has been treated. Stockings may be removed for showering after the fourth postoperative day, but otherwise should be worn continuously.

Complementary sclerotherapy of residual varicosities should be delayed several weeks until postoperative healing is well advanced. Many telangiectasias may progressively and spontaneously regress and disappear following varicose vein removal by ambulatory phlebectomy. Early sun exposure should be avoided, as hyperpigmentation may result. Postoperative care is summarized in Table 22-4. A postoperative patient instruction sheet can be found in Chapter 15 *(Figure 15-8)*.

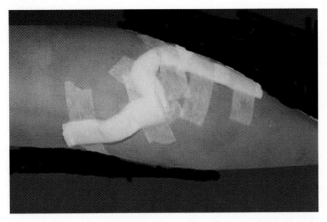

A

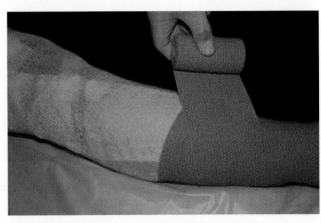

B

C

Figure. 22-6:   Dressing step by step: **(A)** The leg is carefully washed with hydrogen peroxide; the incisions may be covered with a protective film. Selective compression may be achieved applying sterile gauze exactly along the varicose vein pathway. **(B)** The incisions are covered with absorbent pads, which are attached by adhesive plasters and a tubular net dressing. **(C)** A second dressing with a high elasticity bandage achieves compression along operating zones preventing postoperative hemorrhage, pain, and complications. The strip is applied from the toe joints (even if only the thigh has been operated), includes the heel, and extends up proximally to operated areas.

Results

Surgical puncture sites are usually totally invisible after some months, but may persist much longer in younger patients with tighter skin. Patients should be warned about this possibility before the procedure is undertaken. Hematomas rapidly disappear, and pigmentation usually fades in a few weeks. Meticulous application of the postoperative compression dressing diminishes the incidence of bleeding, pain, hematoma, and residual pigmentation. Figures 22-7

Table 22-4
Postoperative Care

No anticoagulation or other medications necessary
Absorbent dressing on the incisions
Elastic bandage (to be loosened during the night!)
Immediate postoperative standing and walking
No loss of time from work in most cases
Dressing changes after 24–48 hours
Daytime compression therapy for 7–14 days (bandages or compression stockings)
Short showers allowed after 4 days
Sclerotherapy of residual varicosities 3 weeks or later

through 22-11 show preoperative and postoperative comparisons in patients with typical varicosities, and Figure 22-12 shows phlebectomy for superficial phlebitis.

Ambulatory Phlebectomy of Body Areas Other than the Legs

This procedure may also be utilized for removing cosmetically unacceptable abnormal dilated periorbital, temporal, or frontal venous networks of the face, as well as venous dilatations of the abdomen, arms, or dorsum of the hands. Removal of nonfunctional refluxing veins always improves residual circulation, but the removal of functional veins for purely aesthetic reasons should not be undertaken lightly. Chapter 17 details phlebectomy of the periorbital reticular vein.

Complications and Their Treatment

Most minor complications are benign and resolve spontaneously, but patients must be warned about their possible occurrence. Complications[8,19,20,21] may be classified as cu-

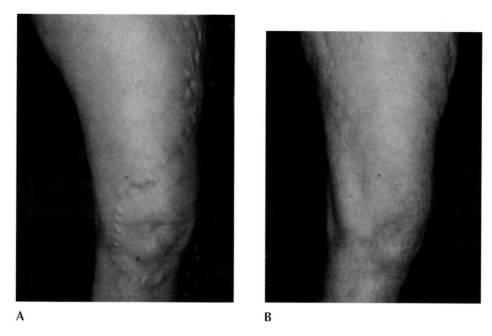

Figure. 22-7 **(A)** Truncal varicose vein (long saphenous accessory). **(B)** Excellent cosmetic result, 5 weeks after Muller's ambulatory phlebectomy.

taneous, vascular, neurological, or general *(Table 22-5)*. Many minor complications are avoidable, and their occurrence may be in many cases ascribed to lack of experience. Recurrences are typically due to incorrect diagnosis of the source of venous reflux *(Figure 22-13)*. Chief among complications are edema, excessive hemorrhage, hematoma formation, scarring, silicotic granulomas, trauma-induced telangiectatic matting, and blisters due to incorrect wound dressings. Other complications, such as occasional nerve injury with sensory disturbances, are relatively unavoidable.[4,21]

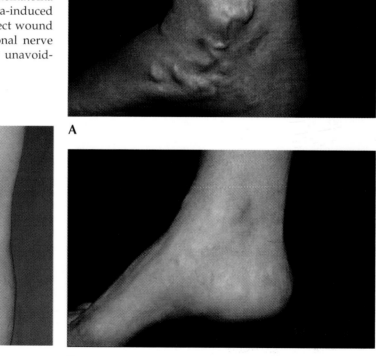

Figure. 22-8 **(A)** Lateral venous system. **(B)** 6 weeks postoperative.

Figure. 22-9 **(A)** Varicose veins of the inner foot. **(B)** 2 months postoperative.

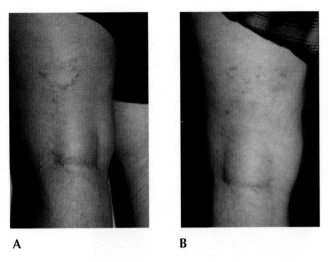

A   **B**

Figure. 22-10   **(A)** Reticular varicose vein of the popliteal fold. **(B)** 6 weeks postoperative.

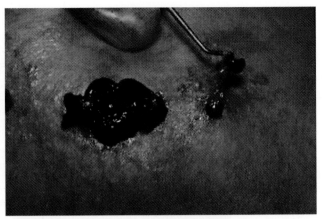

Figure. 22-12   Varicophlebitis. After incision, the clot is expressed and the vein wall may be removed by the hook, assuring a definitive treatment and immediate relief of the pain.

CUTANEOUS COMPLICATIONS

Transitory hyperpigmentation usually fades in a few months without any treatment. Blisters secondary to skin shearing from adhesive tape *(Figure 22-14A)* may induce postbullous depigmentation or transitory hyperpigmentation *(Figure 22-14B)*. Contact dermatitis secondary to antiseptic solutions or adhesives is uncommon, and usually heals quickly with topical steroid application. Wound infection is unusual, and may be treated by local application of Dakin (sodium hypochlorite) solution. Systemic antibiotics generally are not necessary. Keloids and hypertrophic scars are extremely rare because of the minimal size of the incisions. When they do occur, they respond to typical treatment, including intralesional steroids, cryotherapy, and sili-

cone sheet dressings. Tattooing with marking pen ink is unusual. Silicotic granulomas occur several years after the postoperative application of antiseptic powder, and require excision of every foreign body granuloma.[18]

VASCULAR COMPLICATIONS

Superficial hematomas are common. Hematoma formation depends on individual variations in coagulation and on the

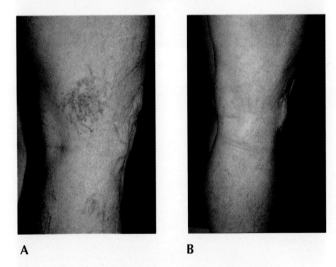

A   **B**

Figure. 22-11   **(A)** Telangiectasias of the knee. **(B)** 1 year after extraction of reticular varicose veins and gentle subcutaneous curettage of telangiectases with the harpoon of the hook, associated with fine needle sclerotherapy (one session).

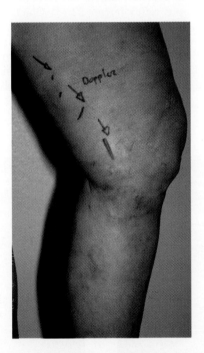

Figure. 22-13   Undesirable outcome due to the incorrect indication and diagnosis. Phlebectomy has been limited to distal saphenous vein without correction of the undiagnosed insufficient proximal part of the vein. This has led to rapid postoperative recurrence of varicosities. *Arrows* indicate reflux as determined by duplex ultrasound.

Table 22-5
Postoperative Complications [21]

Cutaneous frequently
   transient pigmentation
   skin blisters (on sensitive skin after incorrect dressing)
Cutaneous rarely
   contact dermatitis
   infections
   keloids
   tattooing with marking pen
   silicotic (foreign body) granuloma
   necrobiosis lipoidica[22]
Vascular frequently
   hematomas
Vascular infrequently
   postoperative hemorrhages (incorrect dressing)
   neo-telangiectasias (matting)
Vascular rarely
   superficial phlebitis
   edema (frequent after phlebectomy of dorsum of the foot)
   lymphatic pseudocyst
Neurological rarely
   postoperative pain
   concomitant anesthesia of deeper nerves
   carpotarsal syndrome after incorrect compression of the dorsum of the foot
   transitory or definitive sensation defect
   neuroma
General rare
   complications secondary to local anesthesia

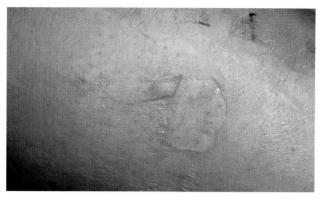

A

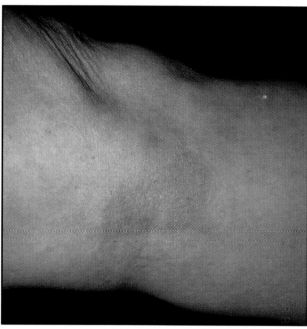

B

Figure. 22-14 Skin complication due to inadequate dressing. **(A)** Blister secondary to skin shearing (adhesive tape). **(B)** Residual (transitory) hyperpigmentation.

effectiveness of the postoperative compression. Hematomas are most common in the popliteal fold, where it is most difficult to achieve good postoperative compression *(Figure 22-15)*.

Some patients complain of persistent subcutaneous nodules, corresponding to deep hematomas in the "tunnel" of the removed vein. When these occur, they will be reabsorbed over a period of several months. Significant delayed postoperative oozing may occur, and for this reason it is wise to reevaluate the postoperative dressing after 30 minutes of walking in or near the office, particularly in patients who may have a long journey home.

Superficial phlebitis of incompletely removed varicose veins or of neighboring veins may occur *(Figure 22-16)*. Treatment of minor cases may be expectant, but progressive phlebitis may require incision and phlebectomy of the inflamed vein. Deep vein thrombosis has not yet been reported after ambulatory phlebectomy, probably because compression bandages and ambulation are effective forms of prophylaxis.

Except on the dorsum of the foot, edema is usually a consequence of an incorrect dressing (tourniquet effect) and usually resolves with proper gradient compression or after

one night without the bandage. Edema may persist for several months after phlebectomy of the dorsum of the foot or of the lesser saphenous vein.

Lymphatic pseudocyst *(Figure 22-17)* may complicate phlebectomy of the ankle, pretibial, or popliteal areas. When a subcutaneous nodule develops rapidly, this lymph collection may be punctured and drained. The best treatment is increased compression along with periodic gentle circular massage. In resistant cases, lymphatic drainage may be required.

Neotelangiectasias ("telangiectatic matting") are the most annoying potential complication of phlebectomy *(Figure 22-18)*. The same complication is seen after classic stripping as well as after sclerotherapy, and the etiology is unclear. In some cases, it seems to be related to a sudden local

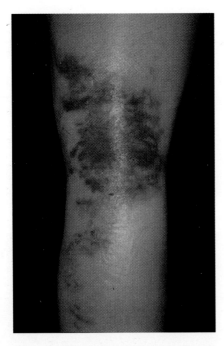

Figure. 22-15   Postoperative hematoma in sensitive skin. A good dressing is very difficult to achieve in the popliteal fold. Such spectacular diffuse hematomas totally disappear in a few weeks.

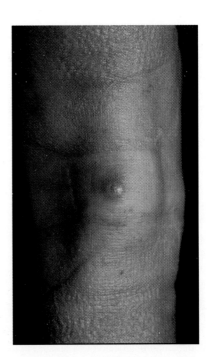

Figure. 22-17   Lymphatic pseudocyst (seen here in the popliteal area) may complicate phlebectomy of the ankle, pretibial, or popliteal areas.

increase in venous pressure or to an area of persistent reflux that remains to be corrected. In others, it may be an abnormal angiogenic response to tissue injury. Some authors have noticed an association with exogenous estrogens, but this

has not been confirmed. Matting usually does spontaneously fade away after several months. In some cases it may be treated with sclerotherapy of the tiniest vessels, but in other cases every attempt to sclerose vessels is met with a

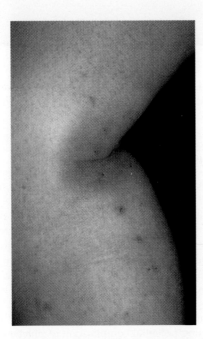

Figure. 22-16   Superficial phlebitis of incompletely removed varicose vein. Rapid healing after incision, expression of the clot, and phlebectomy of the vein.

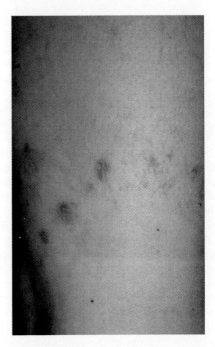

Figure. 22-18   Multiple neotelangiectasias ("telangiectatic matting") after phlebectomy.

new blush of recurrent matting. Laser or high-energy intense pulsed light therapy could also be considered, as discussed in Chapter 20.

Neurological Complications

Anesthetic may diffuse deeply to temporarily affect a motor nerve. This is particularly common when a local anesthetic is used in the external popliteal fold, where a temporary paralysis of the foot may result. It is therefore important to test the mobility of the foot before the patient stands up. This complication usually does not occur in tumescent anesthesia, because the concentration of anesthetic as injected is extremely low.

Although postoperative pain is unusual and analgesics are only required rarely, postoperative pain is more common after surgical removal of varicose veins in patients with lipodermatosclerosis or after removal of veins previously treated by sclerotherapy. Incorrect compression of the dorsum or heel of the foot may cause severe local pain, which will resolve quickly with the removal of compression.

Small cutaneous sensory nerve injury is common when veins are removed under general or regional anesthesia, but is much less common when local anesthesia is used because intraoperative manipulation of a sensory nerve is painful. If the surgeon stops immediately when the patient complains, sensory branches will be left intact.

Small-nerve injury is more frequent in patients previously treated with sclerotherapy because inflammatory fibrous reaction and surrounding tissue adhesions bind the vein to the adjacent sensory nerves. Hyper-, hypo-, or total anesthesia secondary to nerve injury usually resolves within weeks or months. Neuroma is an extremely uncommon complication of peripheral nerve injury.

Altered mental status and even seizures may occur in patients with an unusual sensitivity to lidocaine, if large amounts are accidentally given intravenously, or if the dose recommendations are exceeded. Supportive care is sufficient, as the toxic effects of the drug wear off quickly. This complication is much less likely when a tumescent anesthesia technique is used.

General Complications

Vasovagal reactions sometimes occur, and patients occasionally complain of general vague malaise resulting from local anesthesia. Simple reassurance is usually sufficient to satisfy the patient, and the procedure usually may be continued.

Long-term Results

Long-term results after phlebectomy are excellent when the procedure is performed for appropriate indications, and when high-grade reflux is eliminated prior to phlebectomy. As with any form of therapy, new varicose veins may develop over time, and patients must be informed about the likely evolution and progressive nature of venous insufficiency.

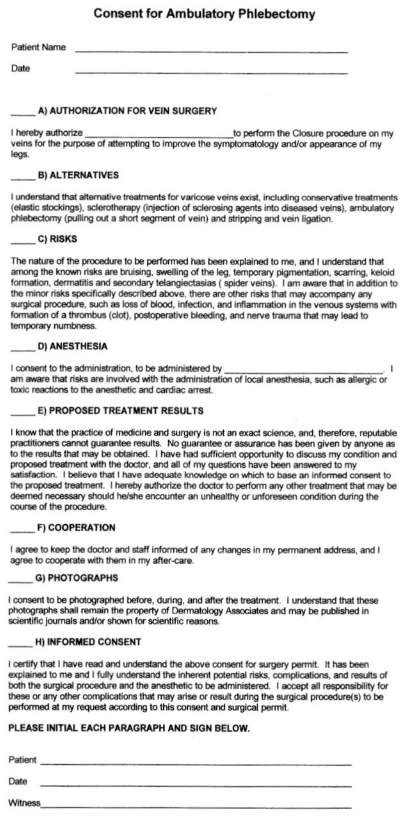

Consent for Ambulatory Phlebectomy

Patient Name ______________________

Date ______________________

____ **A) AUTHORIZATION FOR VEIN SURGERY**

I hereby authorize ______________________ to perform the Closure procedure on my veins for the purpose of attempting to improve the symptomatology and/or appearance of my legs.

____ **B) ALTERNATIVES**

I understand that alternative treatments for varicose veins exist, including conservative treatments (elastic stockings), sclerotherapy (injection of sclerosing agents into diseased veins), ambulatory phlebectomy (pulling out a short segment of vein) and stripping and vein ligation.

____ **C) RISKS**

The nature of the procedure to be performed has been explained to me, and I understand that among the known risks are bruising, swelling of the leg, temporary pigmentation, scarring, keloid formation, dermatitis and secondary telangiectasias (spider veins). I am aware that in addition to the minor risks specifically described above, there are other risks that may accompany any surgical procedure, such as loss of blood, infection, and inflammation in the venous systems with formation of a thrombus (clot), postoperative bleeding, and nerve trauma that may lead to temporary numbness.

____ **D) ANESTHESIA**

I consent to the administration, to be administered by ______________________. I am aware that risks are involved with the administration of local anesthesia, such as allergic or toxic reactions to the anesthetic and cardiac arrest.

____ **E) PROPOSED TREATMENT RESULTS**

I know that the practice of medicine and surgery is not an exact science, and, therefore, reputable practitioners cannot guarantee results. No guarantee or assurance has been given by anyone as to the results that may be obtained. I have had sufficient opportunity to discuss my condition and proposed treatment with the doctor, and all of my questions have been answered to my satisfaction. I believe that I have adequate knowledge on which to base an informed consent to the proposed treatment. I hereby authorize the doctor to perform any other treatment that may be deemed necessary should he/she encounter an unhealthy or unforeseen condition during the course of the procedure.

____ **F) COOPERATION**

I agree to keep the doctor and staff informed of any changes in my permanent address, and I agree to cooperate with them in my after-care.

____ **G) PHOTOGRAPHS**

I consent to be photographed before, during, and after the treatment. I understand that these photographs shall remain the property of Dermatology Associates and may be published in scientific journals and/or shown for scientific reasons.

____ **H) INFORMED CONSENT**

I certify that I have read and understand the above consent for surgery permit. It has been explained to me and I fully understand the inherent potential risks, complications, and results of both the surgical procedure and the anesthetic to be administered. I accept all responsibility for these or any other complications that may arise or result during the surgical procedure(s) to be performed at my request according to this consent and surgical permit.

PLEASE INITIAL EACH PARAGRAPH AND SIGN BELOW.

Patient ______________________

Date ______________________

Witness______________________

Figure. 22-19 Patient consent form used by two of the authors.

Summary

Ambulatory phlebectomy is a safe, economical, and elegant operative procedure for the correction of venous insufficiency below the major junctions, assuring definitive extraction of all types of varicose veins and perforating veins of the legs and other areas of the body. Phlebectomy is also well-suited to the treatment of superficial phlebitis and varicophlebitis. There are many minor pitfalls to be avoided, however, and the technique is best performed by those well trained in its use. A sample patient consent form is shown in Figure 22-19.

References

(1) Scholz A. *Historical aspects*. In Westerhof W, editor. Leg Ulcers. Amsterdam: Elsevier, 1993; 5–18.

(2) Muller R. *Traitement des varices par la phlébectomie ambulatoire.* Bull Soc Fr Phléb 1966; 19:277–279.

(3) Muller R. *Mise au point sur la phlébectomie ambulatoire selon Muller.* Phlébologie 1996; 49:335–344.

(4) Ramelet AA, Monti M. *Phlebology, The guide*. Elsevier: Paris 1999

(5) Ramelet AA. *La phlébectomie selon Muller : technique, avantages, désavantages.* J Mal Vasc 1991; 16:119–122.

(6) Fratila A, Rabe E, Kreysel HW. *Percutaneous minisurgical phlebectomy.* Seminars in Dermatology 1993; 12:117–122.

(7) Muller R, Bacci PA. *La flebectomia ambulatoriale.* Roma: Salus Editrice Internazionale, 1987.

(8) Muller R, Joubert B. *La phlébectomie ambulatoire: de l'anatomie au geste.* Paris: Editions Médicales Innothera, 1994.

(9) Ramelet AA. *Muller phlebectomy, a new phlebectomy hook.* J Dermatol Surg Oncol 1991; 17:814–816.

(10) Weiss RA, Goldmann MP. *Transillumination mapping prior to ambulatory phlebectomy.* Dermatol Surg 1988; 24:447–450.

(11) Larson PO, Ragi G, Swandby M, Darcey B, Polzin G, Carey P. *Stability of buffered lidocaine and epinephrine used for local anesthesia.* J Dermatol Surg Oncol 1991; 17:411–414.

(12) Vidal-Michel JP, Arditi J, Bourbon JH, Bonerandi JJ. *L'anesthésie locale au cours de la phlébectomie ambulatoire selon la méthode de R. Muller.* Phlébologie 1990; 43:305–315.

(13) Krusche PP, Lauven PM, Frings N. *Infiltrationsanästhesie bei varizenstripping.* Phlebol 1995; 24:48–51.

(14) Sommer B, Sattler G. *Tumeszenzlokal anästhesie.* Hautarzt 1998; 49:351–360.

(15) Smith SR, Goldman MP. *Tumescent anesthesia in ambulatory phlebectomy.* Dermatol Surg 1998; 24:453–456.

(16) Ramelet AA. *Die behandlung der besenreiservarizen: indikationen der phlebektomie nach Muller.* Phlebol 1993; 22:163–167.

(17) Ramelet AA. *Le traitement des télangiectasies: indications de la phlébectomie selon Muller.* Phlébologie 1994; 47:377–381.

(18) Ramelet AA. *Une complication rare de la phlébectomie ambulatoire, le granulome silicotique.* Phlébologie 1991; 44:865–871.

(19) Eichlisberger R, Moucka J, Frauchiger B, Jäger K. *Ambulante phlebektomie: das resultat aus der sicht des patienten und des behandelnden arzt.* VASA 1992; 21:453.

(20) Oesch A. *Begleitverletzungen bei den neueren techniken der varizenchirurgie.* VASA 1988; 17:318.

(21) Ramelet AA. *Complications of ambulatory phlebectomy.* Dermatol Surg 1997; 23:947–954,

(22) Vion B, Buri G, Ramelet AA. *Necrobiosis lipoidica and silicotic granuloma on Muller's phlebectomy scars.* Dermatology 1997;194:55–58

CHAPTER 23

RF-Mediated Endovenous Occlusion

Introduction

Radio-frequency (RF) energy can be delivered through a specially designed endovenous electrode to accomplish controlled heating of the vessel wall, causing vein shrinkage or occlusion by contraction of venous wall collagen. With worldwide clinical experience on over 800 patients over 3 years, this technique has rapidly been added to the armamentarium of ways to deal with axial venous reflux. This endovenous occlusion technique is primarily available as an alternative to saphenofemoral ligation and/or stripping, but can serve as a substitute for duplex-guided sclerotherapy and other venous ablation techniques.

Although the concept of endovenous elimination of reflux is not new, previous approaches have relied on electrocoagulation of blood, causing thrombus to occlude the vein. The potential for recanalization of the thrombus is high. Within cardiology, application of radiofrequency directly to tissue, not blood, has been effectively applied for ablation of abnormal conduction pathways for arrhythmias.[1] Venous occlusion by RF by the mechanism of venous blood coagulation has been previously reported, but is different than the modern approach.[2,3] Another term in the medical literature, endovascular diathermic vessel occlusion, is a technique in which a spider-shaped intravascular electrode produces venous occlusion by electrocoagulation with minimal perivascular damage.[4]

Technology

Directing RF energy into tissue to cause its destruction is potentially safer and more controllable than other mechanisms for doing so. Delivered in continuous or sinusoidal wave mode, and using a high frequency between 200 and 3,000 kHz, there is no stimulation of neuromuscular cells. The mechanism by which RF current heats tissue is resistive (or ohmic) heating of a narrow rim (less than 1 mm) of tissue that is in direct contact with the electrode. Deeper tissue planes may be slowly heated by conduction from the small volume region of heating. This is part of the process whereby heat is dissipated by conduction into surrounding normothermic tissue.[5] By carefully regulating the degree of heating with microprocessor control, subtle gradations of ei-

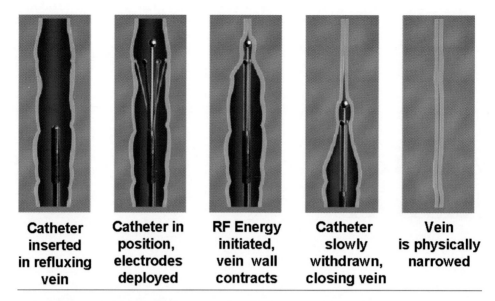

| Catheter inserted in refluxing vein | Catheter in position, electrodes deployed | RF Energy initiated, vein wall contracts | Catheter slowly withdrawn, closing vein | Vein is physically narrowed |

Figure 23-1.   Schematic diagram of use of the Closure™ catheter (Courtesy VNUS Medical Technologies, Sunnyvale, CA).

ther controlled collagen contraction or total thermocoagulation of the vein wall can be achieved.

When carefully feedback-controlled with a thermocouple, this is a relatively safe process since the temperature increase remains localized around the active electrode provided that close, stable contact between the active electrode and the vessel wall is maintained. By limiting temperature to 85°C, boiling, vaporization, and carbonization of the tissues is avoided.[6] Electrode-mediated RF vessel wall ablation is a self-limiting process. As coagulation of tissue occurs, there is a marked decrease in impedance that limits heat generation.[7] Alternatively, if clot builds up on the electrodes, blood is heated instead of tissue, and there is a marked rise in impedance (resistance to RF). The RF generator can be programmed to rapidly shutdown when impedance rises, thus assuring minimal heating of blood, but efficient heating of the vein wall.

Recent technological advances, including introduction of specific application electrodes and accompanying microprocessor-controlled systems to precisely monitor the electrical and thermal effects, have allowed the safe application of this technology. One such system is the Closure™ catheter (VNUS Medical Technologies, Sunnyvale, CA). This device produces precise tissue destruction with a reduction in the occurrence of undesirable effects, such as the formation of coagulum. Immediate evaluation of the anatomic lesional effect by duplex ultrasound is performed. For the Closure™ catheter system, bipolar electrodes are placed in contact with the vein wall. When the vein wall contracts, the electrodes fold up within that vein, allowing maximal physical contraction (Figure 23-1). Selective insulation of the electrodes results in a preferential delivery of the RF energy to the vein wall and minimal heating of the blood within the vessel. Animal experiments (described later) demonstrate endothelial denudation along with denaturation of media

and intramural collagen, with a subsequent fibrotic seal of vein lumen.

The catheter design includes collapsible catheter electrodes around which the vein may shrink, and a central lumen to allow a guidewire and/or fluid delivery structured within the 5-French (1.7-mm) catheter. This permits treatment of veins as small as 2 mm and as large as 8 mm. A larger 8-French catheter allows treatment of saphenous veins up to 1.2 mm in diameter (Figure 23-2). Both catheters have thermocouples on the electrodes embedded in the vein wall which measure temperature and provide feedback to the RF generator for temperature stabilization. The control unit (Figure 23-3) displays power, impedance, temperature, and elapsed time so that precise control may be obtained. The unit delivers the minimum power necessary to maintain the

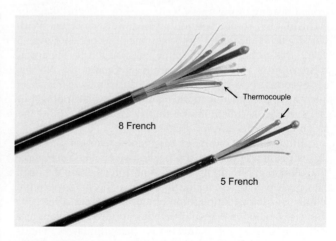

Figure 23-2.   The design of the two sizes of Closure catheters presently available.

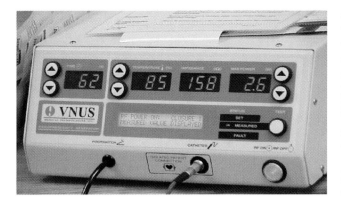

Figure 23-3. Control unit of microprocessor-controlled RF delivery. Note prominent display of (left to right) time, temperature, impedance, watts.

desired electrode temperature. For safety, if a coagulum forms on the electrodes, the impedance rises rapidly and the programmed RF generator automatically cuts off.

Animal Studies

Initial animal studies comparing RF ablation with a potent sclerosing solution were performed on goat rear-limb saphenous veins. Thirteen adult goats were treated by the

endovenous RF occlusion device with a pretreatment mean vein diameter of 5.3 mm. Percutaneous access obtained through a 5-French introducer sheath permits introduction of the RF catheter positioned at the treatment site under fluoroscopic guidance. Blood flow is impeded and as RF is applied the catheter is moved distally along the vein, causing immediate contraction and cessation of flow *(Figure 23-4)*. The electrodes maintain direct contact with the vein wall to maximize vein wall heating and minimize blood coagulation.

Acute observations indicate that 92% of limbs treated had a significant reduction of vein diameter, with a mean diameter reduction of 5.3–1.1 mm. At 6 weeks, persistent occlusion is maintained with no flow through the treatment site. Collateral flow is visible with high-pressure venography. Those veins that did not immediately occlude demonstrated total occlusion within one week. Figure 23-5 summarizes treatment results of RF vein occlusion of goat saphenous vein.

In contrast, sclerotherapy of the posterior-limb saphenous vein from five goats utilizing 0.5–1 cc of 3% sodium tetradecyl sulfate delivered under duplex guidance showed no evidence of occlusion. This was despite compressing the limb for 72 hours, compared with no compression following RF occlusion. Mean diameter change for sclerotherapy was from 5 mm pretreatment to 4 mm posttreatment, with almost no change at 5 weeks follow-up. The goat saphenous vein is a high-flow vessel, and sclerotherapy would not be predicted to be very effective as sclerosing solutions require

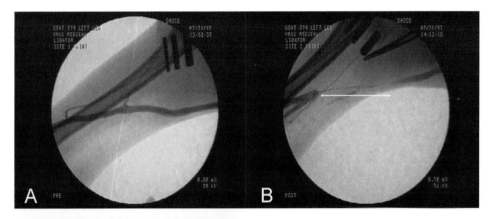

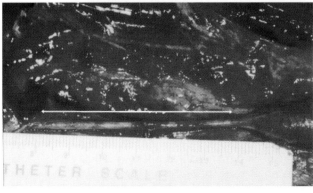

C

Figure 23-4. Fluoroscopic guidance and direct visualization of the Closure™ catheter demonstrates occlusion. **(A)** Injection of radiopaque contrast before treatment **(B)** Immediately posttreatment no flow is seen after injection of contrast material in the segment shown by *arrow*. **(C)** Similar segment seen intraoperatively 6 weeks after RF occlusion. Occluded segment is shown by *arrow*.

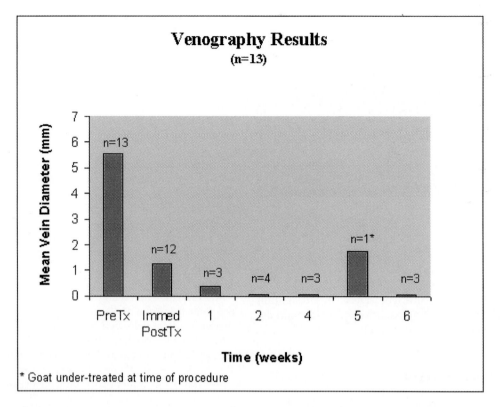

Figure 23-5.   Graph of vein diameter reduction (in mm) as measured by venography. Complete closure is maintained at the conclusion of follow-up at 6 weeks except in one undertreated saphenous vein.

time to interact with the vessel wall, and would be washed away quickly here.[8,9]

Histology

Histologic changes confirm the clinical findings in the animal study. With sclerotherapy, limited endothelial denudation accompanied by some loss of birefringence in vessel wall and 1 mm of surrounding tissue can be seen. No differences between acute and follow-up specimens are noted. For RF occlusion, the acute changes show a 65% reduction in vessel lumen. Acute histologic features include denudation of endothelium, some thrombus formation, thickened vessel walls, denaturation of tissue with loss of collagen birefringence, and neutrophil (PMN) inflamma-tion (*Figure 23-6*). Depth of vein wall damage is limited to 1–2 mm.

Six weeks following RF occlusion chronic histologic changes show further reduction in lumen diameter to complete occlusion. A small residual lumen may be recognized, but occluded by organized fibrous thrombi through the length of treated vein. Thrombus extension did not occur beyond the treatment site. Birefringence is almost fully restored with new collagen growth detected. Electron microscopic findings confirm the light microscopic findings with marked endothelial damage and loss of the endothelium, neutrophils in vessel lumen, and thickened, bulbous collagen fibrils (*Fig-*

ure 23-7). This indicates heat-induced contraction of collagen fibers and is indistinguishable from those changes seen with CO_2 laser-resurfacing-induced collagen contraction.

The conclusion reached from these histologic findings is that acute contraction of myocytes and fibroblasts from thermal denaturation occurs. This is accompanied by acute constriction and folding of intercellular matrix and collagen bundles. Abundant new collagen and intercellular matrix formation appears within several weeks following RF occlusion. The result is a thickened vein wall with further constriction of lumen diameter. The potential safety of this technique is supported by the fact that in animal studies there has been no evidence of thrombus extension, while the zone of thermal damage has been limited to no more than 2 mm beyond the targeted vessel. A high acute success rate of 92% is followed by long-term vessel occlusion.

Clinical Experience

Three years of clinical experience suggest that the Closure™ procedure is effective at occluding saphenous veins and abolishing reflux. Enrollment criteria for the first group of patients was symptomatic saphenous reflux with a saphenous vein diameter of 2–12 mm. The composition of treated patients was 24% male and 76% female. Mean age was 47.2 +/– 12.6, with a mean vein diameter of 7.4 mm.

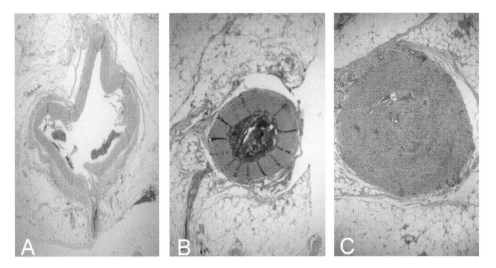

Figure 23-6.   Histology of RF occlusion. **(A)** Before treatment **(B)** Acute histologic features of RF occlusion. **(C)** At 6 weeks demonstrating fibrous cord with no recanalization (H & E 100X).

Most of the veins treated were above-knee greater saphenous (73%), some entire greater saphenous (21%), with the remaining including below-knee greater saphenous, lesser saphenous, and accessory saphenous. Adjunctive procedures performed at the time of treatment were phlebectomy on more distal branches in 61% and high ligation in 21%, but the adjunctive procedures did not affect outcome.

Vein occlusion at 1 week has been documented by duplex ultrasound in 300 out of 308 legs, a success rate of 97%. Occlusion persisted at 6 weeks in 95% and at 6 months in 92%. To date all the patients followed from 6 months to 12 months have remained occluded; in other words, if the saphenous vein is closed at 6 months, this will persist to 12 months and beyond. In our patients, we typically see closure of all the major tributaries at the saphenofemoral junction (SFJ) except for the superficial epigastric, which continues to empty superiorly into the common femoral vein. We believe that there is a high margin of safety by maintaining flow through this tributary. The high flow rate appears to diminish the possibility of extension of any thrombus (in the unlikely event that this would occur) from the greater saphenous vein (GSV). In our personal experience, thrombus has not been observed.

For clinical symptoms, the RF endovenous occlusion procedure rapidly reduces patient pain, fatigue, and aching correlating with a reduction in Clinical, Etiologic, Anatomic, and Pathophysiologic (CEAP) clinical class for symptoms and clinical severity of disease *(Table 23-1)*. When patients have

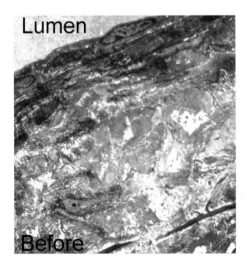 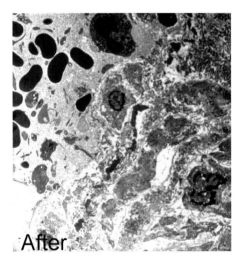

Figure 23-7.   Electron micrographs of histologic appearance before (left) and immediately after (right) RF occlusion of goat saphenous vein. Lumen is on upper left. Note complete destruction of endothelium in the after photograph.

Table 23-1
CEAP Class Description with Findings after Endovenous RF Occlusion

CEAP Clinical class	*Description*
0	Asymptomatic
1	Telangiectasia
2	Varicose veins
3	Edema
4	Skin changes
5	Healed venous ulcer
6	Venous ulcer

	Mean CEAP Class		
Closure Study Population	*Pre-treatment*	*Six weeks*	*Six months*
Pre-treatment, CEAP class = 2	2.0	0.5	0.5
Pre-treatment, CEAP class = 3	3.0	0.5	0.3
Pre-treatment, CEAP class = 4	4.0	2.3	1.4
Total	2.4	0.8	0.6

had surgical stripping on the opposite leg as a comparison, the degree of pain, tenderness, and bruising have been far greater on the leg treated by stripping. Side effects of the Closure™ technique have included thrombus extension from the proximal greater saphenous vein in 0.8% of cases, with one case of pulmonary embolus. Skin burn (prior to the tumescent anesthesia technique) occurs in 2.5%, clinical phlebitis at 6 weeks in 5.7%, and temporary quarter-sized areas of paresthesia in 10%, with most of these occurring immediately above the knee and resolving within 6–12 months. Thus compared to most techniques but in particular traditional surgery of ligation and stripping of similar size saphenous veins, the effectiveness of endovenous RF occlusion is quite high.

Technique of Closure

The patient undergoes the diagnostic process as outlined below. Patients with reflux in the greater or lesser saphenous vein are candidates if the vein size does not exceed 1.2 mm. Reflux may originate at the junction itself, as this region may be safely treated. After eliciting a detailed history as with other venous procedures, and describing alternative procedures such as ligation and stripping in detail, the patient signs the appropriate consent form *(Figure 23-8)*.

The procedure begins with the vein to be treated marked on the skin using duplex ultrasound *(Figure 23-9)*. An appropriate entry point is selected. This is usually just below where reflux is no longer seen in the greater saphenous vein, or where the vein becomes too small to cannulate with a 16-gauge introducer set. For the majority of patients in our series this is at a point just above or below the knee along the course of the GSV. Before proceeding, the patient's feet are wrapped in warm material or socks to minimize vasoconstriction, a heating pad is placed under the thigh, and a small amount of 2% Nitrol paste is rubbed onto the intended entry point to minimize vasoconstriction during the initial cannulation process.

The patient is prepped and draped, and 0.1 cc of 1% lidocaine without epinephrine is injected at the premarked site. With duplex guidance, a 16-gauge needle is inserted

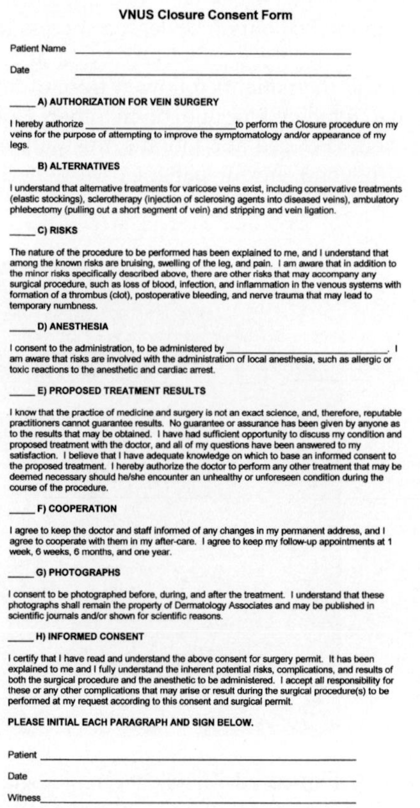

VNUS Closure Consent Form

Patient Name ____________________

Date ____________________

_____ A) AUTHORIZATION FOR VEIN SURGERY

I hereby authorize ____________________ to perform the Closure procedure on my veins for the purpose of attempting to improve the symptomatology and/or appearance of my legs.

_____ B) ALTERNATIVES

I understand that alternative treatments for varicose veins exist, including conservative treatments (elastic stockings), sclerotherapy (injection of sclerosing agents into diseased veins), ambulatory phlebectomy (pulling out a short segment of vein) and stripping and vein ligation.

_____ C) RISKS

The nature of the procedure to be performed has been explained to me, and I understand that among the known risks are bruising, swelling of the leg, and pain. I am aware that in addition to the minor risks specifically described above, there are other risks that may accompany any surgical procedure, such as loss of blood, infection, and inflammation in the venous systems with formation of a thrombus (clot), postoperative bleeding, and nerve trauma that may lead to temporary numbness.

_____ D) ANESTHESIA

I consent to the administration, to be administered by ____________________. I am aware that risks are involved with the administration of local anesthesia, such as allergic or toxic reactions to the anesthetic and cardiac arrest.

_____ E) PROPOSED TREATMENT RESULTS

I know that the practice of medicine and surgery is not an exact science, and, therefore, reputable practitioners cannot guarantee results. No guarantee or assurance has been given by anyone as to the results that may be obtained. I have had sufficient opportunity to discuss my condition and proposed treatment with the doctor, and all of my questions have been answered to my satisfaction. I believe that I have adequate knowledge on which to base an informed consent to the proposed treatment. I hereby authorize the doctor to perform any other treatment that may be deemed necessary should he/she encounter an unhealthy or unforeseen condition during the course of the procedure.

_____ F) COOPERATION

I agree to keep the doctor and staff informed of any changes in my permanent address, and I agree to cooperate with them in my after-care. I agree to keep my follow-up appointments at 1 week, 6 weeks, 6 months, and one year.

_____ G) PHOTOGRAPHS

I consent to be photographed before, during, and after the treatment. I understand that these photographs shall remain the property of Dermatology Associates and may be published in scientific journals and/or shown for scientific reasons.

_____ H) INFORMED CONSENT

I certify that I have read and understand the above consent for surgery permit. It has been explained to me and I fully understand the inherent potential risks, complications, and results of both the surgical procedure and the anesthetic to be administered. I accept all responsibility for these or any other complications that may arise or result during the surgical procedure(s) to be performed at my request according to this consent and surgical permit.

PLEASE INITIAL EACH PARAGRAPH AND SIGN BELOW.

Patient ____________________

Date ____________________

Witness ____________________

Figure 23-8. Consent form for Closure procedure.

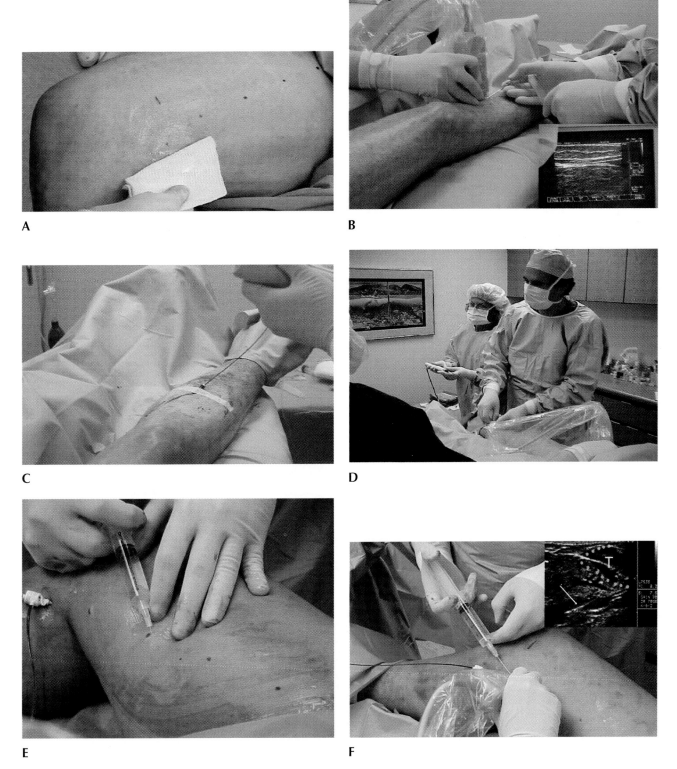

A

B

C

D

E

F

Figure 23-9. How to perform the Closure procedure. **(A)** Marking of the course of the GSV with specific entry point noted by *line*. Nitroglycerine paste is placed on the intended entry point to cause venous dilatation. **(B)** Needle puncture guided by duplex. Entry site monitored on duplex screen showing appearance of 16-gauge needle or angiocatheter (inset). **(C)** Guidewire passed through 16-gauge needle or angiocatheter. **(D)** Closure™ catheter advanced through sheath to saphenofemoral junction. **(E)** Sheath seen on left in skin. Local anesthesia begins once the Closure™ catheter has been correctly placed at the SFJ. **(F)** Tumescent anesthesia may be guided by duplex ultrasound to insure that anesthesia is being placed between the skin and the vein, rather than below the vein. At least 2 cm of space is desirable between the treated vein and the skin to minimize risks to the skin. Inset shows tumescent fluid (*T*) outlined by dots pushing down on the GSV. Catheter in vein is shown by *arrow*.

(continued)

217

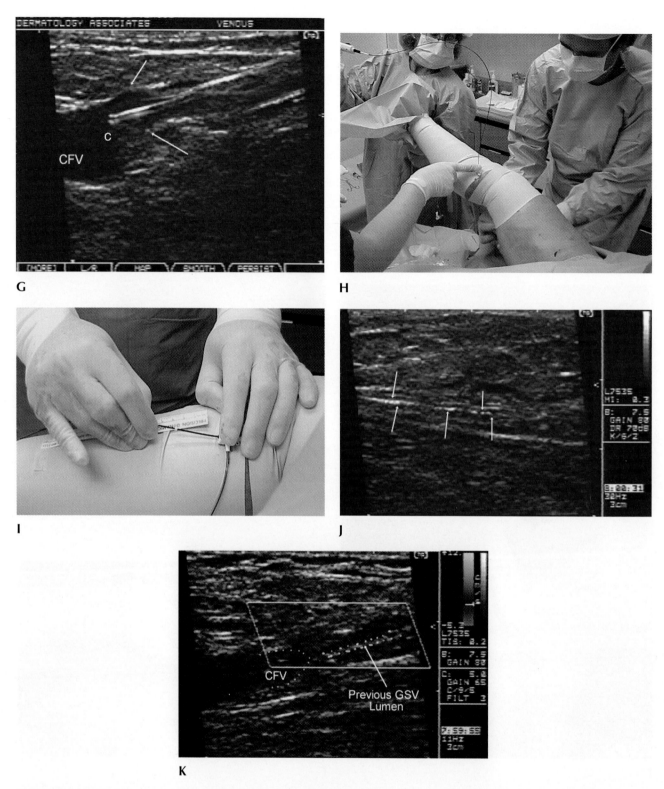

Figure 23-9. *Continued.* How to perform the Closure procedure. **(G)** Correct placement of the catheter at the SFJ (before tumescence). *Arrows* indicate base of terminal valves where electrodes initiate contact for RF occlusion. **(H)** After tumescent anesthesia, the leg is wrapped with a short-stretch bandage to compress the GSV and minimize blood within the vein. **(I)** After reconfirming the tip of the Closure™ catheter, the RF is turned on and slow pullback is initiated guided by a ruler taped to the bandage. Pullback rate is 2–2.5 cm/min. **(J)** After completion of pullback and removal of the catheter, the immediate success of the technique is monitored by duplex ultrasound. This view of the mid-thigh shows the proper endpoint of a thickened cord (*arrows*) with no flow visible and no recognizable or compressible GSV. **(K)** View at the SFJ immediately after RF occlusion. Common femoral vein (*CFV*) has normal flow while the GSV shows shrinkage and no color flow. Previous GSV lumen is occluded. Similar findings are seen in our patients at one year.

through the skin and guided into the saphenous vein *(Figure 23-9)*. When venous return is noted through the attached syringe, the Closure ™ catheter may at this point be placed directly through the needle into the vein. Because this permits some slow leakage of blood around the Closure catheter during the procedure, we prefer to insert a sheath through which the Closure catheter is then advanced. Others prefer gaining entry via a venous cutdown or pulling of the vein close to the surface with an ambulatory phlebectomy hook. Our technique requires one needle puncture only, and is more likely to result in better cosmesis.

In order to place the sheath a guidewire must be first inserted through the 16-gauge needle initially inserted into the skin. The guidewire is passed approximately 5 cm into the GSV. The sheath is then threaded along the guidewire, piercing the skin; its progress is followed by duplex ultrasound until it is seen firmly placed within the lumen of the GSV. After establishing the intraluminal placement of the sheath, the guidewire is carefully withdrawn.

The Closure catheter, with a diluted heparin solution slowly running through a central lumen, is now inserted through the sheath. Its progress up the GSV is monitored by duplex. If the catheter gets hung-up on a valve or slight bend of the GSV, no additional force is used or perforation will occur. Rather, the catheter is twisted or external pressure is applied to the leg to change the shape of the GSV. Sometimes the patient must rotate the leg.

Once the Closure catheter is in place, tumescent anesthesia (consisting of 0.25%–0.5% lidocaine neutralized to pH 7 with sodium bicarb) is injected between the skin and the cannulated GSV. Tumescent anesthesia volume is typically 60–120 cc for the course of the vein along the thigh. Duplex monitoring of the anesthesia injection at the SFJ is recommended as the shape of the SFJ is changed from the round "hook" to a straighter path.

The leg is then wrapped with a short stretch bandage from the ankle to the mid-thigh. This minimizes blood return from the GSV, further diminishing the size of the GSV and reducing the possibility of heating blood rather than vein wall. When the leg wrapping has not been tight enough, we have observed a much higher likelihood of a small coagulum building up at the electrodes of the Closure catheter.

Once the leg is wrapped, the final check of the position of the catheter is made with duplex ultrasound. The tip is positioned with the electrodes deployed. The tips of the electrodes are placed so that they align with the base of the terminal valve cusps. Once positioned, an impedance and temperature check is performed to make sure the catheter is functioning properly. Impedance of the vein wall should be between 200 and 350 ohms, and the thermocouple should transmit a baseline temperature of 33–37°C.

The RF is then applied; the physician monitors the temperature and impedance. Within 15 seconds the target temperature of 85°C should be reached. If this does not occur, the catheter has been mistakenly advanced too far into the common femoral vein. Impedance would most likely rise quickly and the RF generator shut down automatically.

After target temperature is achieved, one waits 10–15 seconds, and then slow withdrawal of the catheter begins. The first 4 cm are treated over 3 minutes, but then the catheter is advanced at a rate of 2.5 cm/min. If the patient experiences a sudden sharp pain, the catheter is pulled 1 mm past that point quickly to minimize the possibility of nerve injury. If a sharp drop in temperature occurs during pullback, this most likely represents a large branch point or perforator, and the catheter is temporarily held in place for 5–10 s until 85°C is reached again.

When the catheter has been pulled back to the introducer sheath site, impedance will suddenly rise and the RF generator cut off. Duplex ultrasound of the SFJ should reveal no flow, except the superficial epigastric emptying into the common femoral vein. The GSV should be more echogenic with thicker-appearing walls. If flow is seen in the GSV, the procedure may be repeated, assuming the Closure catheter can be advanced past the treated distal segment. If one cannot pass the catheter easily no repeat treatment is performed, as vein perforation would be the most likely outcome of such an attempt.

Follow-up Care

Class 2 compression hosiery is worn for 3 days. Patients will note some bruising from the tumescent anesthesia. Anesthesia of the treated portion of the leg may persist for 8–24 hr. To gain experience, we recommend that for the initial cases, one reevaluate the treated veins at three days by duplex ultrasound. This will allow correlation of results with the pullback rate or any difficulty encountered during the procedure. Once comfortable with the procedure, the physician may want to see the patient for a duplex ultrasound follow-up at 6 weeks. At that time, any open segments can be treated by duplex-guided sclerotherapy. It has been our experience that when closed at 6 weeks, the GSV will remain closed, fibrosed, and almost indistinguishable from surrounding tissue at 6 months in all cases. Symptom reduction is rapid, with many patients experiencing relief at 3 days, but some not until 6 weeks *(Figure 23-10)*. Clinical improvement in appearance of varicosities is typically seen within

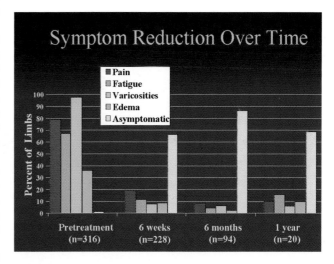

Figure 23-10. Symptom reduction in worldwide clinical data (courtesy of VNUS Medical).

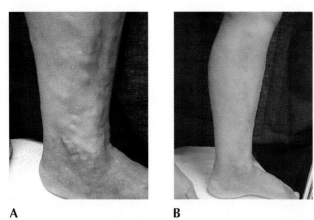
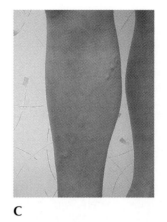
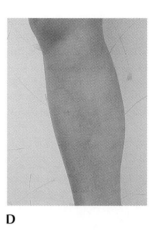

A   B   C   D

Figure 23-11.   Two cases of before and after VNUS Closure™ **(A)** Woman with large varicosities for 20 years and mild changes of chronic venous insufficiency with major reflux originating at the SFJ (before). **(B)** Two weeks after RF occlusion of the GSV along with ambulatory phlebectomy of the veins below the knee. The symptoms and signs of pain, fatigue, and edema resolved totally. **(C)** Young woman, aged 28, with recent onset of small varicosities traced to reflux at the SFJ occurring during her second pregnancy (immediately before treatment). **(D)** Six weeks after treatment showing complete clearance. Only two punctures were necessary for the accompanying ambulatory phlebectomy of small side branches of the incompetent GSV. Treatment resulted in rapid alleviation of symptoms of leg fatigue.

6 weeks as well *(Figure 23-11)*. Although the patient instructions after the Closure™ technique are very straightforward, including 3 days of compression, an instruction sheet is still provided *(Figure 23-12)*.

Side Effects

In our experience, two patients have developed focal numbness 4 cm in diameter on the lower medial leg. This resolved within 6 months. Since adopting the principles of using

POST CLOSURE INSTRUCTIONS

1. Keep bandage and stockings on until bedtime. If your toes turn blue or feel numb, call the doctor immediately.

2. You can resume **normal** activities today (walking is okay).

3. You can resume exercising in 3 days (no weights with the legs for 1 week).

4. You can take a shower this evening but no hot baths for 1 week (the steri-strip needs to stay on for at least one week).

5. Wear your support hose for 3 days, from first thing in the morning (ideally, take a quick 5 minute shower and then put them on before doing the rest of your morning ritual), until last thing at night.

6. Schedule the next follow-up visit in one week.

7. Bruising, local swelling and some tenderness are normal after surgery, but please feel free to call the office if you have any questions.

Figure 23-12.   Postoperative patient instructions for Closure™.

tumescent anesthesia while moving the catheter rapidly distal to any points of sharp pain, no paresthesias have been noted. No skin injury or thrombus has been observed in any of our patients.

Worldwide data indicates thigh paresthesias have not persisted beyond 1 year and usually resolve spontaneously within 6 months. Even when paresthesia occurred, the statistics of satisfaction with the procedure remain unchanged. Ninety-five percent of treated patients would recommend this procedure to a friend (data on file at VNUS Medical). In a few patients who have had bilateral comparison of ligation plus stripping versus endovenous RF occlusion, all the patients reported significantly less side effects with endovenous RF occlusion (data on file at VNUS Medical). A recent study on 10 patients showed no side effects other than erythema and brusing.[10]

Summary

A new technique for endovenous occlusion using radiofrequency ablation catheters offers a less invasive alternative to ligation and stripping, as well as a safer alternative to duplex-guided sclerotherapy of saphenous trunks and junctions. Initial clinical experience in hundreds of patients shows a high degree of success with minimal side effects, most of which can be prevented or minimized with minor modifications of the technique. In the near future, many venous ablative procedures involving saphenous trunks may be replaced or supplemented by this technique.

References

(1) Olgin JE, Kalman JM, Chin M, Stillson C, Maguire M, Ursel P, et al. *Electrophysiological effects of long, linear atrial lesions placed*

under intracardiac ultrasound guidance. Circulation 1997; 96(8):2715–2721.

(2) Van Cleef JF. La "nouvelle electrocoagulation" en phlebologie. Phlebologie (Fr) 1987; 40(2):423–426.

(3) Gradman WS. Venoscopic obliteration of variceal tributaries using monopolar electrocautery. Preliminary report. J Dermatol Surg Oncol 1994; 20(7):482–485.

(4) Cragg AH, Galliani CA, Rysavy JA, Castaneda-Zuniga WR, Amplatz K. Endovascular diathermic vessel occlusion. Radiology 1982; 144(2):303–308.

(5) Haines DE. The biophysics of radiofrequency catheter ablation in the heart: the importance of temperature monitoring. Pacing Clin Electrophysiol 1993; 16(3 Pt 2):586–591.

(6) Haines DE, Verow AF. Observations on electrode-tissue interface temperature and effect on electrical impedance during radiofrequency ablation of ventricular myocardium. Circulation 1990; 82(3):1034–1038.

(7) Lavergne T, Sebag C, Ollitrault J, Chouari S, Copie X, Le HJ, et al. [Radiofrequency ablation: physical bases and principles]. Arch Mal Coeur Vaiss 1996; 89 Spec No 1:57–63.

(8) Goldman MP, Sadick NS, Weiss RA. Cutaneous necrosis, telangiectatic matting, and hyperpigmentation following sclerotherapy, etiology, prevention, and treatment. [review]. Dermatol Surg 1995; 21(1):19–29.

(9) Green D. Mechanism of action of sclerotherapy. Semin Dermatol 1993; 12:88–97.

(10) Goldman MP. Closure of the greater saphenous vein with endoluminal radiofrequency thermal heating of the vein wall in combination with ambulatory phlebectomy: preliminary 6-month follow-up. Dermatol Surg 2000; 26(5):452–456.

PART IV

Problems

CHAPTER 24

Minimizing and Treating Complications

Introduction

The most commonly encountered complications of treatments for venous insufficiency are telangiectatic matting (TM), hyperpigmentation, and cutaneous necrosis. The first two of these problems are minor from a medical standpoint, and hopefully any necrosis would be minor as well, but all can be very distressing to the patient. Fortunately, meticulous technique can keep the incidence and severity of these problems at a very low level. Two additional complications that are not minor are inadvertent arterial injection and in-

advertent nerve injury. Prevention of these serious problems is critical, as there is no treatment that can prevent a bad outcome once these injuries have occurred.

Cutaneous Necrosis

ETIOLOGY

There are several causes of cutaneous necrosis, most common being the extravasation of sclerosant into perivascular tissues. This extravasation necrosis is most common with hypertonic saline, is seen with some regularity with most other agents, and is rare with polidocanol. Extravasation necrosis is rare in experienced hands, but is more common when a practitioner with little experience performs treatment.

A second type of cutaneous necrosis does not arise from extravasation, but rather from back-flow of sclerosant through an unsuspected cutaneous arteriovenous malformation, producing sclerosis of an endarteriole with subsequent necrosis of the cutaneous tissues depending on that arteriole. This type of necrosis can occur with the injection of any sclerosing agent, even under ideal circumstances, and does not necessarily represent physician error. Arteriolar spasm is believed to play a role in many of these cases. Cutaneous necrosis may also result from excessive local compression or from excessive traction on the skin (usually due to tape). Another cause of necrosis, direct intraarterial injection, should be avoidable by proper technique; one should cease injection immediately if a patient complains of sudden severe pain, as arterial puncture is much more painful than venipuncture.

Extravasation

During injection of an abnormal vein or telangiectasia, even the most adept physician may inadvertently inject a small quantity of sclerosing solution into the perivascular tissue. In some cases, sclerosant may flow back out of the vein when the needle is withdrawn. In others, vascular spasm causes the needle tip to pass completely through the small vessel, allowing sclerosant to be deposited in the deep perivenous tissues. Fragile veins may tear during needle placement, allowing immediate leakage during injection.

Sclerosing solutions vary in the degree of cellular necrosis they produce. Hypertonic saline at 23.4% is a caustic sclerosing agent, and when an inexperienced practitioner uses this agent, small spots of superficial epidermal damage often are seen at points of injection where a small bleb of the solution has escaped from the vein.[1]

In contrast to hypertonic saline, polidocanol (POL) was originally intended for subcutaneous injection as a local anesthetic agent, and is only minimally toxic to subcutaneous tissue. Nonetheless, extravasation of POL in sufficient concentration has occasionally been reported to cause necrosis.[2,3] Sodium tetradecyl sulfate is caustic to skin when injected extravascularly, and caution must be exercised with its use in smaller telangiectasias. When injected at concentrations of 0.1%, small amounts of extravasation are unlikely to cause any epidermal injury. High incidences of cutaneous breakdown have been reported with 0.5%–1% concentrations for superficial telangiectasias.[4] Chromated glycerine solutions are extremely weak sclerosants that have only rarely been reported to produce cutaneous necrosis.

Arteriolar injection

Approximately 4% of leg telangiectasia have some communication with a dermal arteriole.[5] Inadvertent flow of sclerosant through this communication is believed to be a cause of cutaneous ulcerations unrelated to extravasation. Excisional biopsies were performed in a small series of patients who developed ulceration after meticulous injection of tiny telangiectasias using low concentrations of POL, and in

every case there was a classic wedge-shaped arterial ulceration with an occluded feeding dermal arteriole at its center (*Figure 24-1*).[6]

Vasospasm

When sclerosant flows into a communicating arteriole, or when sclerosant is extravasated around a dermal arteriole, there is an immediate porcelain-white blanching in a roughly circular pattern. This blanching usually persists for many minutes, and in most cases a hemorrhagic patch forms over the area within 2–48 hours. This patch progresses to a bulla, which usually progresses to an ulcer. In many cases, it appears that arteriolar spasm may play some part in this process, as vigorous local massage and the application of a small amount of 2% nitroglycerin ointment have been reported to prevent the formation of the bulla and the subsequent ulceration.[7]

Excessive compression

Excessive compression of the skin overlying the treated vein may produce tissue anoxia and lead to localized cutaneous ulceration. Subcutaneous tissue flow in the leg is decreased when cutaneous pressure exceeds 20 mm Hg; pressures above 30 mm Hg may even reduce blood flow to the muscle in some patients.[8,9]

Arterial inflow pressure to the legs is highest when the patient is standing and lowest when the patient is recumbent. To avoid tissue ischemia, compression should not exceed 30–40 mm Hg at night, when the patient will be recumbent for many hours.

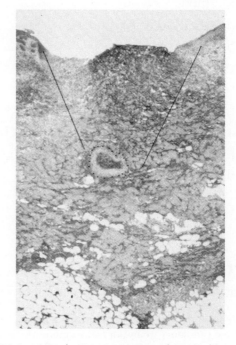

Figure 24-1. Histologic examination of 4-mm diameter ulceration after injection with POL 0.5%. Note wedge-shaped ulceration with a thrombosed artery at the base. (Hematoxylin-eosin x25) (Printed with permission from Mosby.)

If higher levels of compression are needed during periods of ambulation, a double layer of 20–30 mm Hg graduated compression stockings should be used. When the patient is recumbent, the outer stocking is removed, thereby decreasing the cutaneous pressure to 20–30 mm Hg at the ankle. This level of compression is well tolerated by most patients. Compression is further discussed in Chapter 15.

Traction necrosis of the skin occurs when tape exerts a pulling force that interferes with normal cutaneous flow. This most often results from improper application of tape, but can also develop when patient movement puts excessive traction on tape that originally was loosely applied (*Figure 24-2*).

PREVENTION

Meticulous technique is key to prevention of ulceration. Blanching that may indicate cutaneous arteriolar injection or arteriolar spasm is treated with vigorous local massage using a small amount of 2% nitroglycerine ointment. (To avoid a headache, the clinician should wear gloves when applying nitroglycerine ointment.) Careful attention to the application of tape and a compression garment over the tape will help to avoid traction necrosis, and careful selection of the correct size compression garment and the correct amount of compression for each patient will prevent compression necrosis.

If a small bleb of low concentration of solution is extravasated, it can usually be massaged for 1 minute and not cause harm to the skin (although this does not always work with hypertonic saline). It is not known whether extravasated solutions should be diluted by the injection of normal saline. There are case reports of good outcomes when dilution by injection has been performed,[1] but prospectively randomized animal studies suggest that efforts to dilute extravasated sclerosants only leads to an increased incidence of ulcers.[10] If dilution is attempted after hypertonic saline extravasation, it is necessary to inject a volume of normal saline at least 10 times that of the extravasated solution to limit osmotic damage. Detergent sclerosing solutions of high strength, such as concentrated sodium tetradecyl sulfate (STS), are also toxic to subcutaneous tissues if extravasated. Dilution may be attempted, but again, simple dilution has been reported to cause an increase, rather than a decrease, in the incidence of ulceration.

Instead of simple dilution with normal saline, dilution with a hyaluronidase solution has been shown to prevent necrosis in a variety of extravasation situations, including an animal model of sclerosant extravasation.[10] Hyaluronidase enzymatically breaks down connective tissue hyaluronic acid. It is believed that this may disrupt the normal interstitial fluid barrier, allowing rapid diffusion of solution through tissues, thereby increasing absorption. This beneficial effect reduces extravasation injuries from 10% dextrose, calcium and potassium salts, contrast media, sodium bicarbonate, aminophylline, hyperalimentation solution, and doxorubicin.[11,12] There are as yet no published studies with human data on hyaluronidase and reduction of extravasation damage from sclerotherapy solutions.

In addition to its enhanced dilutional ability, hyaluronidase may independently improve healing and cell survival and reduce scarring in a variety of situations.[13] Side effects from hyaluronidase are rare and generally of the urticarial type.[14,15]

If hyaluronidase is to be used, it must be reconstituted with 0.9% sodium chloride immediately before use. The ideal concentration and quantity to inject after extravasation has not been determined, but on an empiric basis, 300 USP units of hyaluronidase may be diluted in 5 ml of 0.9% sodium chloride and injected into the area of extravasation.

TREATMENT

Fortunately, when ulcerations do occur they are usually fairly small, averaging 4 mm in diameter. At this size, primary healing usually leaves an acceptable scar (*Figure 24-3*). Occlusive or hydrocolloid dressings result in an apparent decrease in wound healing time. More importantly, occlusive dressings decrease the pain associated with an open ulcer. Left alone, ulcers may take 4–6 weeks to completely heal. If this is unacceptable, then excision and primary closure is a reasonable alternative, depending on the anatomic location. Excision of the ulcer with split- or full-thickness grafting usually leads to a worse cosmetic result than healing by secondary intention.

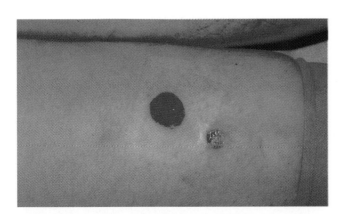

Figure 24-2. Friction blister formed from tape, leading to significant superficial ulceration.

Telangiectatic Matting

Telangiectatic matting™ refers to the appearance of tiny new red (occasionally violaceous) telangiectasias that appear in patients after sclerotherapy or surgical removal of varicose veins or venulectasia. Telangiectatic matting presents as "blush-type" regions containing large numbers of "new" blood vessels less than 0.2 mm in diameter, located in and around the site of treatment (*Figure 24-4*). Telangiectatic matting is often seen on the thighs, medial ankle, and medial and lateral calves. The inner thigh just above the knee is the most common site of telangiectatic matting.[16] This may be due to movement at the knee causing rapid fluctuations in venous pressure or to relative skin anoxia during sleep when the opposite knee in the lateral position compresses

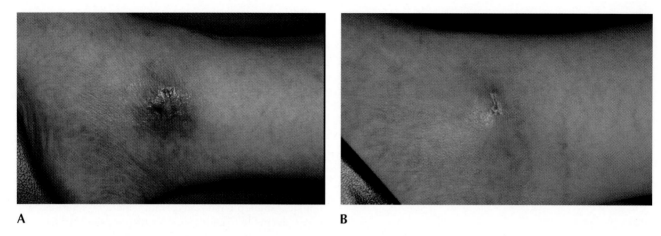

A   B

Figure 24-3. **(A)** Cutaneous ulceration 3 weeks after injection of ankle telangiectasia with POL 0.5%. An AV malformation was suspected. **(B)** After 2 months. Complete healing occurred after 6 weeks of hydrocolloid dressings.

this area. Microvessels that remain after treatment of larger telangiectasias can be confused with early telangiectatic matting. Photographs taken before treatment are helpful in distinguishing the two.

The incidence of TM is between 15% and 24%.[17,18] It is predominantly seen in women, but can also occur in men.[16] Telangiectatic matting may occasionally be associated with intolerable burning pain and leg edema.[19] TM usually resolves spontaneously in 3 to 12 months[17,20]; however, occasionally TM can be permanent, and pretreatment patient information should make this clear in an explicit manner.[21]

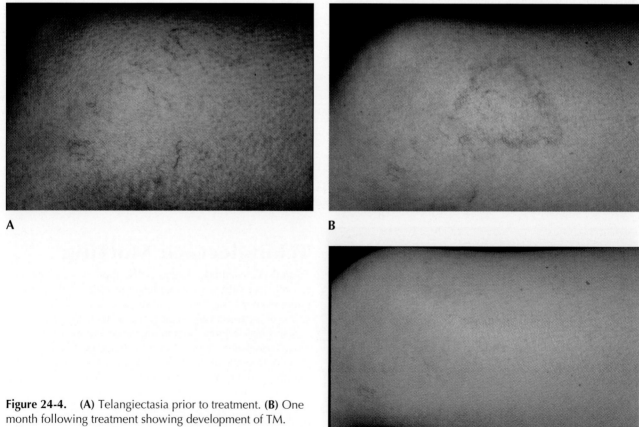

Figure 24-4. **(A)** Telangiectasia prior to treatment. **(B)** One month following treatment showing development of TM. **(C)** Spontaneous resolution at 6 months.

ETIOLOGY

The precise cause of telangiectatic matting remains unknown, and it is not even certain whether the tiny vessels that make up the blush are dilated vessels that already existed, or whether they are new vessels that have grown into the area.

One theory holds that angiogenic and inflammatory processes cause pre-existing subclinical blood vessels to dilate as they carry collateral flow from arteriovenous anastomoses.[22] Another theory maintains that matting represents angiogenesis: new blood vessels grow[23] as a natural reaction to the sclerotic obstruction of existing vessels and to meet increased metabolic demands caused by perivascular inflammation after sclerotherapy.[24,25]

Disruption of endothelial continuity and obstruction of outflow from a vessel (the results of sclerotherapy) are physical factors that are known to trigger angiogenesis. Besides physical factors, more than 40 circulating humoral factors have been implicated in angioneogenesis (Table 24-1). Numerous substances that can inhibit angiogenesis are under active investigation, but none are available for clinical use at this time.[26]

RISK FACTORS

Risk factors for TM have been a subject of great debate in the sclerotherapy literature. It is widely believed (though unproven) that TM is more common when higher infusion pressures, larger volumes, and higher concentrations of sclerosant are used. We have observed that when increased infusion pressure is utilized, resulting in blanching of the entire capillary network of the skin, TM is more likely to occur. Patient factors associated with an increased risk of TM include excessive body weight, a family history of telangiectasias, and longer duration of spider veins.[17] There is a decreased incidence of TM with aging,[27] possibly due to a decrease in dermal venular mast cells.[28]

Exogenous and endogenous increases in estrogen may be an important risk factor for matting,[29] but the mechanism for this is not clear. Estrogen is recognized as a receptor-mediated angiogenic factor in a variety of tumors, but conflicting reports of estrogen and progesterone receptors in telangiectasias make the role of hormones in TM uncertain. Most recently, however, estrogen-receptor levels were re-

ported higher in varicose segments of varicose veins compared with normal veins.[30] In addition, previous studies have shown that human saphenous veins from both sexes express progesterone receptors.[31] Yet when 10 patients with TM were examined for estrogen/progesterone receptors, all were negative. Sadick concluded that although estrogen and progesterone may play an indirect role in the development of postsclerotherapy TM via vasodilatory or secondary angiogenic or cytokine release mechanisms, they do not appear to play a primary role in promoting postsclerotherapy neoangiogenesis.[32]

PREVENTION

Efforts to minimize TM (Table 24-2) are especially important because treatment efforts (other than waiting) are often not successful. Several principles and techniques have been reported to decrease the incidence of TM.[20,33,34] The three most important recommendations are to use the minimal effective concentration of sclerosant for a given vessel, the lowest possible volume of sclerosant to flush the vessel, and the lowest possible infusion pressure to deliver the sclerosant. When a patient who is taking exogenous estrogens demonstrates a tendency toward telangiectatic matting, she may wish to temporarily stop the estrogen during the period of treatment. In the future, telangiectatic matting may be prevented by the addition of antiangiogenic substances to sclerosant solutions.

TREATMENT

The most important first step in treating this complication is to repeat the clinical evaluation of the patient, looking for any previously unrecognized sources of hydrostatic pressure. Transillumination (see Chapter 27 for specific devices) may help locate a previously unseen reticular vein. At the minimum, Doppler examination of the problem areas should be done to listen for unresolved reflux. Much more information can be gained from a duplex ultrasound examination. The duplex study should be performed in the standing position, because previously unrecognized high-pressure reflux from an intermittently incompetent (clinically inapparent) saphenous vein may be the culprit. When the saphenous vein itself is competent, duplex often reveals failed perforators and an unsuspected reticular feeding vessel lying below the subcutaneous tissues. Treatment of this vessel by sclerotherapy or phlebectomy usually causes resolution of the overlying telangiectatic mats (Figure 24-5).

Table 24-1
Biologic Activities of Angiogenic Factors on Endothelial Cells

Factor	Angiogenesis	Proliferation	Matting
Acid FGF	Yes	Yes	Yes
Basic FGF	Yes	Yes	Yes
Angiogenin	Yes	No	N.D.[a]
TGFα	Yes	Yes	No
TGFβ	Yes	Inhibition	No
Wound fluid	Yes	No	Yes
Prostaglandins	Yes	No	No
Adipocyte lipids	Yes	No	Yes

[a]N.D., not determined

Table 24-2
Minimize Occurrence of Telangiectatic Matting

Use minimal sclerosant concentrations.

Limit blanching per injection to an area 1–2 cm in diameter.

Use low injection pressures to avoid back-up of solution into capillaries.

Encourage weight loss prior to institution of therapy.

Consider discontinuing oral contraceptives or hormone replacement therapy for the duration of treatment.

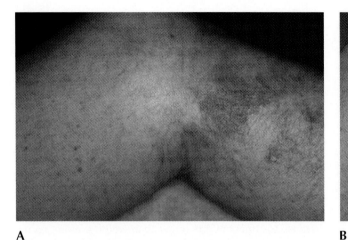
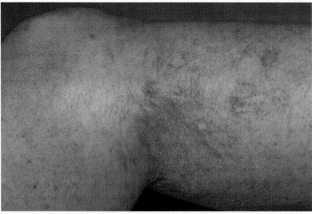

A   B

Figure 24-5. **(A)** Matting below medial knee arising from hidden incompetent saphenous tributary, found by duplex ultrasound. **(B)** Treatment of the refluxing vessel (which was located just proximal to the medial knee) by duplex-guided sclerotherapy resulted in significant clearing within 4 weeks. The matting was also treated with IPL, on the same day as the duplex-guided sclerotherapy.

The second most important part of the treatment plan is simply watchful waiting. The patient is given a mild anti-inflammatory cream to apply to the area, and photographs are taken of the area at 6–8 week intervals until resolution occurs. Patients can be reassured that even the worst matting can resolve completely over time, and are much more tolerant of this waiting period when they have been suitably informed before the start of treatment that TM may occur.

If there is no identifiable feeding vessel and if the matting does not resolve within a reasonable time, then the vessels that make up telangiectatic mats can themselves be treated by sclerotherapy. Disposable insulin syringes and 33-gauge needles can facilitate cannulation of these extremely small vessels. The new double-polariscopic Syris v300 or v600 may enhance visualization of the entry points into matting, facilitating injection even with a 30-gauge needle. In some patients the effort is successful, but in other patients the tiny vessels seem impervious to sclerosing agents. Treatment with high-intensity pulsed light is sometimes effective *(Figure 24-6)* [35], and treatment with pulsed dye laser has also been shown somewhat effective in treating matting that has proven resistant to other therapeutic modalities.[36] The copper bromide and long pulse yellow dye lasers may also turn out to be effective, but have yet to be tested.[37]

Postsclerotherapy Pigmentation

Postsclerotherapy pigmentation is persistent pigmentation (usually brown) along the course of a blood vessel that has been treated by sclerotherapy *(Figure 24-7)*. Pigmentation occurs in 10–30% of patients, and usually is noticed within 4 weeks of sclerotherapy. It often lasts from 6–12 months, in spite of attempts at therapy,[38] and although spontaneous resolution occurs in 70% of patients at 6 months, pigmenta-

tion may persist longer than 1 year in up to 10% of patients.[39]

INCIDENCE

The incidence of hyperpigmentation depends on the sclerosing agent, the concentration, and the technique used. In general, the incidence of hyperpigmentation is higher when a stronger agent is used and when stronger concentrations of an agent are used. Table 24-3 lists the reported range of incidence for various agents.

Table 24-3

Reported Incidence of Hyperpigmentation for Common Sclerotherapeutic Agents

Hypertonic saline[a]	10%–30%
Polidocanol[b]	11%–30%
Sodium tetradecyl sulfate[c]	11%–80%

[a]Based on Duffy DM. *Small vessel sclerotherapy: an overview.* Adv Dermatol 1988; 3: 221–242; Alderman DB. *Surgery and sclerotherapy in the treatment of varicose veins.* Conn Med 1975; 39: 467–471; Weiss RA, Weiss MA. *Resolution of pain associated with varicose and telangiectatic leg veins after compression sclerotherapy.* J Dermatol Surg Oncol 1990; 16: 333–336; Bodian EL. *Techniques of sclerotherapy for sunburst venous blemishes.* J Dermatol Surg Oncol 1985; 11: 696–704; Alderman DB. *Therapy for essential cutaneous telangiectasias.* Postgrad Med 1977; 61: 91–95.
[b]Based on Duffy DM, 1988; Weiss RA, Weiss MA. *Incidence of side effects in the treatment of telangiectasias by compression sclerotherapy: hypertonic saline vs. polidocanol.* J Dermatol Surg Oncol 1990; 16: 800–804; Goldman PM. *Sclerotherapy for superficial venules and telangiectasias of the lower extremities.* Dermatol Clin 1987; 5: 369–379.
[c]Based on Weiss RA, Weiss MA, 1990; Tournay PR. *Traitment sclerosant des tres fines varicosites intra ou saous-dermiques.* [Sclerosing treatment of very fine intra or subdermal varicosities]. Soc Fran de Phlebol 1966; 19: 235–241; Tretbar LL. *Spider angiomata: treatment with sclerosant injections.* J Kansas Med Soc 1978; 79: 198–200; Cloutier G, Sansoucy H. *Le traitement des varices des membres inferieurs par les injections sclerosantes.* L'Union Medicale du Canada 1975; 104: 1854–1863.

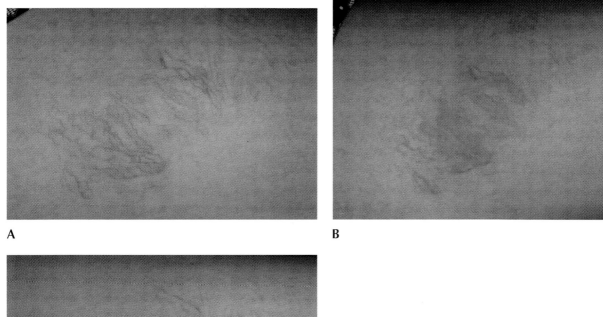

A

B

C

Figure 24-6. Reduction of postsclerotherapy telangiectatic matting by IPL. **(A)** Postsclerotherapy matting, medial thigh. **(B)** Immediately after IPL showing desired urticarial response. **(C)** Improvement at 6 weeks.

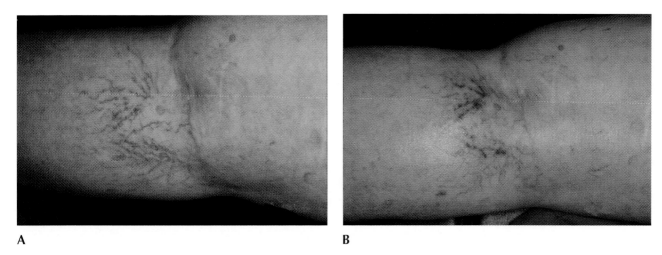

A

B

Figure 24-7. Postsclerotherapy hyperpigmentation. **(A)** Posterior thigh reticular and telangiectatic veins prior to treatment. **(B)** Six weeks following treatment, showing linear hyperpigmentation at the telangiectasia sites. Larger sources of reflux (the reticular veins) were not treated, enhancing hydrostatic pressure and causing leakage of red blood cells leading to pigmentation (hemosiderin deposits) at sites of sclerotherapy. This could have been minimized by injection of the reticular veins at the same time as treatment of the telangiectasias.

In certain patients hyperpigmentation may already be present along the course of superficial varicosities and telangiectasias before any therapy is performed, especially if reflux is long-standing or stasis dermatitis has occurred.[39,40] Careful preoperative documentation, including photographs, is essential to avoid confusion during follow-up patient visits.

ETIOLOGY

The etiology of this pigmentation most likely occurs from a combination of postinflammatory hyperpigmentation as well as direct hemosiderin deposition. Initial histologic examination shows the presence of hemosiderin that is present regardless of sclerosing solution type or baseline pigmentation of the patient.[38] Hemosiderin is an indigestible residue of hemoglobin degraded from red blood cells, which enter the dermis by extravasation after the rupture of treated vessels. Spontaneous hemosiderin pigmentation is also common in patients with chronic venous insufficiency.[41] Red cells also enter the dermal layer by erythrocyte diapedesis, which is triggered by phlebitis and other inflammatory states. Phagocytosis and digestion of red blood cells result in the deposition of hemosiderin in the form of aggregates up to 100 μm in diameter that may contain iron in several forms.[42] In its most insoluble form, iron hydroxide may take years to be eliminated from the dermis. Some speculate that free-radical formation resulting from local iron accumulation may also stimulate melanocytes to produce pigmentation. Several authors have demonstrated melanin incontinence in the presence of venous stasis with extravascular erythrocytes.[43,44]

RISK FACTORS

The risk of hyperpigmentation depends on a large number of factors, including general health, skin type, the size and depth of vessels to be treated, the location of vessels on the body, other medications being taken, and the type and concentration of sclerosant used. It has been suggested to use an individual's response to chromated glycerin injection as a test for susceptibility to pigmentation, since those patients that pigment with this mild sclerosing solution should be treated with only the mildest of solution; inflammatory reactions should be kept to a minimum.[45]

Patient factors

Patient factors play an important role in determining who will get hyperpigmentation after sclerotherapy. Total body iron stores, vessel fragility, increased sensitivity to histamines, elevated ferritin levels, and defects in iron transport have all been associated with an increased risk of postsclerotherapy pigmentation.[46] Hyperpigmentation is more common and more pronounced in patients with dark hair and dark-toned skin; we have observed postsclerotherapy pigmentation in at least one site in every Asian and African-American patient we have treated. This has occurred even with the mildest of sclerosing solutions. Patients with type IV, V, and VI skin are forewarned about the likelihood of temporary, and possibly permanent, hyperpigmentation. These patients need at least 6 months from the last treatment to see clearance.

Vessel depth and size

More superficial veins are more likely to exhibit postsclerotherapy hyperpigmentation than deeper ones for several reasons. Reabsorption of extravasated heme is more efficient in the deeper dermis, and deeper vessels have a more robust perivascular environment that limits extravasation. Hemosiderin pigment is also less visible when it is deposited lower in the dermis. However, the larger the vessel treated, the greater is the potential volume of trapped red blood cells and the greater capacity for hemosiderin deposition. Hyperpigmentation is rare in vessels less than 1 mm in diameter.[20]

Concomitant medications

Patients taking minocycline have been reported to have a higher risk of postsclerotherapy pigmentation.[47] Unlike the golden to deep-brown color typical of sclerotherapy-induced pigmentation, pigmentation in patients taking minocycline may appear blue-grey, and can mimic a blue varicose vein within the dermis. Minocycline hyperpigmentation is due to hemosiderin or some other iron-chelating compound,[48] and can occur in organs other than the skin. It is hypothesized that minocycline or one of its metabolites causes lysosomal disruption, interfering with degradation of hemosiderin and leading to macrophage death and deposition of pigment. If possible, patients should stop taking minocycline while undergoing sclerotherapy, as this blue discoloration may last for years. An example of this is discussed in Chapter 7.

Injection pressure and rate of flow

Excessive intravascular pressure from too-rapid injection may cause vessel rupture. This is particularly true of smaller venules composed essentially of endothelial cells with a thin muscular coat. When too large a volume is injected too quickly, the venule walls overexpand and rupture, leading to escape of red blood cells. It is essential to control the rate of injection, and to inject the tiniest veins as slowly as possible.

Many authors have perpetuated the myth that larger syringes result in lower injection pressures. The most elementary consideration of fluid mechanics shows that this is not true: for a given size needle placed into a given vein, the rate of flow of sclerosant from the needle tip depends *only* on the pressure inside the syringe. For a given rate of flow, the pressure within the syringe of the fluid being injected is identical no matter what type or size of syringe is used. However, it is easier to generate higher flow rates with smaller syringes using less thumb pressure.

Experienced phlebologists choose syringe types and sizes to suit their personal preferences. No one would choose a 60-cc syringe for injecting telangiectasias, but there are those who use syringes as large as 10 cc for this purpose. As a practical matter, there are three reasons why a clinician may prefer smaller 3-cc or 1-cc syringes for injection of the smallest veins:

- When the syringe is larger, the thumb must press harder to achieve the same pressure and the same flow rate. If the piston cross-sectional area is 10 times greater, then the thumb must push 10 times harder to achieve the same flow rate and the same static fluid pressure in the syringe.

- For a given injected volume, the distance moved by the piston is greater for a smaller syringe. Because hand function is optimized over this range of isotonic motion, the opportunity for dynamic control is greater with smaller syringes. It is easier to move the thumb smoothly 1 inch over 2 seconds against a low force than it is to move the thumb smoothly one-tenth of an inch over 2 seconds against a high force.

- Before the piston starts to move, static friction against the wall must be overcome to start the motion. While moving, sliding friction must be overcome to continue the motion. The total amount of friction depends on the surface area of contact between the piston and the syringe. For any given coefficients of static and sliding friction, the total amount of friction will be higher for a larger piston. This is a very real consideration, as the force needed to break the piston free and start it moving can be quite large, especially when sticky or corrosive sclerosants are used. When the piston does break free, the injection pressure will be very high until the hand can react to reduce the pressure to just what is needed to overcome sliding friction. Efforts to inject extremely small volumes can result in alternate sticking and sliding, with jerky alternation of high and low pressures. Friction is a problem in syringes of all sizes, but the magnitude of the problem is much less in smaller syringes because the area of frictional contact is much smaller.

Sclerosing solution

The degree of endothelial destruction depends on the type and concentration of the sclerosing solution used. Excessive vascular injury allows greater extravasation of red blood cells and causes an increase in hyperpigmentation. The minimum effective concentration of the weakest effective sclerosant will minimize the likelihood of hyperpigmentation. Lower flow rates are also less likely to cause vessel rupture, so that minimal thumb pressure is recommended.

There is some disagreement as to which sclerosing agents are most likely to cause hyperpigmentation. Some believe hypertonic saline and sodium tetradecyl sulfate cause a similar incidence of pigmentation,[16] while others report that the incidence is higher with STS.[49] Polidocanol has been reported to have a high incidence of pigmentation when high concentrations are used, but a lower incidence when low concentrations are used.[20,33] Although chromated glycerin (CG) often is said to have an extremely low incidence of hyperpigmentation, one author reports hyperpigmentation in 8% of CG treated patients and in none of POL treated patients.[45]

The selected sclerosing solution probably is less important than the concentration of that solution used for a specific vessel: there is a threefold increase in pigmentation in telangiectasias treated with 1% POL compared with 0.5% POL.[18] A solution that is too concentrated for small vessels

causes too much wall damage and perivascular inflammation, with excessive red blood cell leakage and cutaneous deposition.

Intravascular pressure

Postsclerotherapy pigmentation can occur anywhere on the leg, but appears most commonly in vessels below the thighs, particularly around the knee and ankle.[40] This probably is the result of a combination of increased capillary fragility, increased intravascular pressure, and the difficulty of obtaining constant compression over these irregular and mobile surfaces.

PREVENTION

Treatment of pigmentation is not very effective, thus the utilization of techniques for prevention is of prime importance. Hyperpigmentation depends on leakage of blood cells out of the treated vessels. Risk reduction is accomplished by keeping vessel wall damage to the minimum necessary for effective sclerosis, by reducing the volume of blood trapped within treated vessels, and by reducing the intravascular pressure experienced by treated vessels during treatment and in the postsclerosis period. Table 24-4 summarizes the approach to minimization of postsclerotherapy hyperpigmentation.

A guiding principle to help minimize the intravascular pressure is to always identify and treat proximal reflux points before treating smaller distal veins, and to always identify and treat reticular feeding veins before treating smaller telangiectasias.

Another important fundamental principle is the proper use of graduated compression to help minimize the amount of intravascular coagulum that remains trapped within a vessel. A recent study showed reduced incidence of hyperpigmentation with the use of compression following sclerotherapy.[50] Unfortunately, even optimal external pressure cannot completely occlude the vessel lumen, and a variable amount of thrombus remains within the vessel after sclerotherapy of all veins. The inflammatory process that accompanies resolution of thrombus produces a subacute perivenulitis that can persist for months.[51] This inflamma-

Table 24-4
Ways to Minimize Occurrence of Postsclerosis Pigmentation

Eliminate high-pressure reflux before treating smaller vessels
Minimize risks of vessel rupture
Avoid excessive syringe pressure
Minimize intravascular pressure by elevating leg during treatment
Select a sclerosant with the least inflammatory effects
Use a sclerosant concentration appropriate for vessel size
Apply compression immediately posttreatment
Remove postsclerotherapy coagula as early as possible
Avoid concomitant use of minocycline
Direct treatment at the deepest site in a telangiectatic cluster
Avoid treating patients with known defects in iron transport

---

tory process increases the likelihood of hyperpigmentation, particularly in the presence of continued venous hypertension.

To minimize the risk of pigmentation and to hasten vessel fibrosis, intravascular coagula can be removed by suction extraction using an 18-gauge needle and a 3-cc syringe, followed by manual expression of any residual material within the vein. Many patients require local anesthesia with lidocaine for this procedure. Smaller deposits of coagula can be removed after a 22-gauge needle puncture *(Figure 24-8)*.

TREATMENT

There is no highly effective method for treating hemosiderin hyperpigmentation. Treatments that may have some value include exfoliation, chelation, and laser therapy. Most patients will have spontaneous resolution of hyperpigmentation within 1 year, and watchful waiting with periodic photographic documentation of the pigmentation is satisfactory in most cases. It is important to remind patients to return for drainage if they notice any hyperpigmented firm or nodular areas after treatment, as the duration of hyperpigmentation is lessened by prompt drainage of coagula (preferably within 6 weeks).

Exfoliants such as trichloroacetic acid can reduce hemosiderin staining, but carry the risk of scarring, permanent hypopigmentation, and postinflammatory hyperpigmentation. Traditional bleaching agents such as hydroquinones are ineffective because they work by affecting melanocyte function, while postsclerotherapy pigmentation is composed of hemosiderin.

Chelation of the subcutaneous iron deposition with a 150 mg/ml ointment of disodium ethylenediamine tetraacetic acid (EDTA) has been attempted with some subjective success.[52] Oral stanozolol in combination with graduated elastic compression may reduce the amount of pigmentation from lipodermatosclerosis in patients with varicose veins,[53] leading to speculation that it may also reduce postsclerotherapy pigmentation.

Postsclerotherapy pigmentation is similar to tattooing with hemosiderin, thus it is not surprising that lasers may offer a reasonably effective therapy. It is believed that laser

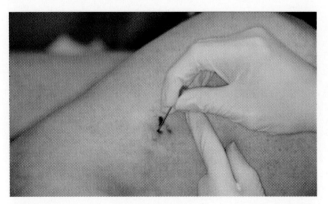

Figure 24-8. Removal of postsclerotherapy coagula with a needle puncture.

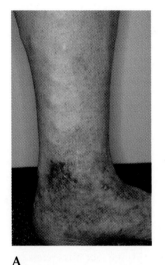 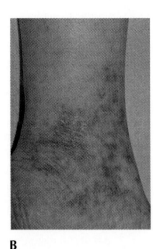

A **B**

Figure 24-9. IPL used on postsclerotherapy hyperpigmentation. **(A)** Patient with saphenofemoral incompetence, GSV varicosity, and severe ankle telangiectasias before treatment. Stasis dermatitis and pigmentation at the ankle were present; this pigmentation increased significantly after sclerotherapy, even though she had saphenofemoral ligation and duplex-guided sclerotherapy prior to treatment of the ankle telangiectasias. **(B)** Good improvement is seen after one IPL treatment of the hyperpigmentation of the ankle.

treatment causes physical fragmentation of pigment granules that are later removed by phagocytosis. A Q-switched laser with nanosecond pulses should theoretically be effective to break hemosiderin particles, with a 1064-nm wavelength reaching to the depth of hemosiderin. The green-yellow light-copper vapor has been reported to hasten resolution of pigmentation.[54] Hemosiderin has an absorption spectrum throughout the visible range, with major peaks at 410–415 nm.[55] Treatment with the copper vapor (CV) laser at 511 nm or the flashlamp-excited pulsed dye (FLPD) laser at 510 nm may be effective. Their disadvantages are that epidermal melanin also has a high absorption at these wavelengths, making the treatment non-specific and raising the possibility of tissue destruction with scarring and inflammatory hyper- or hypopigmentation. Intense pulsed light appears particularly well-suited to treat postsclerotherapy pigmentation, as the IPL spectrum includes yellow, red, and infrared. These are absorbed by hemosiderin and have the ability to penetrate down to the depth of the hemosiderin. Our experience has been good with IPL utilizing the 570-nm filter with a single pulse of 4 ms and 30 J/cm^2 *(Figure 24-9)*.[56]

Arterial and Nerve Injury

Efforts to remove or ablate refluxing veins may lead to injury to nearby structures, most often nerves and arteries. The larger and deeper the vein, the more likely it is to be intimately associated with both arteries and nerves along its course. Injections that cause injury to arteries result in severe necrotic sequelae in the distribution of the injured vessel. Injury to small muscular arteries can lead to compartment syndromes. Injuries to nerves can cause pain, paresthesias, or anesthesia and motor weakness.

The most common site for inadvertent arterial injection is the posterior medial malleolar region, and the artery most often injured is the posterior tibial artery *(Figure 24-10)*.[57] The saphenofemoral and saphenopopliteal junctions are also possible sites for accidental arterial injection, particularly when ultrasound visualization is used to direct needle placement in these high-risk areas.[58,59] At the saphenofemoral junction, a superficial external pudendal artery lies in close proximity to the greater saphenous vein (GSV), and may even bifurcate to enclose the GSV. The saphenopopliteal junction may also have small superficial arteries closely associated with the vein. Gastrocnemius arteries and

a small short saphenous artery may course alongside the lesser saphenous vein (LSV) in the mid-calf. Finally, many perforating veins pass through fascial defects in the company of perforating arteries that can lie very superficially and can curl over and around the perforating vein.

The risk of intraarterial injection can be minimized if the clinician follows a few simple rules. First, one must exercise great caution when injecting veins in locations where arteries lie in close association. Second, consider the use of IV catheters, butterfly catheters, or open needles before every injection to ensure that the needle tip is in a vein rather than in an artery or in the perivenous and periarterial tissues. Third, do not solely rely on two-dimensional ultrasound images to accurately guide needle-tip location in three dimensions when there are delicate structures nearby. The vast majority of intraarterial injections now occur in the hands of experienced practitioners under direct visualization with color-flow duplex. If arterial injection occurs, immediate hospital admission and vascular surgery consultation are indicated. Full-dose heparin should be administered and an intraarterial line may be placed into the affected artery for an infusion of a fibrinolytic agent such as urokinase or tissue plasminogen activator. Newer agents that may prove helpful include drugs directed against "white clot," such as glycoprotein IIb-IIIa inhibitors, which are new antiplatelet agents that should be effective in treatment of intraarterial injections because they prevent platelet sludge from accumulating. They are presently used in chemotherapy-related arterial injury.

Other possible interventions that are of dubious benefit include intravenous dextran, cooling of the extremity, and local injections of procaine. Oral vasodilating agents such as nifedipine have been recommended, but unlikely to be of benefit because spasm plays no role in this syndrome and because arterial occlusion intrinsically produces maximal dilatation of collateral vessels.

Inadvertent neural injury can occur by direct injection into the nerve or by perineural leakage of sclerosant. Nerve injury is most common in the lower leg, where the tibial and sural nerves are intimately associated with the LSV along much of its length. When the LSV has its termination above the knee, joining the GSV in the mid-thigh, it may lie very close to the sciatic nerve. Varicosities in this location may press on the nerve and cause sciatic pain, and careless surgical exploration or leakage of sclerosing agent in this region may cause severe sequelae. Below the level of the knee joint, the GSV is intimately associated with the saphenous nerve throughout its course in the lower leg all the way down to the dorsum of the foot. At times the saphenous nerve may be tightly bound to the GSV, particularly just below the knee and at the medial malleolus. Unfortunately, there is no specific therapy for nerve injury resulting from surgery, phlebectomy, or sclerotherapy.

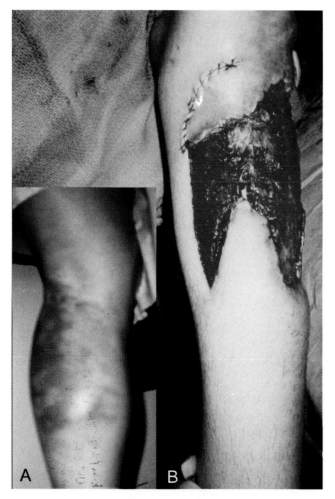

Figure 24-10.   Inadvertent intraarterial injection occurred during duplex-guided sclerotherapy in the popliteal fossa. **(A)** Darkly erythematous, intensely painful area of mottling 2 days post-injection. **(B)** Resulting wound approximately 2 months later, after constant wound care, debridement, and partial grafting. A severe defect in the calf resulted.

Minor Side Effects

URTICATION

Common after injection of all sclerosants, urtication is probably caused by release of perivascular mast cell histamine granules. Polidocanol causes the greatest urtication *(Figure*

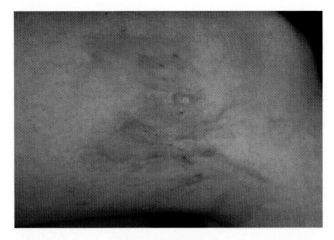

Figure 24-11. Immediate urtication along vessels treated with 0.5% POL.

24-11). It is important to stress to patients that this is not an indication of allergic reaction. Urtication is seen after laser treatment as well. Goldman advises application of a potent topical steroid immediately after treatment that he believes hastens vessel resolution and reduces urtication.[7]

FRICTION BLISTERS

Tape friction blisters typically occur in sites near the knee where cotton balls or rolls have been secured to the skin. Repeated movement causes a bulla that must be distinguished from early necrosis by the fact that purpura is typically absent in a friction blister *(Figure 24-2* and *Figure 24-12).*

ADHESIVE CONTACT DERMATITIS

When cotton balls or other compression methods use adhesive there is a risk of developing a dermatitis consisting of erythema, scaliness, weeping and pruritus. The sites usually correspond to the areas in contact with tape, not the injection sites. Use of a medium-potency topical steroid for one week will result in clearance in most patients. The use of a

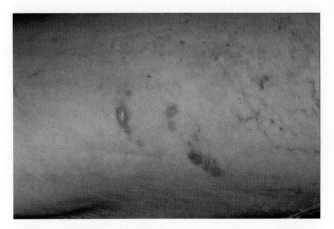

Figure 24-12. Linear bullae from tape.

cohesive, rather than adhesive, dressing for securing compression for the patient's next treatment is advisable.

Systemic Reaction to Sclerosing Agents

Bronchospasm with wheezing has been reported from use of the detergent sclerosing solutions. It usually clears quickly and spontaneously, but asthmatics must be treated appropriately with bronchodilators. These patients must be watched closely for 15 minutes to guard against the possibility of a pending systemic reaction. Accompanying generalized urticaria would be a clue to impending anaphylaxis. Blood pressure is measured; if it is low subcutaneous epinephrine 0.2–0.5 ml 1:1000 should be administered. The patient is transferred to the emergency room setting where appropriate life support can be administered. The most likely agents to cause anaphylaxis are in the detergent class and include sodium morrhuate and ethanolamine oleate. The incidence of reactions to STS is minimized by use of latex-free syringes. Polidocanol may rarely induce systemic urticaria and anaphylaxis. The overall incidence of these severe reactions is estimated at less than 0.01%, but an exact incidence is unknown.

Superficial Thrombophlebitis

Superficial thrombophlebitis is discussed separately in Chapter 25. It is important to distinguish a typical intravascular coagulum following sclerotherapy from true superficial thrombophlebitis *(Figure 24-13).* The postsclerotherapy coagulum is cordlike but non-tender and non-erythematous, while three features characterize superficial phlebitis: heat, erythema, and an intense tenderness with pain induced by the slightest touch.

There can also rarely occur yet another form of postsclerotherapy inflammation that is not well characterized, but presents with a slightly tender or non-tender, erythematous area much larger than the vein itself. This typically occurs within 1–2 days after treatment and resolves with antiinflammatories or no treatment within 3–4 days *(Figure 24-14).* The authors have seen this in rare cases after duplex-guided sclerotherapy; reexamination of the areas with duplex did not show thrombus in any of the cases. This has been ascribed to nonspecific inflammation in response to the 3% sotradecol that was used. Results of treatment were excellent in all the cases.

Summary

Minor and temporary complications are common after therapy for venous insufficiency. Telangiectatic matting and hyperpigmentation are annoying problems that usually resolve without permanent sequelae. Patients are particularly dissatisfied when pigmentation replaces the ectatic veins. Cutaneous necrosis can range from the insignificant to seri-

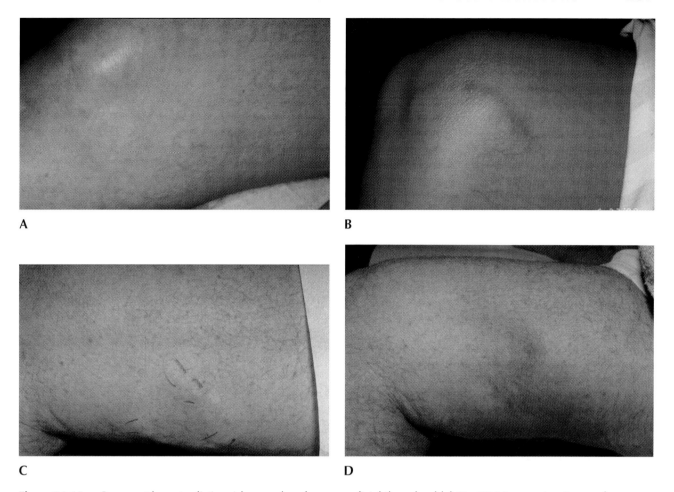

Figure 24-13.   One must learn to distinguish coagulum from superficial thrombophlebitis. **(A)** Minor varicosity near knee before sclerotherapy. **(B)** Sclerotherapy caused this linear, nontender, firm, greenish-brown coagulum, from which was drained very dark-cherry colored blood. **(C)** Larger mid-thigh varicosity before sclerotherapy. **(D)** Tender, red, warm linear area of superficial thrombophlebitis several days postsclerotherapy.

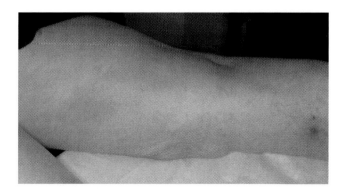

Figure 24-14.   Nonspecific Inflammation. Large erythematous area on posteromedial thigh 2 days following duplex-guided sclerotherapy of deep branch of GSV. No thrombus was present on duplex scan, and the erythema resolved within 4 days.

ous, and these patients must be followed closely with good wound care. Careful attention to diagnostic and treatment protocols will keep the incidence of these minor complications to a minimum. The risks of the much more serious complications of arterial injection and nerve injury can be minimized by experience, caution, and adherence to principles discussed.

In order to completely prevent the most serious risks, relying on external compression alone without performing treatment in patients whose venous problem lies in an anatomically complex area may offer the only protection. Unfortunately, this extremely conservative approach would deprive many patients of symptom relief. Risks of nerve injury are significant with traditional surgery as well. There simply is no risk-free approach to patients with complex problems; a risk–benefit analysis and informed consent must be individualized for each patient.

References

(1) Eaglstein W. *Inadvertent intracutaneous injection with hypertonic saline (23.4%) in two patients without complication.* J Dermatol Surg Onc 1990; 16:878–879.

(2) Goldman MP. *Sclerotherapy: treatment of varicose and telangiectatic leg veins.* 2nd ed. St. Louis: Mosby Year Book, 1995.

(3) Jaquier JJ, Loretan RM. *Clinical trials of a new sclerosing agent, aethoxysklerol.* Soc Fran de Phlebol 1969; 22:383–385.

(4) Shields JL, Jansen GT. *Therapy for superficial telangiectasias of the lower extremities.* J Dermatol Surg Oncol 1982; 8(10):857–860.

(5) deFaria JL, Moraes IN. *Histopathology of telangiectasias associated with varicose veins.* Dermatologica 1963; 127:321–329.

(6) Goldman MP, Weiss RA, Bergan JJ. *Varicose veins and telangiectasias: diagnosis and treatment.* 2nd ed. St. Louis: Quality Medical Publishing, 1999.

(7) Goldman MP. *Complications and adverse sequelae of sclerotherapy.* In: Goldman MP, Weiss RA, Bergan JJ, editors. Varicose veins and telangiectasias: Diagnosis and treatment. St. Louis: Quality Medical Publishing, 1999: 300–379.

(8) Chant ADB. *The effects of posture, exercise, and bandage pressure on the clearance of 24 Na from the subcutaneous tissues of the foot.* Br J Surg 1972; 59:552–555.

(9) Campion EC, Hoffman DC, Jepson RP. *The effects of external pneumatic splint pressure on muscle blood flow.* Australian and New Zealand Journal of Surgery 1968; 38:154–157.

(10) Zimmet SE. *The prevention of cutaneous necrosis following extravasation of hypertonic saline and sodium tetradecyl sulfate.* J Dermatol Surg Onc 1993; 19:641–646.

(11) Zenk KE. *Management of intravenous extravasation.* Infusion 1981; 5:77–79.

(12) Laurie SWS, Wilson KL, Kernahan DA, et al. *Intravenous extravasation injuries: the effectiveness of hyaluronidase in their treatment.* Ann Plastic Surg 1984; 13:191–194.

(13) Grossman JA, McGonagle BA, Dowden RV, et al. *The effects of hyaluronidase and DMSO on experimental flap survival.* Ann Plast Surg 1983; 11:222–226.

(14) Schwartzman J. *Hyaluronidase: a review of its therapeutic use in pediatrics.* J Pediatr 1951; 39:491–502.

(15) Britton RC, Habif DV. *Clinical uses of hyaluronidase. A current review.* Surgery 1953; 33:917–942.

(16) Duffy DM. *Small vessel sclerotherapy: an overview.* Adv Dermatol 1988; 3:221–242.

(17) Davis LT, Duffy DM. *Determination of incidence and risk factors for postsclerotherapy telangiectatic matting of the lower extremity: a retrospective analysis.* J Dermatol Surg Onc 1990; 16:327–330.

(18) Norris MJ, Carlin MC, Ratz JL. *Treatment of essential telangiectasia: effects of increasing concentrations of polidocanol.* J Am Acad Dermatol 1989; 20:683–689.

(19) Ouvry P, Davy A. *Le traitement sclerosant des telangiectasies des membres inferieurs.* Phlebol 1982; 35:349–355.

(20) Weiss RA, Weiss MA. *Incidence of side effects in the treatment of telangiectasias by compression sclerotherapy: hypertonic saline vs. polidocanol.* J Dermatol Surg Onc 1990; 16:800–804.

(21) Puissegur Lupo ML. *Sclerotherapy: review of results and complications in 200 patients.* J Dermatol Surg Onc 1989; 15:214–219.

(22) Merlen JF. *Telangiectasies rouges, telangiectasies bleues.* Phlebol 1970; 23:167–174.

(23) Karosek MA. *Mechanisms of angiogenesis in normal and diseased skin.* Int J Dermatol 1991; 30:831–836.

(24) Barnhill RL, Wolf JE, Jr. *Angiogenesis and the skin.* J Am Acad Dermatol 1987; 16:1226–1229.

(25) Folkman J, Klagsbrun M. *Angiogenic factors.* Science 1987; 235:442–446.

(26) Folkman J, Weisz PB, Jouille MM. *Control of angiogenesis with synthetic heparin substitutes.* Science 1989; 243:1490–1493.

(27) Arenander E, Lindhagen A. *The evolution of varicose veins studied in a material of initially unilateral varices.* Vasa 1978; 7:180–184.

(28) Gilchrest BA, Stoff JS, Soter NA. *Chronologic aging alters the response to ultraviolet induced inflammation in human skin.* J Invest Dermatol 1982; 79:11–15.

(29) Vin F, Allgert FA, Levardon M. *Influence of estrogens and progesterone on the venous system of the lower limbs in women.* J Dermatol Surg Onc 1992; 18:888–892.

(30) Mashiah A, Berman V, Thole HH, Rose SS, Pasik S, Schwarz H, et al. *Estrogen and progesterone receptors in normal and varicose saphenous veins.* Cardiovasc Surg 1999; 7(3): 327–331.

(31) Perrot-Applanat M, Cohen-Solal K, Milgrom E, Finet M. *Progesterone receptor expression in human saphenous veins.* Circulation 1995; 92(10):2975–2983.

(32) Sadick NS, Urmacher C. *Estrogen and progesterone receptors their role in postsclerotherapy angiogenesis telangiectatic matting (TM).* Dermatol Surg 1999; 25(7):539–543.

(33) McCoy S, Evans A, Spurrier N. *Sclerotherapy for leg telangiectasia—A blinded comparative trial of polidocanol and hypertonic saline.* Dermatol Surg 1999; 25(5):381–386.

(34) Sadick NS. *Sclerotherapy of varicose and telangiectatic leg veins. Minimal sclerosant concentration of hypertonic saline and its relationship to vessel diameter* [see comments]. J Dermatol Surg Onc 1991; 17:65–70.

(35) Raulin C, Weiss RA, Schonermark MP. *Treatment of essential telangiectasias with an intense pulsed light source (PhotoDerm VL).* Dermatol Surg 1997; 23(10):941–945.

(36) Goldman MP, Fitzpatrick RE. *Pulsed-dye laser treatment of leg telangiectasia: with and without simultaneous sclerotherapy.* J Dermatol Surg Onc 1990; 16:338–344.

(37) McCoy S, Hanna M, Anderson P, McLennan G, Repacholi M. *An evaluation of the copper-bromide laser for treating telangiectasia.* Dermatol Surg 1996; 22(6):551–557.

(38) Goldman MP, Kaplan RP, Duffy DM. *Postsclerotherapy hyperpigmentation: a histologic evaluation.* J Dermatol Surg Onc 1987; 13:547–550.

(39) Georgiev M. *Postsclerotherapy hyperpigmentations: a one-year follow-up.* J Dermatol Surg Onc 1990; 16:608–610.

(40) Chatard H. *[Post-sclerotherapy pigmentation].* Phlebol 1976; 29:211–216.

(41) Cuttell PJ, Fox JA. *The etiology and treatment of varicose pigmentation.* Phlebol 1982; 35:387–389.

(42) Richter GW. *The nature of storage iron in idiopathic hemochromatosis and in hemosiderosis.* J Exp Med 1960; 11:551–569.

(43) Scott HJ, McMullin GM, Coleridge Smith PD, Scurr JH. *Venous disease: investigation and treatment, fact or fiction?* Ann R Coll Surg Engl 1990; 72:188–192.

(44) Merlen JF, Coget J, Sarteel AM. *Pigmentation et stase veineuse.* Phlebol 1983; 36:307–314.

(45) Georgiev M. *Postsclerotherapy hyperpigmentations. Chromated glycerin as a screen for patients at risk (a retrospective study).* J Dermatol Surg Onc 1993; 19:649–652.

(46) Thibault PK, Wlodarczyk J. *Correlation of serum ferritin levels and postsclerotherapy pigmentation—a prospective study.* J Dermatol Surg Onc 1994; 20(10):684–686.

(47) Leffell DJ. *Minocycline hydrochloride hyperpigmentation complicating treatment of venous ectasia of the extremities.* J Am Acad Dermatol 1991; 24:501–502.

(48) Sato S, Murphy GF, Bernhard JD, et al. *Ultrastructural and x-ray microanalysis observations of minocycline-related hyperpigmentation of the skin.* J Invest Dermatol 1981; 77: 264–271.

(49) Weiss MA, Weiss RA. *Efficacy and side effects of 0.1% sodium tetradecyl sulfate in compression scleortherapy of telangiectasias:*

comparison to 1% polidocanol and hypertonic saline. J Dermatol Surg Onco 1991; 17:90-91. Ref Type: Abstract

(50) Weiss RA, Sadick NS, Goldman MP, Weiss MA. *Post-sclerotherapy compression: controlled comparative study of duration of compression and its effects on clinical outcome.* Dermatol Surg 1999; 25(2):105–108.

(51) Orbach EJ. *Hazards of sclerotherapy of varicose veins—their prevention and treatment of complications.* Vasa 1979; 8:170–173.

(52) Myers HL. *Topical chelation therapy for varicose pigmentation.* Angiology 1966; 17:66–68.

(53) Burnand KG, Clemenson G, Morland R, et al. *Venous lipodermatosclerosis: treatment by fibrinolytic enhancement and elastic compression.* Br Med J 1980; 280:7–11.

(54) Thibault P, Wlodarczyk J. *Postsclerotherapy hyperpigmentation.*

The role of serum ferritin levels and the effectiveness of treatment with the copper vapor laser. J Dermatol Surg Onc 1992; 18:47–52.

(55) Wells CI, Wolken JJ. *Biochemistry:microspectrophotometry of haemosiderin granules.* Nature 1962; 193:977–988.

(56) Weiss RA, Weiss MA. *Use of intense pulsed light therapy for post sclerotherapy pigmentation.* Dermatol Surg 1997; 23:969.

(57) Fegan WG. *The complications of compression sclerotherapy.* Pract 1971; 207:797–799.

(58) Biegeleisen K, Neilsen RD, O'Shaughnessy A. *Inadvertent intra-arterial injection complicating ordinary and ultrasound-guided sclerotherapy.* J Dermatol Surg Onc 1993; 19:953–958.

(59) Benhamou AC, Natali J. *[Complications of sclerosing and surgical treatment of leg varices. Apropos of 90 cases].* Phlebologie 1981; 34(1):41–51.

CHAPTER 25

Thrombophlebitis and Venous Thromboembolism

Introduction

Venous thrombophlebitis is a life-threatening complication of many medical conditions and surgical interventions. The problem is neither rare nor limited to those with recognizable risk factors: Fully 30% of patients in the ICU develop thrombophlebitis that progresses to involve the deep veins.[1]

Properly treated, superficial thrombophlebitis can be benign. Unfortunately, clinical examination cannot tell whether a patient with superficial vein phlebitis also has deep vein thrombosis (DVT), which is related to a high morbidity and mortality. Superficial vein thrombosis can progress to the deep veins at any time because the deep and superficial systems communicate through hundreds of perforating veins up and down the leg.

Depending on the clinical setting, up to 45% of patients with what appears to be purely superficial phlebitis also have an associated deep vein thrombosis.[2-7] Approximately 10% of hospitalized patients who develop superficial phlebitis progress to develop DVT and pulmonary embolism (PE), with a 20% death rate in the group with PE.[8-10]

Superficial thrombophlebitis, deep vein thrombosis, and pulmonary embolism are all manifestations of a single clinical entity, venous thromboembolism (VTE). The major sequelae of VTE are chronic venous insufficiency (CVI), chronic cor pulmonale, and death from massive pulmonary embolism.[11] Most venous thromboses result in some degree of pulmonary embolism, but the diagnosis of PE is missed in approximately 80% of cases.

Epidemiology

The true incidence of DVT and PE in the population at large is generally underestimated because most incidence studies depend on the clinical diagnosis of clinically apparent disease. This doesn't work well for venous thromboembolism (VTE) because the clinical diagnosis is notoriously unreliable.

CLINICALLY RECOGNIZED VTE

For clinically recognized disease, the best epidemiological evidence comes from the 30-year prospective study of men born in 1913.[12] This study found an incidence of 387 cases of recognized venous thrombosis, of which 285 cases had a diagnosis of PE and 107 suffered fatal PE. This translates into 39 cases and 11 deaths per year in a practice of 10,000 patients. This same study found that one out of every nine people will develop DVT before age 80, and that clinically recognized VTE accounts for one out of every 20 deaths after age 50.

Clinical estimates of the incidence of deep venous thrombosis and pulmonary thromboembolism always underestimate the problem when compared with prospective studies and with autopsy findings.[13] This is true because non-obstructing thrombus does not cause any symptoms and because the symptoms that occur with obstructing thrombus are often vague and nonspecific. Clinical signs and symptoms are insensitive and nonspecific for venous thrombosis.

Table 25-1
Incidence of Phlebitis in Selected Populations

Patient population	Incidence of DVT	Citation
After venography	7%	22
General surgery	12%	20
Medical patients at bedrest	13%	23,24
Pulmonary patients at bedrest	26%	24,25
ICU patients at bedrest	33%	1,23
Acute myocardial infarction	40%	26–28
Coronary artery bypass	48%	29
Hospital autopsies	60%	30
Surgery for fractured hip	70%	31

Even when venous thrombosis is strongly suspected on the basis of classical signs and symptoms, the clinical diagnosis is only accurate half of the time.[14,15] The presence of tenderness, erythema, edema, or a palpable cord on examination of the lower extremities does not prove thrombophlebitis, nor does their absence rule it out. It is an unfortunate fact that half of the patients with DVT and PE have no symptoms of DVT whatsoever.

TRUE INCIDENCE OF VTE

Most cases of DVT and PE are never clinically recognized, even if the patient dies from the disease. About 60% of all autopsies show that the patient has had DVT and PE, but the diagnosis has been missed in about 80% of the cases.[16-18] In the Framingham study, autopsies showed that 16% of all deaths were caused by PE.[19]

The true incidence of DVT during life depends on the clinical setting, and is best estimated from screening studies that do not depend on clinical symptoms. Table 25-1 shows the frequency of DVT in a range of clinical situations, with an incidence of DVT ranging from about 10% in general medical ward patients to about 70% in patients admitted for a fractured hip.

Postoperative deep venous thrombosis complicates surgical procedures so frequently that routine perioperative anticoagulation is recommended for any major surgery and for a number of selected types of minor surgery.[20,21]

Mechanisms

In the normal course of life, microthrombi are continually formed and dissolved in a dynamic balance of hemostasis without intravascular thrombosis. In 1846 the German pathologist Virchow demonstrated that venous stasis, hypercoagulability, or injuries to the vessel wall can disturb this balance, causing clinical thrombosis. Venous stasis and vessel injury are easily understood as physical phenomena, but coagulability depends on a complex mixture of coagulation factors, circulating anticoagulants, and fibrinolytic mechanisms.

Hypercoagulability alone does not cause venous thrombosis, but any amount of vascular endothelial injury will trigger immediate thrombus formation. When endothelium is injured, platelets immediately aggregate at the site and activate circulating factor X, triggering the entire clotting cascade. This type of thrombin-mediated platelet aggregation is not inhibited by aspirin or nonsteroidal anti-inflammatory agents, thus these drugs are not effective in preventing or treating venous thrombosis.

The three factors that retard and prevent propagation of thrombus are blood flow, natural anticoagulants, and natural thrombolytics. Blood flow normally carries activated coagulation factors away from the growing thrombus, but if blood flow is impeded, these coagulation factors can accumulate to cause thrombus propagation. The natural anticoagulant proteins antithrombin III, protein C, and protein S work together to prevent runaway thrombosis, but a deficiency or a resistance to any one of these proteins can cause thrombus to propagate where it is not wanted. The fibrinolytic system normally ensures that thrombus is lysed where it is not needed, but defective or inhibited fibrinolysis can allow thrombus to persist in these locations.

With the exception of trauma patients and pregnant patients, DVT nearly always starts in the calf veins. Venographic studies show that symptomatic DVT includes the calf veins 99% of the time. It is isolated to the calf veins in 12% of cases, includes both calf and proximal deep veins in 87%, and is isolated to proximal deep veins in only 1%.[32]

Risk Factors for Thrombophlebitis

Some patients are at special risk for VTE because of a hypercoagulable state, which may be temporary or permanent. These patients may develop DVT after minor surgery, prolonged travel, bedrest, minor injury, or any other situation that causes endothelial injury or venous stasis. Special precautions should be taken if sclerotherapy or venous surgery is to be performed in patients at high risk for DVT. It is noteworthy that varicosities themselves may be a marker for increased risk of DVT: patients below age 60 are three times more likely to develop DVT if they have preexisting varicosities.[33,34]

Because DVT is a disease of recurrences, a past history of DVT is a special "red flag" that often indicates a high risk because of an underlying coagulopathy: persons with a past history of venous thrombosis are five times more likely to have a new DVT than those who have not had prior episodes.[33-35] A past history of DVT raises the likelihood of new postoperative venous thrombosis from 26% to 68%, while a past history of both DVT and PE raises the likelihood of new postoperative venous thrombosis to 100%.[33]

Intrinsic coagulopathy is another common and serious problem. Congenital or acquired abnormalities can affect any component of the coagulation, anticoagulation, or thrombolytic systems. The most common congenital coagulopathy is an inherited abnormality in factor V (factor V Leyden) that makes it resistant to activated protein C. Factor V Leyden is found in 7% of the general population and accounts for about half of all cases of DVT that were previously considered "idiopathic;" congenital deficiencies of protein C, protein S, or antithrombin III each account for about 5% of the cases of DVT.

Besides intrinsic hypercoagulability, many medical illnesses and procedures can increase the risk of DVT by affecting blood coagulability, the vascular endothelium, or flow rates. Acquired antithrombin III deficiency can be caused by liver disease, and deficiency of protein C or protein S can be caused by cancer, chemotherapy, vitamin K deficiency, oral anticoagulants, surgery, and disseminated intravascular coagulation. A list of commonly recognized risk factors for venous thromboembolism is found in Table 25-2.

Adverse Sequelae of DVT

The principal adverse sequelae of venous thrombosis are death from pulmonary embolism, chronic cor pulmonale from pulmonary embolism, and chronic venous insufficiency from venous valve damage.

PULMONARY EMBOLISM

Of all patients with deep vein thrombosis, 60% to 80% also develop detectable pulmonary embolism, although the majority are clinically unrecognized.[36-38] Pulmonary embolism follows acute myocardial ischemia and cerebrovascular accident as the third most common fatal cardiovascular disease, causing more than 200,000 deaths in the United States annually *(Figure 25-1)*. The diagnosis is missed in approximately 70% of cases.[30,39-41]

In patients with DVT, the presence of pulmonary signs and symptoms makes the diagnosis of pulmonary thromboembolism a virtual certainty. The absence of chest symptoms in a patient with DVT does not rule out PE, because only 15–20% of pulmonary emboli produce recognizable symptoms.[38,42-47]

Thrombus can embolize from any site. Upper extremity thrombosis often causes PE. Calf vein thrombosis often embolizes and often is lethal.[18,27,44,48] At autopsy, more than 35% of patients with pulmonary emboli have isolated calf vein thrombosis.[18]

Without treatment, the mortality is approximately 35%. Prompt diagnosis and treatment can reduce the mortality to 10% or less.[49-51] Recurrence is common, and up to 70% of patients with recurrent pulmonary embolism will develop chronic pulmonary hypertension with chronic cor pulmonale.[52,53]

PHLEGMASIA DOLENS

Severe proximal obstruction of the venous system can produce a dramatically swollen, painful, leg. Thrombosis of all venous channels in the leg can produce a painful and pulseless leg that simulates primary arterial blockage.

VENOUS INSUFFICIENCY

Recanalization of thrombosed veins *(Figure 25-2)* often results in a valveless channel, leading to chronically elevated ambulatory venous pressure within the legs and clinical postphlebitic syndrome.[54] This postphlebitic syndrome is responsible for chronic pain, edema, hyperpigmentation, and ulceration *(Figure 25-3)*, as well as many cases of recurrent DVT and pulmonary embolism.[55] The vast majority of venous ulcers, however, are caused by superficial venous insufficiency (see Chapter 26).

Table 25-2
Recognized Risk Factors for Venous Thrombosis
and Pulmonary Embolism

Acute myocardial infarction
AIDS (lupus anticoagulant)
Antithrombin III deficiency
Behcet's disease
Blood type A
Burns
Chemotherapy
Congestive heart failure
Disorders of plasminogen activators
Drug-induced lupus anticoagulant
Dysfibrinogenemia
Dysplasminogenemia
Estrogen replacements
Familial hyperlipidemias
Fractures
Hemolytic anemias
Heparin-induced thrombocytopenia
Homocysteinuria
Immobilization
Increasing age
In-dwelling venous infusion catheters
Intravenous drug abuse
Malignancy
Multiple trauma
Obesity
Oral contraceptives
Phenothiazines
Polycythemia
Postoperative (especially pelvic and orthopedic procedures)
Postpartum period
Postvenography
Pregnancy
Previous history of deep venous thrombosis
Protein C deficiency
Protein S deficiency
Resistance to activated protein C
Significant varicosities
SLE (systemic lupus erythematosus)
Thrombocytosis
Ulcerative colitis
Venous pacemakers
Warfarin (first few days of therapy)

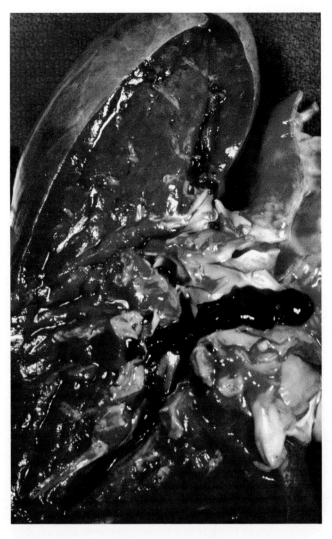

Figure 25-1. Fatal pulmonary embolism after a missed diagnosis of DVT and PE. Note thrombus filling the main pulmonary artery.

MONDOR'S DISEASE

Thrombophlebitis of a subcutaneous vein leading from the breast to the axilla is known as Mondor's disease. This entity is painful and can be disfiguring, since spontaneous fibrosis of the vessel often leads to retraction of subcutaneous tissues, with puckering and hardening of one quadrant of the breast.

Tests for Deep Vein Thrombosis

Outflow obstruction caused by deep vein thrombosis may be diagnosed by any of the invasive or noninvasive tests described earlier. The usefulness of venous testing depends both upon the skill and experience of the operator and upon the patient population in which the tests are used. False-

Thrombotic damage to a single perforating valve at any level can release high pressure into the superficial system and produce chronic venous insufficiency. More than 60% of those with isolated popliteal valve failure develop severe signs of chronic venous insufficiency,[56] and isolated calf vein thrombophlebitis results in clinical postphlebitic syndrome in 20–40% of cases.[57,58]

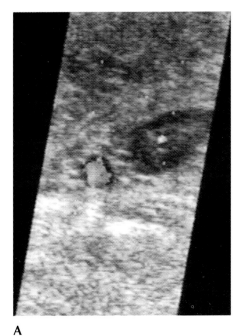

A

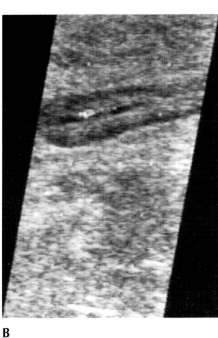

B

Figure 25-2.   Color-flow duplex ultrasound image showing early recanalization of thrombus in the femoral vein: **(A)** transverse and **(B)** longitudinal views.

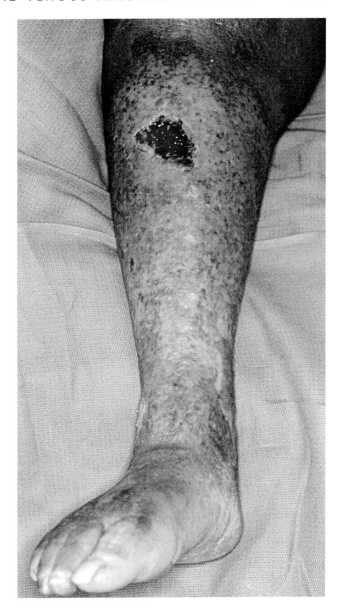

Figure 25-3.   Postphlebitic syndrome: chronic pain, swelling, discoloration, and ulceration in a patient with persistent partial outflow obstruction and chronic deep system reflux after DVT.

positive and false-negative results are quite common for all venous tests.[59]

Plethysmographic and rheographic tests of venous function fail to detect most cases of DVT, since physiologic changes measured by these devices may be subtle in DVT. Contrary to the claims of some equipment sales agents, functional tests can only detect thrombus that is large and obstructing. These tests miss 86% of all cases of DVT in a high-risk population,[60] and have largely been replaced by duplex ultrasound.

Duplex ultrasound imaging is neither perfectly sensitive nor specific. Results depend on the skill of the technician. Some studies show that duplex ultrasound can miss nearly 40% of proximal deep vein thrombi.[61] Duplex ultrasound is more accurate when the patient has an acutely swollen leg, and less accurate when the leg is not swollen or painful. Even when the leg is swollen, duplex frequently is unable to detect DVT above the groin or below the knee.[62]

When duplex ultrasound fails to confirm a suspected diagnosis of DVT, magnetic resonance venography (MRV) may provide a diagnosis. This non-invasive test is as sensitive and specific for DVT as invasive contrast venography, and may provide an alternate diagnosis when the symptoms are not due to DVT.[63]

Prevention of DVT

AVOIDANCE OF STASIS

Venous stasis is an important risk factor for thrombosis. Many cases of thrombophlebitis can be attributed to long rides in a car or airplane, or to prolonged bedrest. Patients undergoing vein treatments, whether by surgery, sclerotherapy, or other means, should therefore remain ambulatory to avoid venous stasis.

EXOGENOUS HYPERCOAGULANTS

Smoking and exogenous estrogens are common avoidable causes of a general hypercoagulable state. Fatal pulmonary embolism in a patient shortly after a sclerotherapy treatment has been attributed to concomitant oral contraceptive use,[64] but this is most likely coincidental, as hundreds of thousands of patients have undergone sclerotherapy without incident while taking exogenous estrogens.

ANTICOAGULATION

Patients with prior venous thrombosis or known hypercoagulable states should have prophylactic anticoagulation before undergoing surgery or prolonged immobilization. Low-molecular-weight heparin (LMWH) is a safe and effective form of prophylaxis that has become the method of choice because it is safer and more effective than unfractionated heparin, can be given subcutaneously, and does not require monitoring. Like all forms of heparin, LMWH increases the risk of bleeding at any site. Dosage regimens for LMWH are discussed in the section following on treatment of acute DVT.

VENA CAVA FILTER

In patients with DVT who cannot be anticoagulated, a vena cava filter, such as the Greenfield filter, may reduce the risk of fatal pulmonary embolism by trapping large clots in the vena cava before they can reach the lung. PE often occurs in spite of a filter because small thrombi pass easily through the loose mesh, while large thrombi may form above the filter or may pass around it.[65] Filters do not prevent DVT, and anticoagulation is recommended whenever possible.

COMPRESSION THERAPY

Venous stasis is reduced when venous tone is increased by external compression or any other method.[66-68] Gradient compression stockings can increase the velocity of flow in the deep veins by a factor of five or more,[66,69-71] and can significantly reduce the incidence of DVT and PE in many clinical settings.[21,72]

Effective compression requires at least a 30–40 mm Hg pressure gradient. Jobst, JuZo, Medi, Venosan, and Sigvaris are among the manufacturers of commonly available effective gradient compression hose (Chapter 15). The "Ted hose" that are often used as an antiembolic stocking provide

only symbolic compression, and are ineffective in preventing stasis. Compression stockings should be at least thigh-high, and must be properly fitted at the ankle, calf, and thigh. They should include a waist strap or a garter belt to prevent a tourniquet effect due to rolling of the stocking top.

Treatment of Acute Thrombosis

ANTICOAGULATION

Unfractionated heparin

Effective anticoagulation with heparin reduces the mortality of PE from 30% to less than 10%. Heparin works by activating antithrombin III to slow or prevent the progression of deep venous thrombus and to reduce the size and frequency of pulmonary emboli.[73-75] Heparin does not dissolve existing clot. Anticoagulation is essential, but anticoagulation alone does not guarantee a successful outcome. Recurrence or extension of deep venous thrombosis and pulmonary embolism may occur despite full and effective heparin anticoagulation.[76]

An activated partial thromboplastin time (aPTT) of at least 1.5 times the control value is necessary for a therapeutic heparin effect. Recurrence of DVT and PE is 15 times more frequent if the APTT is not therapeutic in the first 48 hours.[77] To be effective, unfractionated heparin must be given intravenously in adequate doses. Table 25-3 gives an appropriate dosing schedule for full-dose unfractionated intravenous heparin. Low-dose subcutaneous unfractionated heparin should not be used, as it is not an effective therapy for DVT nor an effective prophylaxis against recurrence.[78]

Low-molecular-weight heparins

With proper dosing, several low-molecular-weight heparin (LMWH) products have been found safer and more effective than unfractionated heparin both for prophylaxis and treat-

Table 25-3
Unfractionated Heparin for Venous Thrombosis

- In the absence of contraindications, anticoagulation should be started at the first suspicion of thromboembolic disease, without waiting for the results of diagnostic tests.
- The initial bolus of intravenous heparin should be at least 10,000 U.
- The initial infusion of intravenous heparin should be approximately 20 U/kg/hr.
- The APTT should be checked every 6 hours until stable, and heparin dosing should be adjusted as follows:

  If the APTT is subtherapeutic (less than 1.5 times the control value) rebolus with 5000 U and increase the drip by 10%

  If the APTT is supratherapeutic (more than 2.5 times the control value) decrease the drip 10%

  If the APTT is extremely high (> 100 s) hold the heparin drip for 1 hour and decrease the drip 10%

ment of DVT and PE.[79] It is not necessary nor useful to monitor the aPTT when giving LMWH, because the drug is most active in a tissue phase, and does not exert most of its effects on coagulation factor IIa.

There are many different low-molecular-weight heparin products available around the world, and because of pharmacokinetic differences, dosing is highly product-specific. At this writing, there are three LMW heparin products available in the United States: enoxaparin (Lovenox™), dalteparin (Fragmin™), and ardeparin (Normiflo™). Enoxaparin is the only one of these currently approved for treatment of DVT. Each has been approved at a lower dose for prophylaxis, but all appear to be safe and effective at some therapeutic dose in patients with active DVT or PE.

Enoxaparin (Lovenox™) is administered by subcutaneous injection. The recommended adult dose for treatment of DVT or PE is 1 mg/kg given every 12 hours, or 1.5 mg/kg given every 24 hours. The recommended adult dose for prophylaxis is 30 mg given every 12 hours. In patients undergoing abdominal surgery, the dose for prophylaxis is 40 mg once daily, with the first dose given 2 hours prior to surgery. Enoxaparin is available in prefilled syringes, designed to allow patient self-administration at home. If necessary, 1 mg protamine can neutralize 1 mg of enoxaparin.

Dalteparin (Fragmin™) is also administered by subcutaneous injection using prefilled syringes. Dalteparin has been approved for postoperative DVT prophylaxis in abdominal surgery with once daily dosing of 2500 U SQ. If necessary, 1 mg protamine can neutralize 100 U of dalteparin.

Ardeparin (Normiflo™) is another subcutaneous LMWH that was recently released in the United States for DVT prophylaxis in patients undergoing hip and knee surgery. The prophylactic dose is 50 U/kg given every 12 hours. If necessary, 1 mg protamine can neutralize 100 U of ardeparin.

Warfarin

Warfarin competitively inhibits the regeneration of the reduced active form of vitamin K, thus interfering with the action of the vitamin K dependent clotting factors II, VII, IX, and X, as well as the action of the anticoagulant factors protein C and protein S. Warfarin anticoagulation is usually effective when the International Normalized Ratio (INR) is above 2.5, but patients with thrombosis due to a hypercoagulable state require a higher INR (above 3.0) to prevent recurrent thrombosis.[80,81]

Heparin should always be given when starting warfarin. Starting warfarin without heparin increases the early incidence of death from PE. Extension of DVT occurs in 40% of patients started on coumadin alone, compared with only 8% of those treated with heparin and coumadin together.[82] Early warfarin hypercoagulability also causes the syndrome of warfarin skin necrosis, in which large areas of skin and portions of the distal extremities become gangrenous and may require amputation.

All anticoagulants cause an increased risk of bleeding. If major hemorrhage occurs, the warfarin effect may be reversed within a few hours by giving fresh frozen plasma and parenteral vitamin K (10 mg given SQ or IM). Warfarin is teratogenic and should not be used in pregnancy. It is se-creted in breast milk in small quantities, but may nonetheless be used in nursing mothers.

Duration of anticoagulation

Most patients with DVT should be anticoagulated for 6 months.[83,84] Long-term anticoagulation is indicated for patients with recurrent venous thrombosis or with an irreversible underlying risk factor.[75] No matter how long anticoagulation is continued, most recurrences of DVT and PE occur shortly after stopping therapy.[79,83,85]

Complications of anticoagulation

Unfractionated heparin causes bleeding complications in 10–15% of patients.[86,87] Aspirin and other platelet inhibitors increase the risk. Fresh frozen plasma and platelet transfusions are ineffective when excessive bleeding is due to heparin, but heparin anticoagulation is reversed by protamine sulphate (15 mg infused over 3 minutes). Table 25-4 lists the commonly recognized contraindications to anticoagulation.

Heparin-associated thrombocytopenia (HAT) is an immune-complex disease that causes increased venous and arterial thrombosis, and can be fatal. Two-thirds of patients with HAT do not have a cross-reaction to the low-molecular-weight heparin enoxaparin.

Heparin is not teratogenic and may be used in pregnancy, but there is a 20% incidence of fetal demise and a 14% incidence of premature delivery in pregnant women on heparin. Heparin does not cross the placenta, nor is it secreted in breast milk.[88]

SUPERFICIAL VENECTOMY

Ascending superficial phlebitis may propagate into the deep veins via perforating veins at any level, but is most worrisome when it progresses along the greater saphenous vein (GSV) and approaches the level of the saphenofemoral junction (SFJ) at the groin. Once superficial thrombus reaches the saphenofemoral junction, the incidence of DVT without intervention is 100%. Therapy for ascending greater saphenous phlebitis in the thigh should include full heparin anticoagulation and intravenous antibiotics. Surgical interruption of the saphenofemoral junction and removal of the phlebitic saphenous vein has long been recommended, but may not result in a decreased incidence of DVT. Fibrinolytic agents may be effective in dissolving the thrombus.

AMBULATION VERSUS BEDREST FOR DVT AND PE

Ambulation is absolutely indicated for DVT prophylaxis, but ambulation in the treatment of acute DVT is controversial. The traditional American medical opinion has been that early ambulation increases the risk of embolization of a fragment of thrombus to the pulmonary circulation. The European medical opinion has been that stasis was part of the original cause of the thrombus, and that bedrest to produce further stasis will only cause more thrombus to develop and propagate, with a further increased risk of embolization from fresher, softer thrombus. In patients at bedrest, heparin anticoagulation slows, but does not prevent, the progression of thrombus. Recent prospective studies lend sup-

Table 25-4
Contraindications to Thrombolytic or Anticoagulant Therapy

Clinical Setting	Fibrinolysis	Heparin
Active major external bleeding	Absolute	Absolute
Active internal bleeding (even if minor)	Absolute	Absolute
Recent neurosurgery (past 8 weeks)	Absolute	Relative
Recent hepatic or renal biopsy	Absolute	Relative
Recent ocular surgery (past 8 weeks)	Absolute	Relative
Severe heparin-induced thrombocytopenia	Not contraindicated	Absolute
Recent major trauma	Relative	Relative
Recent surgery (including organ biopsy)	Relative	Not contraindicated
Recent major vessel puncture (current cannula acceptable)	Relative	Not contraindicated
Immediately postpartum	Relative	Relative
Recent past history of GI bleeding	Relative	Relative
HTN uncontrolled at the time of fibrinolysis	Relative	Relative
Longstanding diastolic HTN over 110 T	Relative	Relative
Recent prolonged cardiovascular resuscitation	Relative	Relative
Current pregnancy	Relative	Not contraindicated
Diabetic retinopathy with recent hemorrhage	Absolute/Relative	Relative
Bacterial endocarditis	Relative	Not contraindicated
Mild heparin-associated thrombocytopenia	Not contraindicated	Relative
Central nervous system cancer	Relative	Relative

HTN = hypertension

port to the European viewpoint, and the modern American trend is to recognize the overwhelming contribution that stasis makes to thrombogenesis, and to keep patients ambulatory in compression hose from the first day of recognized onset.

FIBRINOLYSIS FOR DVT

Anticoagulants do not dissolve existing thrombus, thus anticoagulation alone is not an optimal treatment for DVT. At least 65% of patients treated with heparin and warfarin for lower-extremity deep vein thrombosis develop persistent deep vein valve incompetence and altered venous return. More than half suffer a lifelong "postphlebitic" chronic venous insufficiency (CVI) syndrome of recurrent pain, swelling, stasis dermatitis, ulceration, and recurrent DVT.[55] Fifty to eighty percent of patients with DVT treated by anticoagulation will develop a venous ulcer within 10 years.[89,90] These sequelae are common after isolated calf vein thrombosis as well as after proximal thrombosis.[91]

Fibrinolytic therapy has intrinsic appeal because it is intuitively obvious that it is preferable to remove an abnormal clot rather than to allow it to remain in place. Besides the obvious advantage of restoring a widely patent outflow channel, fibrinolysis can preserve and restore normal venous valve structure and function if performed early enough in the course of the disease process.[92,93]

A convincing body of evidence supports the routine use of fibrinolytic therapy for patients with DVT, and many cen-

ters have developed extensive experience with a variety of techniques for dissolving thrombus within the deep veins. The number of reported single cases and small series with markedly improved outcomes after fibrinolysis is itself impressive, and several prospective randomized trials add additional support to the practice.

In one study of patients randomized to receive heparin alone or heparin plus urokinase or streptokinase, 6% of the heparin group had normal plethysmography results after 24 hours, compared to 70% with normal results in the fibrinolytic therapy group.[94] At follow-up there were 25% normal studies in the heparin group, compared to 75% normal studies in the fibrinolysis group. This demonstrates the ability of fibrinolysis to maintain and restore normal physiologic function of the venous system of the leg, when anticoagulation alone fails to do so in the vast majority of cases.

Another study of patients randomized to receive either heparin alone or heparin together with a lytic agent demonstrated symptomatic CVI in 56% of those who had "poor" clot resolution, but in only 25% of those who obtained "good" clot resolution.[95]

A six-year follow-up of 35 patients randomized to lytic therapy or to heparin alone demonstrated that in the heparin group, no patient had a normal venogram and 67% had clinical symptoms of CVI.[96] In the group of patients who had received lytic therapy, 41% had normal venograms and only 24% had symptoms of CVI.

Yet another study compared patients receiving only warfarin, heparin plus warfarin, or lytic agents plus warfarin. The incidence of CVI was 80% in the warfarin-only group, 40% in the heparin–warfarin group, and 0% in the lytics–warfarin group.[97]

The cumulative evidence is fairly strong that compared with anticoagulation alone, lytic therapy for DVT produces more rapid clot resolution, more complete clot resolution, a marked reduction in late symptoms, and a reduced likelihood of recurrent deep vein thrombosis.[96,98-100] The dose, the agent, and the method of administration used for lytic therapy in published studies varies widely, but in every case, it appears that the greater the reduction in amount of intravenous thrombus and the earlier it can be accomplished, the greater the benefit to the patient.

When compared to systemic infusions, transcatheter techniques for delivery of fibrinolytic agents directly into the bulk thrombus have a significantly higher success rate with fewer systemic effects.[101-103] This technique is now being used routinely at many centers for all patients with iliofemoral DVT, and a multicenter patient registry has been established to aid in retrospective analysis of outcomes. Most interventional radiologists now are prepared to carry out catheter-directed fibrinolysis on a routine basis.

FIBRINOLYSIS OF CATHETER-ASSOCIATED THROMBUS

Untreated, the syndrome of catheter-induced thrombosis of the axillary and subclavian vein is neither benign nor self-limited. In patients undergoing chemotherapy, thrombus extends from the subclavian vein to produce obstruction of the superior vena cava in more than 10% of cases.[104] Permanent outflow obstruction or chronic upper extremity venous insufficiency are seen in up to 90% of patients treated by anticoagulation alone.[105-108] Pulmonary embolism has been found in more than 30% of the patients with catheter-associated subclavian vein thrombosis treated with heparin alone.[105,109,110]

For all of these reasons, fibrinolysis has become the standard of care for catheter-induced thrombosis of the deep veins of the upper extremity. Catheter-associated femoral, axillary, or subclavian vein thrombosis may be treated by infusion of low-dose thrombolytic agents directly into the thrombus through the central venous catheter, already in place. Complete lysis of thrombus is achieved without a systemic lytic state in the majority of cases where direct intrathrombus infusion is possible.

THROMBOLYTIC AGENTS

The relative benefits of one thrombolytic agent over another have been debated in the literature at great length, and will not be considered here. The agents available today include two forms of recombinant tissue plasminogen activator (PA), urokinase, anisoylated purified streptokinase activator complex (APSAC), and streptokinase itself. Another agent, pro-urokinase, is now undergoing clinical trials.

Tissue-type plasminogen activators are physiologic human thrombolytic agents that are not antigenic and may be readministered as necessary. They are much faster-acting than other available fibrinolytic agents, and are to be preferred over other agents in the setting of pulmonary em-

bolism. The two drugs currently available are alteplase (tPA, Activase™) and reteplase (rPA, Retavase™). Alteplase is widely used for catheter-directed treatment of DVT. Dosing usually includes a bolus of 5 mg alteplase followed by a continuous intrathrombus infusion of 1 mg/hr or up to 0.05 mg/kg/hr.[112] The systemic dose of alteplase for patients with PE is 100 mg infused over 2 hours. The systemic dose of reteplase for patients with PE is 10 mg as an IV bolus, with a second bolus given 30 minutes later. There is no published recommendation for dosing of reteplase for catheter-directed fibrinolysis of DVT.

Urokinase is a physiologic human thrombolytic agent that rarely produces allergic reactions. The usual systemic dose of urokinase for deep venous thrombosis and pulmonary embolism is 4400 U/kg (2000 U/lb) as an IV bolus, followed by a maintenance drip of 4400 U/kg/hr. The drip is continued for 1 to 3 days, until clinical or laboratory investigation demonstrate thrombus resolution. When direct intrathrombus delivery is possible, a systemic lytic state may be avoided if urokinase is given without a bolus at an initial infusion rate of 500 U/kg/hr. If clot lysis is inadequate, the infusion rate is gradually increased up to 2000 units/kg/hr.[111] Other regimens are under investigation.

Streptokinase is a streptococcal fibrinolytic that has a high antigenicity and results in high levels of antistreptococcal antibodies. It cannot be safely administered a second time within six months. The usual systemic dose regimen for deep venous thrombosis and pulmonary embolism is an IV bolus of 250,000 U followed by a maintenance drip at 100,000 U/hr. The drip is continued for 1 to 3 days, until clinical or laboratory investigation demonstrate thrombus resolution. Unfortunately, adverse reactions to streptokinase often force cessation of therapy prior to completion of lysis.

Anisoylated purified streptokinase activator complex (APSAC) is a newer modified form of streptokinase that does not require free circulating plasminogen for its effectiveness. It has many theoretical benefits over streptokinase, but suffers antigenic problems similar to those of the parent compound. The effective dose for deep venous thrombosis and pulmonary embolism has not been established.

Complications of fibrinolysis

The incidence of systemic bleeding complications is roughly the same for lytic agents and for heparin, but lytic agents cause more bleeding at the site of invasive procedures,[113] and about 0.5% develop intracranial bleeding.[114,115]

Bleeding from a compressible site can be managed with compression, but bleeding at a noncompressible site requires that the infusion of lytic agent be stopped. Fresh frozen plasma and cryoprecipitate will reverse the lytic state. Aminocaproic acid (AMICAR), an inhibitor of plasminogen activators, is effective as a 5 gm IV loading dose over 30 minutes followed by a drip of 1 gm/hr as long as bleeding continues.

Contraindications to fibrinolysis

Venous thrombosis is most often recognized in patients with underlying disease and in postoperative patients, thus many patients have contraindications to fibrinolytic or anti-

Table 25-5
Practical Management of Patients with Thrombophlebitis

Duplex Ultrasound Finding	Management
Superficial thrombus not involving the GSV above the knee, in a patient without special risk factors.	• Nonsteroidal anti-inflammatories • Compression hose (30–40 mm Hg or 40–50 mm Hg) • Increased ambulation • Repeat ultrasound every 72 hrs until regression of thrombus is noted
Superficial thrombus involving the GSV above the knee, but not yet close to the SFJ, or any superficial thrombophlebitis in a patient with special risk factors.	• Prophylactic doses of LMWH • Consider antibiotic coverage for streptococcus and staphylococcus • Compression hose (30–40 mm Hg or 40–50 mm Hg) • Increased ambulation • Repeat ultrasound every 24-72 hrs until regression of thrombus is noted
Superficial thrombus involving GSV above the knee, extending into the SFJ.	• Admit to hospital • Therapeutic doses of LMWH or full-dose intravenous heparin • Antibiotic coverage for streptococcus and staphylococcus • Compression hose (30–40 mm Hg or 40–50 mm Hg) • Increased ambulation • Repeat ultrasound every 24 hrs until regression of thrombus is noted • Consider surgical interruption of GSV with or without excision of the vein
Small amounts of deep vein thrombus limited to saccular soleal or peroneal plexus in the calf.	• Prophylactic doses of LMWH • Compression hose (30–40 mm Hg or 40–50 mm Hg) • Increased ambulation • Repeat ultrasound every 24 hrs until some regression of thrombus is noted
Deep vein thrombosis in the calf, involving anterior or posterior tibial veins, or involving the peroneal vein near the popliteal trifurcation.	• Admit to hospital • Therapeutic doses of LMWH or full-dose intravenous heparin • Consider fibrinolysis • Compression hose (30–40 mm Hg or 40–50 mm Hg) • Increased ambulation • Repeat ultrasound every 24–72 hrs until regression of thrombus is noted • Maintain anticoagulation with oral warfarin or subcutaneous LMWH for 3–6 months
DVT at or above the knee (involving the popliteal or more proximal veins)	• Admit to hospital • Therapeutic doses of LMWH or full-dose intravenous heparin • Fibrinolysis recommended if no contraindications • Consider thrombectomy • Consider vena cava filter • Compression hose (30–40 mm Hg or 40–50 mm Hg) • Increased ambulation (European model) or decreased ambulation (older American model) • Repeat ultrasound every 24-72 hrs until regression of thrombus is noted • Maintain anticoagulation with oral warfarin or subcutaneous LMWH for 3–6 months

coagulant therapy.[116,117] Table 25-4 lists the most important recognized contraindications to anticoagulation and fibrinolysis.

Practical Treatment of Phlebitis

A rational approach to the initial treatment of phlebitis can be based on the patient's history and risk factors, together with the results of a detailed ultrasound examination. The clinical impression is absolutely unreliable, and management of phlebitis should never be attempted without a definitive diagnostic test (duplex ultrasound, venography, or magnetic resonance venography).

UNCOMPLICATED SUPERFICIAL THROMBOPHLEBITIS

A patient without any known risk factors and with no prior thromboembolic history who develops purely superficial phlebitis that does not involve the GSV above the knee will usually respond to nonsteroidal antiinflammatory agents, strict compression hose, increased ambulation, and early repeat examination. Bedrest is absolutely contraindicated in this setting.

SUPERFICIAL THROMBOPHLEBITIS IN PATIENTS AT SPECIAL RISK

Prophylactic dosing with subcutaneous LMWH is the appropriate therapy for a patient with superficial phlebitis who has a prior history of deep thrombophlebitis, any known irreversible risk factors for venous thrombosis, decreased mobility, or involvement of the GSV above the knee. Antibiotics should be used if there is any clinical evidence that phlebitis may be septic, and in every case in which the GSV is involved in the proximal thigh. Fibrinolytic therapy or surgical interruption of the SFJ (with or without removal of the saphenous vein) must be considered if greater saphenous phlebitis approaches the SFJ.

LIMITED SOLEAL OR PERONEAL VEIN INVOLVEMENT

An outpatient regimen of prophylactic doses of subcutaneous LMWH, compression hose, increased ambulation, and early repeat duplex ultrasound is probably safe for patients with superficial phlebitis that has passed through calf perforators but involves only small venous channels in the peroneal and soleal plexus. If outpatient treatment is attempted, these patients should be followed with frequent serial duplex exams (repeated every 24–72 hours and with any change in symptoms) until the thrombus is seen to regress.

TIBIAL VEIN, POPLITEAL VEIN, OR FEMORAL VEIN THROMBOPHLEBITIS

Deep vein thrombophlebitis involving the tibial veins carries nearly the same risk of pulmonary embolism as deep vein thrombus in the popliteal and more proximal thigh veins. Standard therapy for these patients includes hospitalization and full-dose intravenous unfractionated heparin anticoagulation. Therapeutic off-label doses (as distinct from prophylactic doses) of LMWH may be substituted for unfractionated heparin. Strict gradient compression therapy is essential. Ambulation (as opposed to bedrest) is required in Europe and is coming into favor in the United States.

It is not yet known whether outpatient therapy using LMWH is as safe as inpatient therapy, but it must be remembered that most patients with DVT will develop PE, and that hemodynamic collapse can be quite sudden.

The potential risks and benefits of intravenous fibrinolytic therapy should be considered. Many believe that patients with femoropopliteal or iliofemoral thrombosis will benefit from immediate referral to an interventional radiologist for catheter-directed fibrinolytic therapy.

Table 25-5 provides a summary overview of modern treatment recommendations based upon an ultrasonic localization of thrombus. More frequent duplex ultrasound examinations are needed in higher risk cases when the therapy being used is less than maximal.

Summary

The past few years have brought significant improvements in the diagnosis and treatment of venous thromboembolism. Duplex ultrasound and magnetic resonance venography have largely replaced plethysmography and contrast venography. Low-molecular-weight heparins are replacing unfractionated heparins. Compression therapy has been recognized as an effective means of prophylaxis and an important adjunct to treatment. Early fibrinolysis has come into focus as an important way to restore normal structure and function to vein valves.

References

(1) Hirsch DR, Ingenito EP, Goldhaber SZ. *Prevalence of deep venous thrombosis among patients in medical intensive care.* JAMA 1995; 274:335–337.

(2) Becker F. [*Superficial venous thrombosis of the lower limbs*]. Rev Prat 1996; 46(10): 1225–1228.

(3) Chengelis DL, Bendick PJ, Glover JL, Brown OW, Ranval TJ. *Progression of superficial venous thrombosis to deep vein thrombosis.* J Vasc Surg 1996; 24(5):745–749.

(4) Jorgensen JO, Hanel KC, Morgan AM, Hunt JM. *The incidence of deep venous thrombosis in patients with superficial thrombophlebitis of the lower limbs.* J Vasc Surg 1993; 18(1):70–73.

(5) Bergqvist D, Jaroszewski H. *Deep vein thrombosis in patients with superficial thrombophlebitis of the leg.* Br Med J (Clin Res Ed) 1986; 292(6521):658–659.

(6) Skillman JJ, Kent KC, Porter DH, Kim D. *Simultaneous occurrence of superficial and deep thrombophlebitis in the lower extremity.* J Vasc Surg 1990; 11(6): 818–824.

(7) Prountjos P, Bastounis E, Hadjinikolaou L, Felekuras E, Balas P. *Superficial venous thrombosis of the lower extremities co-existing with deep venous thrombosis. A phlebologic study on 57 cases.* International Angiology 1991; 10:63–65.

(8) Zollinger RW, Williams RD, Briggs DO. *Problems in the diagnosis and treatment of thrombophlebitis.* Arch Surg 1962; 85:18.

(9) Guilmot J-L, Wolman F, Lasfargues G. *Thromboses veineuses superficielles.* Rev Prat 1988; 38:2062.

(10) Zollinger RW. *Superficial thrombophlebitis.* Surg Gynecol Obstet 1967; 124:1077.

(11) Kakkar VV. *Prevention of venous thrombosis and pulmonary embolism.* Am J Cardiol 1990; 65(6):50–54.

(12) Hansson PO, Welin L, Tibblin G, Eriksson H. *Deep vein thrombosis and pulmonary embolism in the general population.* 'The Study of Men Born in 1913.' Arch Intern Med 1997;157:1665–1670.

(13) Karwinski B, Svendsen E. *Comparison of clinical and postmortem diagnosis of pulmonary embolism.* J Clin Pathol 1989;42:135–139.

(14) Haeger K. *Problems of acute deep venous thrombosis. The interpretation of signs and symptoms.* Angiology 1969; 20:219–223.

(15) Richards KL, Armstrong JD, Jr., Tikoff G, Hershgold EJ, Booth JL, Rampton JB. *Noninvasive diagnosis of deep venous thrombosis.* Arch Int Med 1976;136:1091–1096.

(16) Gibbs NM. *Venous thrombosis of the lower limbs with particular reference to bedrest.* Brit J Surg 1957;45:209–236.

(17) Roberts GH. *Venous thrombosis in hospital patients: A postmortem study.* Scot Med J 1963; 8:11.

(18) Havig O. *Deep vein thrombosis and pulmonary embolism. An autopsy study with multiple regression analysis of possible risk factors.* Acta Chir Scand 1977; 478:1–120.

(19) Goldhaber SZ, Savage DD, Garrison RJ, Castelli WP, Kannel WB, McNamara PM, et al. *Risk factors for pulmonary embolism. The Framingham study.* Am J Med 1983; 74:1023–1028.

(20) Collins R, Scrimgeour A, Yusuf S, Peto R. *Reduction in fatal pulmonary embolism and venous thrombosis by perioperative administration of subcutaneous heparin.* N Engl J Med 1988; 318:1162–1173.

(21) Consensus Statement. *National Institutes of Health consensus development conference statement: Prevention of venous thrombosis and pulmonary embolism.* JAMA 1986; 256:744–749.

(22) Hull RD, Hirsh J, Sackett DL, Taylor DW, Carter C, Turpie AG, et al. *Clinical validity of a negative venogram in patients with clinically suspected venous thrombosis.* Circulation 1981; 64:622–625.

(23) Cade JF. *High risk of the critically ill for venous thromboembolism.* Crit Care Med 1982; 10:448–450.

(24) Kierkegaard A, Norgren L, Olsson CG, Castenfors J, Persson G, Persson S. *Incidence of deep vein thrombosis in bedridden non-surgical patients.* Acta Med Scand 1987; 222:409–414.

(25) Ibarra-Perez C, Lau-Cortes E, Colmenero-Zubiate S, Arevila-Ceballos N, Fong JH, Sanchez-Martinez R, et al. *Prevalence and prevention of deep venous thrombosis of the lower extremities in high-risk pulmonary patients.* Angiology 1988; 39:505–513.

(26) Simmons AV, Sheppard MA, Cox AF. *Deep venous thrombosis after myocardial infarction. Predisposing factors.* Brit Heart J 1973; 35:623–625.

(27) Murray TS, Lorimer AR, Cox FC, Lawrie TDV. *Leg vein thrombosis following myocardial infarction.* Lancet 1970; ii:792–793.

(28) Nicolaides AN, Kakkar VV, Renney JT, Kidner PH, Hutchinson DC, Clarke MB. *Myocardial infarction and deep vein thrombosis.* Brit Med J 1970; 1:432–434.

(29) Reis SE, Polak JF, Hirsch DR, Cohn LH, Creager MA, Donovan BC, et al. *Frequency of deep venous thrombosis in asymptomatic patients with coronary artery bypass grafts.* Am Heart J 1991; 122:478–482.

(30) Coon WW. *Spectrum of pulmonary embolism: Twenty years later.* Arch Surg 1976; 111:398–402.

(31) Stamatakis JD, Kakkar VV, Sagar S, Lawrence D, Nairn D, Bentley PG. *Femoral vein thrombosis and total hip replacement.* Brit Med J 1977; 2:223–225.

(32) Cogo A, Lensing AW, Prandoni P, Hirsh J. *Distribution of thrombosis in patients with symptomatic deep vein thrombosis.* Implications for simplifying the diagnostic process with compression ultrasound. Arch Intern Med 1993; 153:2777–2780.

(33) Kakkar VV, Howe CT, Nicolaides AN, Renney JT, Clarke MB. *Deep vein thrombosis of the leg: Is there a "high-risk" group?* Am J Surg 1970; 120:527–530.

(34) Nicolaides AN, Irving D. *Clinical factors and the risk of deep venous thrombosis.* In: Nicolaides AN, editor. Thromboembolism: Aetiology, Advances in Prevention and Management. Lancaster, England: MTP Press, 1975.

(35) Janssen HF, Schachner J, Hubbard J, Hartman JT. *The risk of deep venous thrombosis: A computerized epidemiologic approach.* Surgery 1987; 101:205–212.

(36) Moser KM, Fedullo PF, LitteJohn JK, Crawford R. *Frequent asymptomatic pulmonary embolism in patients with deep venous thrombosis.* JAMA 1994; 271:223–225.

(37) Monreal M, Ruiz J, Olazabal A, Arias A, Roca J. *Deep venous thrombosis and the risk of pulmonary embolism. A systematic study* [see comments]. Chest 1992; 102:677–681.

(38) Huisman MV, Buller HR, Ten Cate JW, van Royen EA, Vreeken J, Kersten MJ, et al. *Unexpected high prevalence of silent pulmonary embolism in patients with deep venous thrombosis.* Chest 1989;95:498–502.

(39) Freiman DG, Suyemoto J, Wessler S. *Frequency of pulmonary thromboembolism in man.* N Engl J Med 1965; 272:1278–1280.

(40) Coon WW, Willis PW, Keller JB. *Venous thromboembolism and other venous disease in the Tecumseh Community Health Study.* Circulation 1973; 48:839–846.

(41) Coon WW. *Venous thromboembolism—prevalence: risk factors and prevention.* Clin Chest Med 1984;5:391.

(42) Kistner RL, Ball JJ, Nordyke RA, Freeman GC. *Incidence of pulmonary embolism in the course of thrombophlebitis of the lower extremities.* Am J Surg 1972; 124:169–176.

(43) Hull RD, Hirsh J, Carter CJ, Jay RM, Dodd PE, Ockleford PA, et al. *Pulmonary angiography, ventilation lung scanning, and venography for clinically suspected pulmonary embolism with abnormal perfusion lung scan.* Ann Intern Med 1983;98:891–899.

(44) Moreno-Cabral R, Kistner RL, Nordyke RA. *Importance of calf vein thrombophlebitis.* Surgery 1976;80:735–742.

(45) Partsch H, O'Burger K, Mostbeck A. *Frequency of pulmonary emboli in walking patients with pelvic vein thrombosis.* Proc Am Venous Forum 1992;4:60. (abstract)

(46) Anderson DR, Lensing AW, Wells PS, Levine MN, Weitz JI, Hirsh J. *Limitations of impedance plethysmography in the diagnosis of clinically suspected deep-vein thrombosis.* Ann Intern Med 1993;118:25–30.

(47) Ginsberg JS, Wells PS, Hirsh J, Panju AA, Patel MA, Malone DE, et al. *Reevaluation of the sensitivity of impedance plethysmography for the detection of proximal deep vein thrombosis.* Arch Intern Med 1994;154:1930–1933.

(48) Monreal M, Lafoz E, Ruiz J, Valls R, Alastrue A. *Upper-extremity deep venous thrombosis and pulmonary embolism. A prospective study.* Chest 1991; 99:280–283.

(49) Bell WR, Simon TL. *Current status of pulmonary thromboembolic disease.* Am Heart J 1982;103:239–262.

(50) Dalen JE, Alpert J, Paraskos J. *Resolution of acute pulmonary embolism in man.* New Engl J Med 1969; 280:1194–1199.

(51) Dalen JE, Alpert JS. *Natural history of pulmonary embolism.* Prog Cardiovasc Dis 1975; 17:257–270.

(52) Riedel M, Stanek V. *Long term follow-up of patients with pulmonary thromboembolism.* Chest 1982;81:151–158.

(53) De Soyza NDB, Murphy ML, De Soyza ND. *Persistent post-embolic pulmonary hypertension.* Chest 1972; 62 (6):665–668.

(54) Immelman EJ, Jeffrey PC. *The postphlebitic syndrome: Pathophysiology, prevention and management.* Clin Chest Med 1984; 5:537–550.

(55) Hirsh J, Genton E, Hull RD. *Venous thromboembolism.* New York: Grune & Stratton, 1981.

(56) Shull KC, Nicolaides AN, Fernandes J, Miles C, Horner J, Needham T, et al. *Significance of popliteal reflux in relation to ambulatory venous pressure and ulceration.* Arch Surg 1979; 114:1304–1306.

(57) Browse NL, Clemenson G, Thomas ML. *Is the postphlebitic leg always postphlebitic? Relation between phlebographic appearances of deep vein thrombosis and late sequelae.* Brit Med J 1980;281:1167–1170.

(58) Lindhagen A, Bergqvist D, Hallbook T, Efsing HO. *Venous function five to eight years after clinically suspected deep venous thrombosis.* Acta Med Scand 1985; 217:389–395.

(59) Schiff MJ, Feinberg AW, Naidich JB. *Noninvasive venous examinations as a screening test for pulmonary embolism.* Arch Int Med 1987;147:505.

(60) Agnelli G, Cosmi B, Ranucci V, Renga C, Mosca S, Lupatelli L, et al. *Impedance plethysmography in the diagnosis of asymptomatic deep vein thrombosis in hip surgery. A venography-controlled study.* Arch Intern Med 1991;151:2167–2171.

(61) Borris LC, Christiansen HM, Lassen MR, Olsen AD, Schott P. *Comparison of real-time B-mode ultrasonography and bilateral ascending phlebography for detection of postoperative deep vein thrombosis following elective hip surgery.* Thromb Haemost 1989; 61:363–365.

(62) Lensing AWA, Prandoni P, Brandjes D. *Detection of deep-vein thrombosis by real-time B-mode ultrasonography.* N Engl J Med 1989; 320:342–345.

(63) Carpenter JP, Holland GA, Baum RA, Owen RS, Carpenter JT, Cope C. *Magnetic resonance venography for the detection of deep venous thrombosis: comparison with contrast venography and duplex Doppler ultrasonography.* J Vasc Surg 1993; 18:734–741.

(64) Jones HO, Townsend JCF, Roberts JT. *Varicose veins, oral contraceptives, and thromboembolism.* Brit Med J 1967; 2:637–638.

(65) Gomez GA, Cutler BS, Wheeler HB. *Transvenous interruption of the inferior vena cava.* Surgery 1983; 93:612–619.

(66) Sigel B, Edelstein AL, Savitch L, Hasty JH, Felix WR. *Type of compression for reducing venous stasis: A study of lower extremities during inactive recumbency.* Arch Surg 1975; 110:171–175.

(67) Lewis CE, Antoine J, Mueller C, Talbot WA, Swaroop R, Edwards WS. *Elastic compression in the prevention of venous stasis: A critical appraisal.* Am J Surg 1976; 132:739–743.

(68) Husni EA, Ximenes JO, Goyette EM. *Elastic support of the lower limbs in hospital patients: A critical study.* JAMA 1970;214:1456–1462.

(69) Horner J, Fernandes E, Nicolaides AN. *Value of graduated compression stockings in deep venous insufficiency.* Brit Med J 1980; 280:820.

(70) O'Donnell TF, Jr., et al. *Effect of elastic compression on venous hemodynamics in postphlebitic limbs.* JAMA1979; 242:2766.

(71) Norgren L, Austrell C, Nilsson L. *The effect of graduated elastic compression stockings on femoral blood flow velocity during late pregnancy.* Vasa 1995;24(3):282–285.

(72) Kierkegaard A, Norgren L. *Graduated compression stockings in the prevention of deep vein thrombosis in patients with acute myocardial infarction.* Eur Heart J 1993; 14(10):1365–1368.

(73) Barritt DW, Jordan SC. *Anticoagulant drugs in the treatment of pulmonary embolism: A controlled trial.* Lancet 1960;1:1309–1312.

(74) Pollak CW, Sparks FC, Barker WF. *Pulmonary embolism: An appraisal of therapy in 516 cases.* Arch Surg 1973;107:66.

(75) Petitti DB, Strom BL, Melmon KL. *Duration of warfarin anticoagulant therapy and the probabilities of recurrent pulmonary embolism.* Am J Med 1986; 81:255.

(76) UPET. *The Urokinase Pulmonary Embolism Trial: A national cooperative study.* Circulation 1973;47 (Supp II):1–108.

(77) Hull RD, Raskob GE, Hirsh J. *Continuous intravenous heparin compared with intermittent subcutaneous heparin in the initial treatment of proximal-vein thrombosis.* N Engl J Med 1986;315:1109–1114.

(78) Hull RD, Delmore T. *Warfarin sodium versus low-dose heparin in the long-term treatment of venous thrombosis.* N Engl J Med 1979;301:855.

(79) Levine MN, Hirsh J, Gent M. *Optimal duration of oral anticoagulant therapy: a randomized trial comparing four weeks with three months of warfarin in patients with proximal deep vein thrombosis.* Thromb Haemost 1995; 16(2):321–8.

(80) Cannegieter SC, Rosendaal FR, Wintzen AR, van der Meer FJ, Vandenbroucke JP, Briet E. *Optimal oral anticoagulant therapy in patients with mechanical heart valves* [see comments]. N Engl J Med 1995; 333:11–17.

(81) Rosove MH, Brewer PM. *Antiphospholipid thrombosis: clinical course after the first thrombotic event in 70 patients.* Ann Intern Med 1992;117:303–308.

(82) Brandjes DPM, Heijboer H, Buller HR, De Rijk M, Jagt H, Wouter Ten Cate J. *Acenocoumarol and heparin compared with acenocoumarol alone in the initial treatment of proximal-vein thrombosis.* N Engl J Med 1992; 327:1485–1489.

(83) Schulman S, Rhedin AS, Lindmarker P, Carlsson A, Larfars G, Nicol P, et al. *A comparison of six weeks with six months of oral anticoagulant therapy after a first episode of venous thromboembolism. Duration of Anticoagulation Trial Study Group* [see comments]. N Engl J Med 1995; 332:1661–1665.

(84) BritThoracSoc. *Optimum duration of anticoagulation for deep-vein thrombosis and pulmonary embolism. Research Committee of the British Thoracic Society.* Lancet 1992; 340:873–876.

(85) Safavi K. *Letter regarding "Duration of anticoagulant therapy for venous thrombosis."* N Engl J Med 1995; 333:1288–1289.

(86) Mant MJ, Thong KL. *Hemorrhagic complications of heparin therapy.* Lancet 1977; i:1133–1135.

(87) Porter J, Jick H. *Drug-related deaths among medical inpatients.* JAMA 1977;237:879–881.

(88) Hall JH, Paule RM, Wilson KM. *Maternal and fetal sequelae of anticoagulation during pregnancy.* Am J Med 1980; 68:122–140.

(89) Bauer G. *A roentgenological and clinical study of the sequels of thrombosis.* Acta Chir Scand 1942; 86:1.

(90) O'Donnell TF, Browse NL, Burnand KG. *The socioeconomic effects of an ileofemoral venous thrombosis.* J Surg Res 1977; 22:483–488.

(91) Widmer LK, Zemp E, Widmer MR. *Late results in deep vein thrombosis of the lower extremity.* Vasa 1985; 14:264.

(92) Kakkar VV. *Natural history of postoperative deep-vein thrombosis.* Lancet 1969; ii:230–232.

(93) Hermans H, Eisenbud DE, Cluley S, Brener BJ, Russel H, Villanueva A, et al. *Valvular function and prostacyclin production following clot lysis and balloon thrombectomy in thrombosed canine veins.* Proce. Am. Venous Forum 1992; 4:35. (abstract)

(94) Sharma GVRK. *Thrombolytic therapy of deep vein thrombosis.* In: Thrombolysis and Urokinase. New York: Academic Press, 1977.

(95) Turpie AG, Levine MN, Hirsh J, Ginsberg JS, Cruickshank M, Jay R, et al. *Tissue plasminogen activator (rt-PA) vs heparin in deep vein thrombosis. Results of a randomized trial.* Chest 1990; 97:172S–175S.

(96) Arneson H, Hoseth A. *Streptokinase or heparin in the treatment of deep vein thrombosis, follow-up results of a prospective study.* Acta Med Scand 1982; 211:65.

(97) Bieger R, Boekhout-Mussert RJ, Hohmann F, Loeliger E. *Is streptokinase useful in the treatment of deep vein thrombosis?* Acta Med Scand 1976; 199:81–88.

(98) Comerota AJ. *Deep vein thrombosis: to treat or not to treat using lytic therapy.* In: Comerota AJ, editor. Latest concepts and management of acute venous thromboembolic disease. Coronado: Abbott Pharmaceuticals, 1992:8–15.

(99) Jeffrey PC, Immelman E, Amoore J. *Treatment of deep vein thrombosis with heparin or streptokinase: long-term venous function assessment.* Proceedings of the second International Vascular Symposium (London) 1986; S20.3 (abstract)

(100) Elliot MS, Immelman EJ, Jeffrey PC, Benatar SR, Funston MR, Smith JA, et al. *A comparative randomized trial of heparin versus streptokinase in the treatment of acute proximal venous thrombosis: an interim report of a prospective trial.* Brit J Surg 1979; 66:838–843.

(101) Comerota AJ, Katz ML, Hashemi HA. *Venous duplex imaging for the diagnosis of acute deep venous thrombosis.* Haemostasis. 1993; 23 Suppl 1:61–71.

(102) Druy EM. *Thrombolytic therapy in the treatment of axillary and subclavian vein thrombosis.* J Vasc Surg 1985; 2:821–827.

(103) Schulman S, Lockner D. *Local venous infusion of streptokinase in DVT.* Thromb Res 1984;34:213.

(104) Lokich JJ, Becker B. *Subclavian vein thrombosis in patients treated with infusion chemotherapy for advanced malignancy.* Cancer 1983;52:1586–1589.

(105) Harley DP, White RA, Nelson RJ, et al. *Pulmonary embolism secondary to venous thrombosis of the arm.* Am J Surg 1984; 147:221–224.

(106) Drapanas T, Curran WL. *Thrombectomy in the treatment of "effort" thrombosis of the axillary and subclavian veins.* J Trauma 1966;6:107–119.

(107) Hughes ESR. *Venous obstruction in the upper extremities (Paget-Schrotter's syndrome). Review of 320 cases.* Int Abst Surg 1949; 88:89–127.

(108) Crowell DL. *Effort thrombosis of the subclavian and axillary veins: Review of the literature and case report with two-year follow-up with venography.* Ann Intern Med 1960; 52:1337–1343.

(109) Swinton NW, Edgett JW, Hall RJ. *Primary subclavian vein thromboses.* Circulation 1968; 38:737–745.

(110) Adams JT, McEvoy RK, DeWeese JA. *Primary deep venous thrombosis of upper extremity.* Arch Surg 1965; 91:29–41.

(111) Fraschini G, Jadeja J, Lawson M, Holmes FA, Carrasco HC, Wallace S. *Local infusion of urokinase for the lysis of thrombosis associated with permanent central venous catheters in cancer patients.* J Clin Oncol 1987; 5:672–678.

(112) Kessler CM. *Anticoagulation and thrombolytic therapy: Practical considerations.* Chest 1989;95(5) Supp:245S–256S.

(113) Stein PD, Hull RD, Raskob G. *Risks for major bleeding from thrombolytic therapy in patients with acute pulmonary embolism. Consideration of noninvasive management.* Ann Intern Med 1994; 121:313–317.

(114) Heit J. *Thrombolytic agent dosage for pulmonary embolism: Current research and clinical experience.* In: Comerota AJ, editor. Latest Concepts and Management of Acute Venous Thromboembolic Disease. Coronado: Abbott Pharmaceuticals, 1992:24–33.

(115) Goldhaber SZ, Kessler CM, Heit J, Markis J, Sharma GVRK, Dawley D, et al. *Randomized controlled trial of recombinant tissue plasminogen activator versus urokinase in the treatment of acute pulmonary embolism.* Lancet 1988; 2:293–298.

(116) Terrin M, Goldhaber SZ, Thompson B. *Selection of patients with acute pulmonary embolism for thrombolytic therapy: the Thrombolysis In Pulmonary Embolism (TIPE) patient survey selection of patients with acute pulmonary embolism for thrombolytic therapy. Thrombolysis in pulmonary embolism (TIPE) patient survey. The TIPE investigators.* Chest 1989; 95:279S–281S.

(117) Brown WD, Goldhaber SZ. *How to select patients with deep vein thrombosis for tPA therapy.* Chest 1989; 95:276S–278S.

CHAPTER 26

Leg Ulcers

Non-healing Leg Ulcers

GENERAL APPROACH

When a patient presents with a nonhealing lower-extremity ulcer, local wound care may be initiated based upon the appearance and behavior of the wound, but a rational and comprehensive treatment plan requires a firm diagnosis in order to address the underlying etiology. Although many conditions can lead to chronic nonhealing ulcers of the lower extremities, the initial clinical history should permit the clinician to focus on a fairly small group of differential diagnoses. A comprehensive examination will almost always narrow the choices to only a few alternatives. After an initial evaluation has established a clinical differential, directed diagnostic testing will provide a definitive diagnosis in most cases.

Although not every ulcer has a venous etiology, venous disease must be investigated in every case of new or acutely worsening lower extremity ulceration. Even minor superficial venous insufficiency may trigger skin breakdown in a patient whose non-venous underlying disease is otherwise well compensated, and virtually every cause of lower extremity ulceration is associated with one or more risk factors for venous thrombosis. In clinical practice, more than half of patients who present with non-healing ulcers do have a venous component, and many have isolated superficial reflux that is eminently treatable. In the 25% of the population with clinical evidence of venous disease of the lower extremities, up to 2% have been reported to develop venous stasis leg ulcers.[1] Approximately 1–2 million persons in the United States at any time have ulceration due to superficial venous disease, and approximately one out of ten is classified as "disabled" due to the condition.[2]

The classification of possible etiologies for nonhealing ulcers is quite extensive. Table 26-1 lists the major classes of diseases that cause nonhealing ulceration of the lower extremity, together with the most commonly recognized etiologies for each class. Two primary mechanisms for pathogenesis of ulceration in chronic venous insufficiency have been proposed. The first one relates to increased venous

Table 26-1
Differential Diagnosis for Nonhealing Ulceration of the Lower Extremity

---

Infectious conditions
  Treponemal/spirochetic (esp. syphilitic)
  Mycobacterial (m. leprae, lupus vulgaris, atypical tuberculosis, tuberculids)
  Fungal (sporotrichosis, histoplasmosis, coccidiomycosis)
  Bacterial
Malignancy
  Basal cell carcinoma (may occur in transformation of preexisting chronic ulcer)
  Squamous cell carcinoma
  Kaposi's sarcoma
  Lymphoma
  Mycosis fungoides
Large vessel arterial insufficiency
  Arteriosclerotic (including arteriosclerosis obliterans)
  Traumatic
  Thrombotic
Small vessel arterial insufficiency
  Diabetes mellitus
  Hypertension
  Thromboangiitis obliterans
  Raynaud's and livedo reticularis
Deep venous blockage or insufficiency
  Thrombotic obstruction
  Extrinsic compression
  Deep valvular insufficiency (especially postphlebitic)
Superficial venous insufficiency
  Saphenofemoral insufficiency
  Saphenopopliteal insufficiency
  Perforator insufficiency

Lymphatic obstruction
  Venolymphatic disease (pure overload)
  Primary lymphatic insufficiency syndromes
  Lymphangiosarcoma
Intrinsic circulatory insufficiency (hematologic abnormalities)
  Anemias (especially sickle-cell disease)
  Polycythemias
  Dysproteinemias
Collagen vascular disorders
  Systemic lupus erythematosus
  Scleroderma
  Polyarteritis nodosum
  Wegener's granulomatosis
Trophic causes
  Diabetic neuropathy
  Alcoholic neuropathy
  Decubitus
  Bone spurs
Miscellaneous
  Pyoderma gangrenosum
  Gout
  Porphyria
  Ergotism
  Drug abuse
  Radiation necrosis

---

pressure leading to distention of the capillary bed with an enhanced permeability and leakage of macromolecules, particularly fibrinogen, into the dermis. This fibrinogen polymerizes to form fibrin cuffs around the capillaries, creating a barrier to the diffusion of oxygen and other nutrients, ultimately leading to ulceration.[3] The second mechanism proposed is that "trapped" leukocytes occlude capillaries, resulting in cutaneous ischemia, leading to ulceration.[4] A schematic for venous ulceration pathogenesis is shown in Figure 26-1.

Evaluation

At the first visit, a comprehensive clinical evaluation should be performed, including a detailed history and physical examination with continuous wave Doppler ultrasound evaluation of the limbs. Prior records should be obtained and blood tests should be ordered, including a VDRL, CBC, comprehensive chemistry panel, chest X-ray, PPD, and a tangential x-ray of the ulcer base. At this visit, routine

wound care should be based upon the appearance of the severity of the wound.

Further diagnostic tests are selected based on the comprehensive clinical evaluation and on the results of previous studies. Each component of the investigation is intended to help diagnose or rule out one or more of the most common causes for non-healing ulcers of the lower extremities. There are no idiopathic lower extremity ulcers, thus the diagnostic process is not complete until the underlying etiology has been discovered. Table 26-2 lists useful tests that can help to direct this process.

Clinical Presentation

Chronic venous obstruction and chronic venous insufficiency are very common causes of lower extremity ulcerations. In patients with impaired venous circulation, ulceration follows after a series of clinical manifestations that have become part of the overall classification of chronic venous disease known as the CEAP classification (Table 26-3).[5]

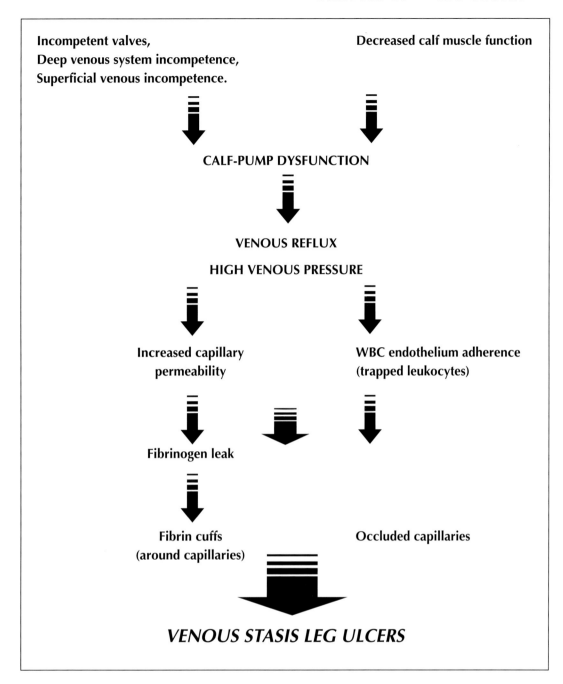

Figure 26-1. Possible mechanism of ulceration in chronic venous insufficiency (Adapted from Falanga V. Chronic wounds: Pathophysiologic and experimental considerations. Prog Dermatol 1992; 26 (4): 1–8)

Treatment is aimed at ameliorating the symptoms and, whenever possible, at correcting the underlying abnormality.

The progressive clinical findings observed in chronic venous hypertension include: edema, eczematous dermatitis, brown hyperpigmentation, induration of the subcutaneous tissue (lipodermatosclerosis), and ulceration. The initial clinical feature of patients with chronic venous insufficiency is mild edema of the lower extremities, which typically worsens with dependency and hot temperatures. These patients typically complain of dull pain of the limbs that worsens at the end of the day. This pain typically distinguishes venous versus arterial etiologies (Table 26-4).

The eczematous dermatitis, also known as stasis dermatitis, consists of erythema, scaling, oozing, and pruritus (Figure 26-2). Lichenified plaques and hyperpigmentation are also present in chronic lesions. Hyperpigmentation appears golden-brown surrounded by petechiae. Extravasation of red blood cells and hemosiderin deposition are responsible for this pigmentation. The most chronic mani-

Table 26-2
Diagnostic Tests that May Reveal the Cause of Nonhealing Ulcerations

Large-vessel arterial insufficiency	Infections
Bidirectional Continuous Wave Doppler	Fungal or bacterial cultures of the ulcer
Ankle-brachial index	Quantitative tissue bacterial cultures
Duplex ultrasound	Coagulation disorders
Magnetic resonance angiogram	Factor V Leiden mutation
Contrast angiogram	Activated protein C resistance
Transcutaneous tissue PO_2	Protein C antigen and functional assay
Small-vessel arterial insufficiency	Protein S antigen and functional assay
Transcutaneous tissue PO_2	Anti-thrombin III antigen and functional assay
Laser Doppler	Homocysteine blood levels
Venous outflow obstruction	Lupus anticoagulant assays: APPT, RVVT.
Maximum venous outflow (plethysmography)	Anticardiolipin antibodies with isotypes (IGG, IgM, IgA), anti-beta 2 glycoprotein 1 antibodies, anti-prothrombin antibodies, and anti-annexin v antibody
Calf muscle pump ejection fraction (plethysmography)	
Duplex ultrasound	
Contrast computerized tomography	Nutritional
Magnetic resonance venogram	Serum albumin
Contrast venogram	Serum amino acids
Deep and superficial venous valvular insufficiency	Zinc
Venous refilling time (plethysmography) with and without tourniquets	Vitamins
	Biopsy
Duplex ultrasound	Persistent ulcers or unresponsive to therapy
Collagen vascular disease, hematologic disorders	
Antinuclear antibody	
Rheumatoid arthritis prep	
Serum complement	

festation is lipodermatosclerosis, or sclerosing panniculitis, consisting of bound-down, indurated plaques.

The incidence of chronic contact dermatitis in these patients is greatly increased, as the ulcers are frequently exposed to a variety of different topical agents.[6] This often complicates the clinical picture, as application by the patient of lanolin and topical antibiotics is very common, yet can make the ulceration worse.

The base of a venous ulcer is typically exudative and covered with a thick layer of fibrinous material *(Figure 26-3)*. The borders of the ulcer are ragged and erythematous. Rare complications of chronic venous ulcers are the development

Table 26-3
CEAP Classification of Chronic Lower Extremity Venous Disease

C—clinical signs	Grade 0–6, supplemented by A for asymptomatic and S for symptomatic
E—etiologic classification	Congenital, primary or secondary
A—anatomic distribution	Superficial, deep or perforator, alone or in combination
P—pathophysiologic dysfunction	Reflux or obstruction, alone or in combination
Clinical signs grading by number	
0	No visible or palpable signs of venous disease
1	Telangiectasias, reticular veins, malleolar blush
2	Varicose veins
3	Edema without skin changes
4	Skin changes ascribed to venous disease (Chapter 1, Table 1–3)
5	Skin changes as above with healed ulceration
6	Skin changes as above with active ulceration

TABLE 26-4
Signs and Symptoms of Arterial Versus Venous Disease of the Leg

Sign and Symptom	Arterial Disease	Venous Disease
Pain		
Muscle contraction	Worsens	Improves
Limb dependency	Improves	Worsens
Location	Calf or foot	Diffuse aching, focal burning at varicosity site
Compression hose use	Worsens	Improves
Limb temperature	Cool	Warm
Ulceration sites	Distal toes, dorsum foot extending up ankle	Medial ankle (GSV), Lateral ankle (LSV)
Ulceration characteristics	Black eschar, extensive necrosis, sharp margin	Erythematous border, moist, ragged margin
Skin findings	Atrophic, dry, shiny, decreased hair, dystrophic nails	Leg/ankle edema, dermatitis, hyperpigmentation, lipodermatosclerosis

Adapted from ref 8.

of Marjolin's ulcer (squamous cell carcinoma), chronic osteomyelitis, secondary amyloidosis, and angiosarcoma in patients with concomitant chronic lymphedema.

Management

COMPRESSION

Gradient compression hose are the cornerstone of the modern treatment of venous insufficiency (Chapter 15). Properly fitted, these stockings provide 30–40 mm Hg or 40–50 mm Hg of compression at the ankle, with gradually decreasing compression at more proximal levels of the leg. This amount of gradient compression is sufficient to restore normal venous flow patterns in many or most patients with superficial venous reflux, and to improve venous flow even in those patients with severe deep vein incompetence. Some elderly patients with venous ulceration are not strong enough to pull up such tight compression, and they may use two additive stockings or a zippered stocking with inner liner such as the Jobst Ulcer-Care Kit.

The compression gradient is extremely important, since non-gradient stockings or high-stretch elastic bandages ("ace wraps") will cause a tourniquet effect with worsening of the venous insufficiency. The so-called "anti-embolic" stockings commonly available in American hospitals do not

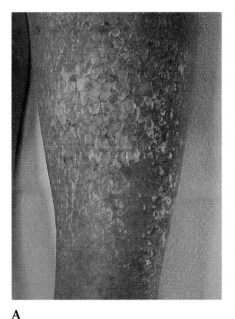
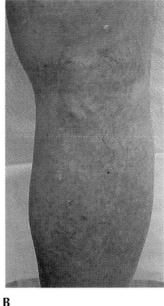

A   B

Figure 26-2. **(A)** Stasis dermatitis of one year's duration. **(B)** Physical examination of this patient reveals large vein in popliteal fossa with accompanying marked reflux of the lesser saphenous vein by CWD. PPG examination reveals a refill time of 15 seconds.

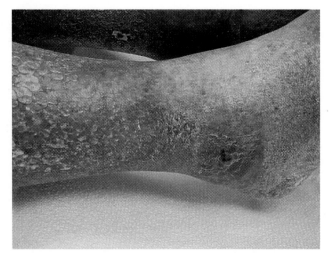

Figure 26-3. Same patient with ulcer on the lateral ankle, the zone of influence and drainage of the LSV. Most venous ulcers due to greater saphenous reflux occur on the medial ankle.

provide sufficient compression to improve venous return from the legs. No patient with symptoms due to venous insufficiency should be without gradient compression hose.

WOUND CARE

While compression treats the underlying problem of venous hypertension, local wound care must simultaneously be carried out on a regular basis. Additional therapy, such as antibiotic therapy or hyperbaric oxygen therapy, is ordered as indicated. The primary goal of local wound care is to allow for a warm, moist and clean environment that is ideal for reepithelialization. A hydrocolloid foam dressing (Cutinova™ or Allevyn™ foam) provides a soft surface, wicking away exudate in which bacteria and harmful waste products may accumulate, but allowing growth factors to remain in contact with the skin.[7] Different categories of wound dressings are summarized in Table 26-5.

When a large wound is clean and adequately vascularized and has developed a good bed of granulation tissue,

the possibility of skin grafting is considered. This is rarely absolutely necessary, but in some cases may significantly decrease time lost from work. The majority of chronic non-healing ulcers can be made to heal with constant meticulous wound care and compression. Typically healing is seen within 10–20 weeks, but unless the underlying cause is addressed, the ulcer will recur in a very short time.

TREATMENT OF DEEP VEIN OBSTRUCTION

If the underlying etiology for the ulceration is chronic venous obstruction, there is no widely accepted treatment approach to offer the patient. Venous to venous bypass is an option, and when postoperative thrombosis can be avoided, the symptoms may be markedly improved. Thrombectomy or endovenectomy is rarely successful because the incidence of postoperative thrombotic reocclusion is very high, and because even when patency is restored, the valveless channel causes deep venous insufficiency that may be just as symptomatic as the original obstruction.

TREATMENT OF DEEP VEIN REFLUX

Deep vein valvular incompetence severe enough to produce ulcers is extremely difficult to treat. Valvuloplasty has occasionally been carried out successfully, but is accompanied by a very high incidence of postoperative deep vein thrombosis. Venous bypass has been reported to be successful in selected patients. External vein valve banding devices and endovenous radiofrequency (RF) narrowing are undergoing clinical trials. At this time, restoration of valvular function to incompetent deep veins remains a "holy grail" for vascular physicians.

TREATMENT OF SUPERFICIAL REFLUX

Ulceration most often occurs when the total amount of deep and superficial reflux is greater than 15 ml/sec. It is much easier to treat superficial venous reflux than deep reflux, because any refluxing superficial vessel can be safely removed or ablated without sequelae (as long as the deep system is patent). A refluxing vessel has already proven itself unnecessary, because it is carrying venous blood incorrectly in a retrograde direction. If removal or sclerosis of a superficial vessel can reduce the total venous reflux below 10 ml/sec,

Table 26-5
Categories of Wound Dressings

Dressing Type	Advantages	Disadvantages
Hydrocolloids—absorbent with polyurethane coating	Debrides wound, easy use	Leakage of fluid, maceration
Hydrogels—semitransparent gel-like	Debrides wound, absorbant	Maceration, expense
Granules (dextranomer, copolymer, or hydroactive)	Absorbant, debride wounds, easy to apply	May dry, difficult to remove
Films—thin, transparent, polyurethane	Adherent, visualize wound	Maceration, pull cells off
Alginates (biodegradable)	Absorbant, hemostatic	Fibers in wound bed, thick to place under compression
Foam (microporous polyurethane foam)	Absorbant, cushions external trauma	Adheres to wound
Laminates—silicone with collagen	Absorbant	More occlusion, less oxygen exchange

most venous ulcerations will heal and patient symptoms will be resolved. Therefore, *never* assume that a patient with venous ulceration cannot be helped by elimination of superficial varicosities.

Non-venous Ulcers

Many of the common causes for ulcers can be treated once the diagnosis is made. When the ulcer is not caused by venous disease, referral to an appropriate specialist is often necessary. Patients with diabetic ulcers are referred to a diabetologist. If poor local tissue care is suspected, a social services referral should be made, and home-care arrangements investigated. If drug abuse or factitious ulceration are suspected, a psychiatric consultation is necessary. Sickle-cell disease or circulating factor abnormalities warrant a hematologic referral. If a trophic ulcer due to chronic underlying bony abnormalities is suspected, a podiatric or orthopedic referral should be made. Osteomyelitis will require orthopedic consultation, often resulting in placement of a long-term catheter and arrangements with a home-infusion nurse for daily antibiotics. If malignancy is suspected, a biopsy should be performed and referral and treatment based on the results.

Summary

Chronic non-healing leg ulcers are a serious and common problem. Good local wound care is helpful, but long-term healing usually requires that the underlying problem be identified and treated. Many diseases that cause ulceration cannot be cured, but in many cases, even a minor amelioration may permit the ulcer to heal. Ulcers caused by venous disease may respond rapidly to gradient compression alone. It is reasonable to treat superficial venous reflux even in the presence of chronic obstruction or deep system reflux, because venous ulcers will heal if the total impairment to circulation is brought below a critical threshold.

References

(1) Biland L, Widmer LK. *Varicose veins (VV) and chronic venous insufficiency (CVI). Medical and socio-economic aspects, Basle study.* Acta Chir Scand Suppl 1988; 544:9–11.

(2) Coon WW, Willis PW, Keller JB. *Venous thromboembolism and other venous disease in the Tecumseh community health study.* Circulation 1973; 48:839–846.

(3) Browse NL, Burnand KG. *The cause of venous ulceration.* Lancet 1982; 2(8292):243–245.

(4) Coleridge Smith PD, Thomas P, Scurr JH, Dormandy JA. *Causes of venous ulceration: a new hypothesis.* Br Med J (Clin Res Ed) 1988; 296(6638):1726–1727.

(5) Kistner RL, Eklof B, Masuda EM. *Diagnosis of chronic venous disease of the lower extremities: the "CEAP" classification* [see comments]. Mayo Clin Proc 1996; 71(4):338–345.

(6) Wilson CL, Cameron J, Powell SM, Cherry G, Ryan TJ. *High incidence of contact dermatitis in leg-ulcer patients—implications for management.* Clin Exp Dermatol 1991; 16:250–253.

(7) Weiss RA, Weiss MA, Ford RW. *Randomized comparative study of Cutinova foam and Allevyn with Jobst UlcerCare stockings for the treatment of venous stasis ulcers.* Phlebology 1996; 1(Supp):14–16.

(8) Weiss RA. *Vascular studies of the legs for venous or arterial disease.* [review]. Dermatol Clin 1994; 12(1):175–190.

PART V

Practice

CHAPTER 27

Outfitting the Phlebology Practice

Introduction

The physical infrastructure of a phlebology practice is critically important for its success. The right equipment, supplies, and management are essential to the health of the patient and the viability of the practice. Even the seasoned practitioner who has an active ongoing practice in another specialty will need to make a special effort to understand the administrative nuances of a phlebology practice.

Diagnostic equipment is perhaps the most important of all investments to be made in a phlebology practice. The safety and efficacy of sclerotherapy has made it one of the most popular cosmetic procedures worldwide, but major complications, including anaphylactic reactions, intraarterial injections, deep venous thromboses, and pulmonary emboli have all been reported. Minor complications, such as telangiectatic matting, ulcerations, pigmentation stains, and early recurrences can be extremely annoying. Thorough diagnostic evaluation and adherence to meticulous technique will help to keep complications to an absolute minimum. Diagnostic reevaluation during the course of treatment or on patients' return visits may often be necessary.

Forms, Documents, and Patient Information

Patient education and information forms are very important to the success of a phlebology practice. Brochures are useful to answer the most common questions asked by patients and by referring physicians. Medical fact sheets can help patients to understand their disease process in more detail. Pre- and post-treatment instruction sheets will help to ensure that the patient is prepared for treatment and will comply with post-treatment directions. Appendix A offers samples. Appendix B includes sources for patient brochures. Many physicians have found that a patient-oriented educational videotape helps increase patient understanding. Trained staff can review all of this information thoroughly with the patient before the physician sees the patient. This allows the physician to more efficiently concentrate on evaluation of the patient and development of a treatment plan. However, the physician should always review the patient's understanding of the proposed treatment and risks before actually beginning treatment. When patients return for maintenance treatment after 1–2 years, it is advisable to again review the information; after lengthier intervals between treatments, one may consider having the patient also re-sign consent forms.

Patient Chart

A properly designed phlebology chart will greatly facilitate record keeping and improve the management of patients being treated for venous disease. These documents should be grouped separately from unrelated treatment records in the patient's chart. Table 27-1 lists the key components of the phlebology chart, and samples of these documents are found in Appendix A.

Table 27-1
Components of the Phlebology Chart

Registration form
History and physical exam
Assessment and plan
Photographic documentation
Treatment estimate
Diagnostic testing results
Treatment and progress notes
Consent form

Bookkeeping and Insurance Considerations

For bookkeeping purposes any ready made accounting package can be used. Quickbooks® is an intuitively easy and comprehensive package. A "superbill" or "encounter form" is used to provide the patient with a receipt for services rendered and as a primary source for financial record keeping (see Appendix C for appropriate procedural terminology codes). The universal HCFA 1500 form is used for insurance billing. Computerized medical billing systems are evolving at too rapid a rate to allow us to make specific recommendations.

The decision to bill an insurance company or the patient for sclerotherapy of varicose veins depends on two major factors: physician participation and medical necessity. If a physician does not "participate" by contract with an insurance company, then the patient can be charged directly and then file for reimbursement using a copy of the encounter form. Payment at the time of service is strongly recommended, but it is good public relations to assist patients in obtaining reimbursement by promptly providing the insurance company with any required information (exam notes, photographs, test results). Because most insurance companies are increasingly restricting or eliminating coverage of sclerotherapy of varicose veins, it is crucial to know the specific guidelines of each plan with which the physician participates. At the initial consultation, patients can be informed if there is a chance of reimbursement.

If insurance coverage is being considered, it is imperative to obtain written, specific preauthorization of the planned treatment. This administrative burden can be eased somewhat through use of a word-processing template letter that can be easily individualized. For preauthorization, most insurance companies require pretreatment photographs that show the varicose veins to be treated. Unfortunately, many varicosities do not photograph well, especially in overweight patients. In this situation, supporting abnormal test data is crucial to document the patient's problem. The number of allowed treatment sessions should be noted in the chart, as well as the expiration date of the authorization. The insurance company's decision should be reviewed with the patient so that they have a full understanding of their financial obligation. Because regulations and insurance company guidelines vary on a state-to-state basis and can change frequently, the authors recommend that physicians apply due diligence in understanding their individual situations.

Even when insurance approves coverage, reimbursement in the United States usually falls far short of a nonparticipating physician's fee. For those physicians still participating with insurance companies, the low reimbursement for medically indicated sclerotherapy or ambulatory phlebectomy of varicose veins might lead to the decision to drop insurance contracts as the proportion of phlebology cases rises in their practice. Many in-office practices devoted to phlebology do not participate in insurance.

If the veins do not "qualify" for coverage (for example, being too small or asymptomatic), then the office does not usually need to attempt preauthorization even if they participate with a particular plan. The cosmetic treatment of telangiectasias is not covered by almost all insurance companies. Such treatments must be clearly coded with the appropriate CPT procedure code and ICD-9 diagnosis (see Appendix C) to distinguish their treatment from that of varicose veins. Patients need to understand their probable costs before they begin treatment.

Pretreatment Evaluation

PHYSIOLOGIC TESTING

The basic tests to be considered are the continuous-wave Doppler ultrasound, the venous refilling time, the calf muscle pump ejection fraction, and the maximum venous outflow. A handheld Doppler unit is sufficient for the first of these, and any plethysmographic or rheographic equipment may be used for the latter three. Typically, a handheld Doppler will be the first device purchased as a physician progresses from the occasional treatment of isolated telangiectasias to treatment of reticular and varicose veins. The understanding and use of Doppler is critical to making the leap from sclerotherapy novice to skilled practitioner.

The Doppler is as essential to the physician practicing sclerotherapy, as a stethoscope is to an internist. Several manufacturers make combined units that will perform all four of these tests. Typical units are shown in Figure 27-1. Vendors are easily found at the Annual Congress and regional symposia of the American College of Phlebology. Appendix B includes a list of manufacturers.

For those physicians who are treating smaller vessels, the natural order of equipment acquisition is Doppler followed by photoplethysmograph. The photoplethysmograph (PPG) allows the physician to assess venous function. With digital PPG (DPPG), trained office staff can easily do this and the results are accurate, quantified, and reproducible. As physicians progress to treating larger veins and varicosities, the PPG is very helpful to gauge the severity of the patient's venous insufficiency. An abnormal PPG is a warning signal to evaluate the patient thoroughly, and is usually followed by duplex evaluation. The PPG is inexpensive compared to duplex, and most insurance companies will pay for the test. In the United States, one must check current HCFA and other insurance company guidelines to determine how many types of vascular tests may be done at one visit.

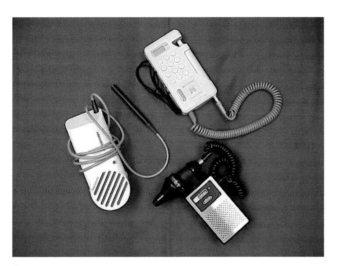

A

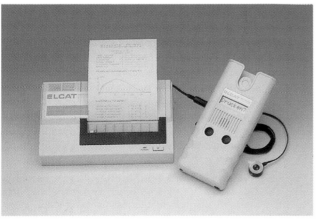

B

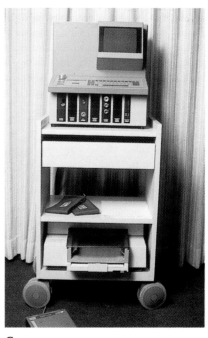

C

Figure 27-1. Typical equipment used for diagnostic physiologic testing. **(A)** Three inexpensive handheld Doppler units, by Huntleigh, Imex, and Elcat. **(B)** Digital photoplethysmograph (DPPG) (photo courtesy of Elcat GmBH). **(C)** Combination unit by Imex.

ANATOMIC IMAGING

Duplex ultrasound adds an important dimension to the phlebology practice, and is essential for any practice that is completely specialized in phlebology. Duplex ultrasound is used for venous mapping, for diagnosis of complex or refractory cases, and to guide injections in selected cases of large varices, incompetent perforators, and feeding vessels that may not be visible from the surface. Postoperatively, the duplex ultrasound exam is the best routinely available non-invasive test for evaluating patients for possible DVT.

Purchase or leasing of a duplex ultrasound machine is a major financial commitment, and many physicians performing sclerotherapy will not need to make the investment if they do not choose to treat those vessels that require duplex-guided injection. However, in these situations, it is imperative to develop a close, cooperative relationship with a vascular laboratory that has a technician who is trained in the subtleties of venous disease. Otherwise, the typical report after venous duplex examination in a vascular laboratory is "no evidence of deep venous thrombosis," with no examination of the actual varicosities for the highest point of reflux—the target area for treatment. Such a report is useless for treatment guidance.

Without a duplex examination that can identify reflux points, one must rely on a skilled and complete Doppler exam to identify the highest point of reflux. This is especially important when there are varicosities of the medial leg in the region of greater saphenous vein influence. The accuracy of this exam is greatly dependent on both the experience of the physician and the size of the patient; a patient's body fat can easily obscure the origin of the reflux. One then runs the risk of incomplete closure of the varicosities by missing the highest reflux point. If treatment is not optimally successful, then one must refer the patient for a duplex examination by a physician who can perform a detailed duplex mapping and duplex-guided injection, if necessary.

Although the skilled clinician can make good use of a grayscale duplex device, color-flow duplex ultrasound offers many added benefits. A videotape recorder, a frame-grabber, and a color printer are essential components of a duplex ultrasound setup. A typical color-flow duplex ultrasound unit is shown in Figure 27-2. Technological advances in duplex ultrasound are occurring rapidly, and smaller, less expensive units will soon be available.

PHOTOGRAPHY

All patients should have pre- and posttreatment photographs. These photographs are extremely helpful in judging treatment progress and evaluating the evolution of minor side effects. During the course of treatment, many patients forget the original severity of their problem. Patients may even come to believe that longstanding scars, moles, birthmarks, and other skin landmarks have actually been caused by their treatment. Regular review of pretreatment photographs is the best way to keep patients oriented to the reality of the process. Midtreatment photographs of problem areas such as matting or pigmentation can be helpful. When patients return after intervals of months or years for mainte-

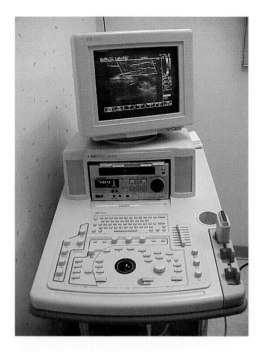

Figure 27-2. Hewlett Packard color-flow duplex ultrasound unit.

nance therapy, it is important to photograph at that time to document their current condition.

A secondary reason to take photographs is for insurance purposes. Despite the fact that photographs show only what is on the surface of the skin, many insurance companies require initial photographs for predetermination of benefits, and final payment is often approved or denied based on how impressive the veins appear to a reviewer in the photographs.

All pictures should be taken using standard positioning and lighting. It is helpful to photograph an entire anatomic area in one shot (e.g., anterior thigh), but also to take areas of particular interest at a closer range for more detail. With experience, common photographic mistakes, such as shooting from too far away, will be overcome. Views of varicose veins taken with the patient standing typically are much more representative of the true size of the veins, but views of areas of spider veins taken with the patient lying both prone and supine on the exam table are very helpful as well.

Any 35 mm camera with a macro lens may be used. Digital cameras with more than 1.5 million pixels also provide adequate resolution. With the newest digital cameras, image quality has greatly improved to the point where available picture resolution far exceeds the quality necessary for documentation. The practitioner does not need to purchase a digital camera capable of high-quality 5x7 prints for his or her practice. The authors successfully use a consumer-oriented digital camera (Sony Mavica MVC-FD-91 or FD-95), widely available from catalogues, retail, and Internet photographic outlets. Actual prints are only made when needed for specific purposes such as patient request or insurance. Those made by color printers have a high enough quality for submission to insurance companies when necessary. Patients can have their own labeled inexpensive disc, easily stored in the chart without adding significant bulk. At subsequent visits the visual images can be quickly reviewed with the patient when necessary by inserting the disc into the camera. The savings in film/slide development over time are considerable, as the discs can be bought in bulk at very low cost.

In contrast, when 35-mm slides are used, a photo logbook must be carefully maintained to use for slide labelling when the film has been developed. The possibility of loss of the film in transport or development exists. Typically such slides are filed in clear vinyl slide-holder sleeves that are kept alphabetically in notebooks, as keeping them in a patient's chart makes the chart much thicker than desirable. Staff time for slide/photo retrieval from storage areas is significant in a busy phlebology practice; this is eliminated by use of the digital system.

Ideally, a staff person can be trained to take the photos to save the physician's time, but this can prove difficult with 35 mm cameras, where one has no idea if the image is satisfactory (correct distance, area, and focus) until the film has returned from development. By that time, treatment has typically started, and if the original slides or photos are unsatisfactory there is no way to redo them. The cost of "instant" photos is prohibitive, and the quality unsatisfactory. With the digital system, however, the physician can immediately review the images taken by the assistant and take new ones if necessary. Such review is usually only necessary during the training period of the assistant who, once trained, can review the images themselves. Unsatisfactory images can be deleted from the disc without cost in film. Multiple digital image computerized filing systems have also been developed for physicians who choose to centralize their image storage.

Treatment

SUPPLIES

Table 27-2 provides a checklist of the minimum sclerotherapy supplies that are needed for a phlebology practice equipped to treat a wide variety of diseased veins (Table 27-2). Figure 27-3 shows a typical tray set up for routine sclerotherapy in one of the author's practices. Appendix B lists suppliers.

Needles

When butterfly catheters are used, a 27-gauge needle is preferred. The length of tubing is also important for ease of infusion: tubing that is too short is difficult to manipulate, while tubing that is too long clutters the area and will encumber multiple injection sites.

Nearly all phlebologists use a 30-gauge needle for injection of telangiectasias. Some physicians prefer a 31-gauge or 33-gauge needle, but these highly flexible needles are not stiff enough to allow for controlled cannulation. A 30-gauge needle is quite sufficient to allow even the smallest telangiectasia to be cannulated, while retaining a stiffness that permits great control over the placement of the tip. Reusable fine-gauge needles dull quickly and are not generally recommended in this era of bloodborne pathogens.

Table 27-2
Medical Supplies Needed

- ❏ 27G × ½" winged infusion set with tubing
- ❏ 18G × 1 ½" needles
- ❏ 21G × 1 ½" needles
- ❏ 30G × ½" needles
- ❏ Metal cup for used needles and syringes
- ❏ 1cc syringes
- ❏ 3cc syringes
- ❏ 5cc syringes
- ❏ Vacutainer tubes without silicone lining
- ❏ Exam gloves (nonsterile), including non-latex gloves
- ❏ Large cotton balls
- ❏ Cotton rolls
- ❏ ½" paper tape
- ❏ 1" Transpore™ tape
- ❏ Rubbing alcohol
- ❏ Alcohol dispenser bottle
- ❏ Plastic cup with cotton balls soaked in alcohol
- ❏ Band-Aids™
- ❏ Disposable exam shorts (or patients can bring their own)
- ❏ Sundry jars (cotton jars)
- ❏ Pillows
- ❏ Disposable pillow covers
- ❏ Disposable drapes

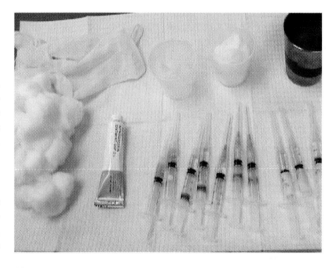

Figure 27-3. The typical sclerotherapy tray is prepared with multiple strips of Transpore™ or paper tape, nonsterile cotton balls, a plastic cup with alcohol-soaked cotton balls, a plastic cup with extra disposable 30-gauge plastic-hub needles, a metal cup to put empty syringes and needles in before final disposal, nonsterile gloves, labeled syringes of sclerosing solution, and a timer (if desired). A tube of nitrol® ointment is in every treatment room, and often put on the tray.

Syringes

A 3-cc syringe is ideal for the butterfly technique, as it contains an appropriate volume of solution to be infused and is still easy to handle. For fine spider veins, either a 1-cc or a 3-cc syringe may be used (the authors are divided in their personal preferences). When using the 3-cc syringe, that author prefers that it be filled with only 1½ cc of solution, to allow more comfortable hand positioning. Several syringes should be tested to find the one that best meets the injection needs of the practitioner. Testing suggests that Terumo® latex-free brand syringes may be preferred because they tend to have lower coefficients of starting friction and sliding friction than do the plastic syringes made by Becton Dickson (B-D®). Because sotradecol at concentrations of 0.5% or greater can begin to break down the rubber in the syringe over time, those concentrations are not stored in the syringes.

Solution dilution and storage vials

One of the authors recommends that to avoid any possibility of cross-contamination, opened medications always be discarded once they have been taken into a treatment room with a single patient. This author does not take multidose vials into a treatment room; instead, single-dose vials are used whenever possible, and dilutions are made in single-patient containers. A convenient single-patient container for dilutions is a special redtop vacutainer tube that is glycerin-lined rather than silicone-lined. These can be specifically ordered by asking for redtop tubes #6442.

Another authors' practice utilizes a different system for solution dilution. A specially trained nursing assistant injects 1% sotradecol ampules into sterile glass vials with the appropriate amount of diluent to form concentrations of 0.1% and 0.2%. Table 27-3 lists instructions for dilution of Sotradecol. The glass bottles are labelled, and multiple 3-cc syringes are filled with 1½ cc of solution. Each syringe is immediately marked with a printed, color-coded label of the solution and concentration. Small plastic boxes containing an assortment of clearly labelled dilutions, as well as glass vials of 1% and 0.5% sotradecol, are kept refrigerated, and brought out daily for use. The assistant withdraws from the 1% and 0.5% vials only as specifically requested by the physician, and labels that syringe before it is placed on the tray. Because a sterile, unopened syringe is used only once to draw up the 1½ cc amount from the multidose vial, risk of cross-contamination is eliminated. Ampules of 3% sotradecol are used only for duplex-guided solution, and are stored separately. Syringes are filled with 1 cc of 3% sotradecol at the time of injection.

The essentials of dilution are that it be done without contamination and that solutions be clearly labelled to minimize risk of inadvertent use of inappropriate concentration of solution. Sclerosing solutions must obviously be kept separated from other injectables, such as lidocaine, so as to eliminate the possibility that a sclerosing solution be injected instead of a local anesthetic. Table 27-4 lists the formula for mixing saline and dextrose, as found in Sclerodex™.

Table 27-3
Instructions for Diluting Sotradecol™

1% Sotradecol	1 part of 3% Sotradecol
	2 parts of 0.9% sodium chloride injectable
Example	2 cc of 3% Sotradecol
	4 cc of 0.9% sodium chloride injectable
0.5% Sotradecol	1 part of 3% Sotradecol
	5 parts of 0.9% sodium chloride injectable
Example	2 cc of 3% Sotradecol
	10 cc of 0.9% sodium chloride injectable
0.25% Sotradecol	1 part of 1% Sotradecol
	3 parts of 0.9% sodium chloride injectable
Example	0.5 cc of 1% Sotradecol
	1.5 cc of 0.9% sodium chloride injectable
0.2% Sotradecol	2 parts of 1% Sotradecol
	8 parts of 0.9% sodium chloride injectable
Example	0.2 cc of 1% Sotradecol
	0.8 cc of 0.9% sodium chloride injectable
0.1% Sotradecol	1 part of 1% Sotradecol
	9 parts of 0.9% sodium chloride injectable
Example	0.1 cc of 1% Sotradecol,
	0.9 cc of 0.9% sodium chloride injectable

Gloves

Non-latex gloves for patients or staff with latex rubber allergies should be kept on hand. Typically, nonsterile gloves are used for sclerotherapy; obviously, sterile gloves are used when sterile technique is necessary, as in ambulatory phlebectomy, surgery, and VNUS Closure™.

Cotton rolls and foam pads

Foam pads often are used to provide extra compression directly over a treated vessel (*Figure 27-4*). These foam pads contain latex, and can produce serious allergic reactions even in patients who are not known to have any prior history of latex allergy. Even in the absence of a true allergy, there is a tendency for skin breakdown at the corners of these pads. An alternative is to use cotton strips rolled and custom-shaped into a cylinder. These cotton rolls may be placed along a treated varicose vein in a tortuous course, and can be tolerated even in difficult areas such as behind the knee.

Table 27-4
Formula for Dextrose/Saline Solution

Formula: Amount to prepare	5 × 50 cc
Dextrose USP	62.5 grams
Sodium chloride	25 grams
Propylene glycol	25 mls
Phenyl ethyl alcohol	2 mls
Sterile water for injection	QS to 250 ml

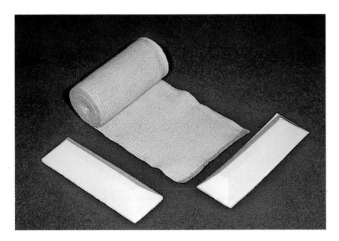

Figure 27-4.   STD foam pads, sizes large and small, with wrapping (photo courtesy of Delasco).

Tape

Surgical tape, Transpore™, or paper tape is used to hold cotton balls and cotton rolls or foam pads in place. Tape should always be applied in such a way as to avoid any traction on the skin, as skin traction can produce impressive blisters and skin breakdown in a very short time. Patients are reminded that they can remove the tape if it causes irritation (Figure 27-5 shows an example of taping).

Alcohol

Isopropyl alcohol is used to swab each area to be injected. A non-contact alcohol dispenser is preferred, as back-contamination has been observed when a bloodstained cotton ball was inadvertently reapplied to a contact-type alcohol dispenser. Alternatively, an inexpensive disposable plastic cup filled with alcohol-soaked cotton balls can be placed on the tray for each patient.

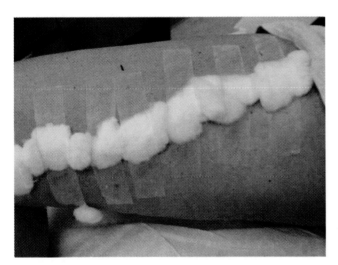

Figure 27-5.   Cotton balls are applied along the course of the treated vessel with overlying tape.

Cotton balls

Cotton balls are used to clean the skin in areas to be injected, and are also taped into place as a means of increasing local compression at the site of injection. Real cotton balls are better tolerated than synthetic puffs for this purpose.

Adhesive strips

When cotton balls or rolls are not applied over an injection site that will come into contact with clothing, an adhesive strip (such as Band-Aid ™ brand strips) should be applied to the injection sites to avoid any staining of the patient's clothes.

Exam shorts

Although patients are requested to bring a pair of loose-fitting shorts to each examination and treatment session, patients often are unable to do so. Disposable paper shorts provide an excellent option that prevents accidental reuse of dirty clothing and removes the need for laundry services.

Pillows

Many patients with curvature of the upper spine cannot lie flat at all, and many who can lie flat are uncomfortable in that position after only a few minutes. For these patients, a normal-sized bed pillow with a disposable single-use pillowcover is an important addition to every treatment room.

Graduated compression hose

Graduated compression hose are used to enhance treatment results and reduce complications. Thigh-high compression stockings are more useful than calf-high stockings, because full-leg compression offers proven protection against venous thrombosis and reduces superficial reflux through the whole leg. It is critically important that compression hose not be permitted to roll down or to bunch up, because rolling or bunching will cause a tourniquet effect that can cause significant distal edema and can increase the risk of deep vein thrombosis.

Waist-high (pantyhose-style) stockings are the most effective way to avoid slipping and rolling, but are poorly tolerated by most men. Thigh-high stockings with a waistband attachment are well tolerated, but double waistbands can become bulky when these stockings are used on both legs at once. A wide, stiff, silicone-lined band has been added to the top of several brands of stockings as an "integrated retention device." This is an effective way to keep the stocking up and to prevent rolling in many patients, but does not work well in patients who have a large thigh-to-knee ratio or in those who have very soft and compressible thighs. A special stocking glue ("It-Stays," MEDI USA, LP, Arlington Heights, IL) is available to keep stockings from slipping or rolling, and can be very effective in patients with firm upper legs. A traditional garter belt is an effective alternative solution when none of the above solutions proves satisfactory. Women may use a standard garter belt available in lingerie shops, but heavy, white medical garter belts have proven more acceptable to men.

Table 27-5
Compression Hose

Pantyhose
Thigh-high with waist attachment
Thigh-high with silicone top band
Thigh-high without silicone top band
Knee-high socks for men

A well-stocked office will maintain an inventory of each of the above stocking styles in small, medium, and large sizes, as well as medical garter belts and "It-Stays" for use in selected patients. Patients appreciate the convenience as well as proper fitting that the well-trained staff can provide. Table 27-5 lists the type of hose that should be stocked.

EQUIPMENT
Magnifiers
All varicose and reticular veins and most telangiectasia are easily visualized for treatment with the naked eye. The smallest telangiectasia may be too small to be easily treated without magnification, and when treating these vessels, eye loupes can be very helpful. Headband magnifiers are less expensive than loupes, but are less well-suited to clear, distortion-free magnification. They offer the advantage that they can be worn over regular prescription glasses.

Double-polarized light and magnification device
A recently developed headpiece *(Figure 27-6)* that combines magnification with double-polarized light greatly facilitates the visualization of reticular veins and the cannulation of tiny telangiectasias.

Transillumination
The new Venoscope® transilluminator *(Figure 27-7)* allows the physician to noninvasively locate, evaluate, and assess the patient's peripheral venous network. It can help visualize hidden reticular "feeder" veins and is useful for vein mapping prior to ambulatory phlebectomy.

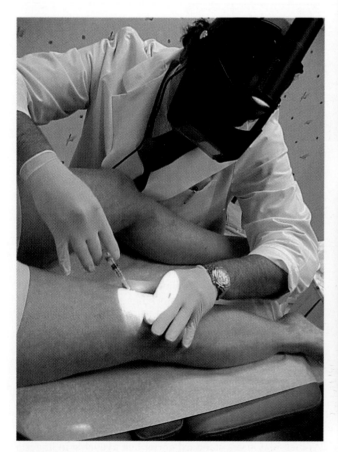

Figure 27-6.   One of the authors using the double-polarized light and magnification device for sclerotherapy of telangiectasias.

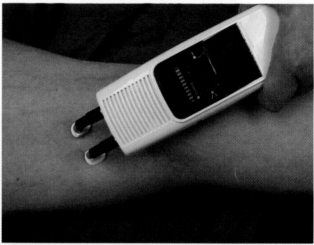

A

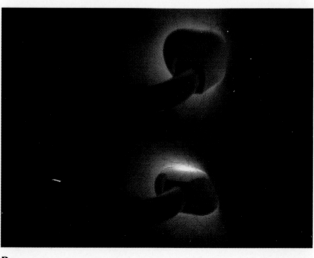

B

Figure 27-7.   **(A)** Venoscope® transillumination device, **(B)** In use in the darkened room (different leg, varicosity in middle).

The VeinLite also uses a transilluminating technique for visualizing veins, but from the side. The variable halogen light source is channeled through a flexible fiberoptic guide to the specially designed light ring where it is directed in to the skin. While the authors do not yet have personal experience with this device, it is reported to help ease venous access, mapping, and finding reticular veins.

Phlebectomy tools

Stab avulsion phlebectomy equipment is discussed in detail in Chapter 22, including manufacturer's addresses. A complete set of tools is necessary in order to carry out the procedure with a high degree of success. Table 27-6 contains a list of instruments and materials typically needed for this procedure.

Autoclave

If phlebectomy is to be performed, an autoclave is essential for sterilization of the various instruments used. Small mosquito forceps ("snaps") are often useful for stabilization of needles and catheters during duplex-guided injections, which also must be sterilized after each use.

MEDICATIONS

Medications stocked in a phlebology office fall into three categories: sclerosants, ancillary agents used in routine phlebology, and emergency medications, which are rarely used.

Sclerosants

Most sclerotherapy in the United States is carried out using the detergent sclerosants sodium tetradecyl sulfate, polidocanol, the osmotic agent hypertonic saline, or a mixture of dextrose and hypertonic saline (*Table 27-7*). These and other sclerosants are discussed extensively in the chapter devoted

Table 27-6
Material for Phlebectomy

Indelible marking pen or KMnO4 (7.5%)
Antiseptic solution
Disposable facemask
Sterile gloves
Local anesthetic, saline or Ringer solution
Syringes
Needles
Resuscitation material
Clamps, sterile gauzes
18-Gauge needle
11 scalpel
Mosquito forceps
Hydrogen peroxide (for postoperative washing of the leg)
Absorbent dressings
Tubular dressings
Elastic bandages
Phlebectomy hooks

Table 27-7
Sclerosants commonly used in the United States

Sodium tetradecyl sulfate
Polidocanol (Laureth-9)
Hypertonic saline
Mixture of saline and dextrose

to sclerosants. The distributors of sclerosing medications are listed in Appendix B.

Ancillary medications

Ancillary agents used in a phlebology practice include normal saline for dilution, EMLA® or ELAMAX® creams for patients who are needle-phobic or extremely sensitive, and lidocaine for local anesthesia where needed. For tissue dilution some physicians use hyaluronidase after inadvertent extravasation of concentrated caustic solutions. Nitrol ointment should be available to be applied in the rare instances when immediate, persistent tissue blanching indicates that anastamotic arteriolar injection or spasm may have occurred. Nonsteroidal antiinflammatory agents and acetaminophen are also very useful medications to have on hand. Ammonia ampoules may be useful when patients have syncope or near-syncope from vasovagal reactions to the sight or sound of blood or from prolonged standing. Starter doses of subcutaneous low-molecular-weight heparin are very useful when a patient has progressive superficial phlebitis or when a decision is made to treat deep vein thrombosis on an outpatient basis. Antibiotics may be useful when there is any question of infection related to non-healing ulcers or to puncture sites. Ancillary agents are listed in Table 27-8.

Emergency medications

A crash cart is useful in case of unanticipated anaphylactic reactions. Table 27-9 lists equipment and medications that may be helpful. At the minimum, epinephrine and diphenhydramine for injection should be immediately available. All staff should be familiar with emergency plans for patient transfer to the appropriate facility in the very unlikely event that this should become necessary.

Table 27-8
Ancillary Medications

0.9% Sodium chloride (normal saline) (injectable)
EMLA® cream, ELAMAX® cream
Lidocaine (1% and 2% with and without epinephrine)
Hyaluronidase (Wydase®, lyophilized, 150 USP u/ml, Wyeth, Philadelphia, PA)
Nitrol® ointment
Nonsteroidal antiinflammatory agents
Acetaminophen
Low-molecular-weight heparin
Oral antibiotics

Table 27-9
Suggested Medications and Equipment for Crash Kit

Epinephrine
Cimetidine
Diphenhydramine
Solumedrol
Intubation kit or airway
Oxygen
Defibrillator
Ambu-Bag
50% Dextrose

SAFETY CONCERNS

Blood is present during every procedure and is found in all waste materials after a procedure, and sharps are present during procedures and enter the disposal system afterwards. For these reasons, every member of a phlebology staff should receive immunization against hepatitis B. An easy-to-use eyewash station should be provided in a readily accessible place. Protective garments should be used wherever blood exposure is expected. In the United States, physicians and their staff must comply with current OSHA bloodborne pathogen guidelines. Elsewhere, following these guidelines offers patients and staff the highest levels of safety.

STAFFING

Staffing requirements will vary based on the particular organization of each individual office. In addition to a receptionist and a competent billing person or a billing service, an active phlebology practice requires at least one clinical support person (RN, LPN, PA, or MA) for every clinician who will be performing evaluations and treatments. An experienced clinical team can manage approximately three treatments per hour during the busy season. Every physician should remember that a patient's first encounter with the practice would be through the staff, so that a thoroughly trained and friendly staff is a top priority.

Some offices use a dedicated ultrasound technician, while others prefer to cross-train doctors and nurses in vascular ultrasound. Regulations for billing are changing often requiring an RVT (registered vascular technologist) to perform the exam. A simple bilateral "hospital-style" examination to rule out large deep vein thrombosis above the knee can be carried out in about 15 minutes by an experienced ultrasonographer. A complete examination to rule out any deep venous thrombosis in the iliac veins and in the leg both above and below the knee can require an hour or more, depending on the patient's body habitus and anatomy. Ultrasound mapping of reflux requires from 30–60 minutes per leg, depending on the complexity of the findings. After

mapping, experienced practitioners may be able to complete an ultrasound-guided injection session within 15 minutes of ultrasound time.

ROOMS AND TABLES

For an individual practitioner, anything less than 1500 square feet will result in a cramped practice environment. It is difficult to establish an active and successful phlebology practice with fewer than three examination rooms, even if diagnostic equipment is mounted on a cart and rolled from room to room. Duplex ultrasound requires a dedicated room. A separate medication storage and preparation area is essential.

Any exam table with an adjustable back may be used for diagnostic examination and treatment. Various types of stools or steps may be used to place the standing patient at a height comfortable for the examining physician, but there should be adequate supports for the patient to feel secure from falling. An adjustable power table can add a great deal in terms of speed of treatment, flexibility, and patient comfort. Physicians and staff work much more comfortably with power tables; consideration of proper ergonomics will benefit all concerned.

Marketing

Any phlebology practice will depend on referrals from physicians and patients for growth. Appropriately increasing the visibility of the practice within the medical and lay community will develop these patient sources and reach out to interested potential new patients. Marketing endeavors must follow the principles of professional medical integrity, and it is important to check with the State Board of Medicine and the Federal Trade Commission about physician-marketing regulations. Every marketing expenditure of time or money requires careful tracking and analysis to determine whether ongoing efforts of a similar nature are justified. Remember that satisfied patient word-of-mouth remains the single most important factor in practice development. The authors encourage beginning physicians to read and learn as much as they can from the many professional sources available on this subject.

Summary

Besides special knowledge and training, a successful phlebology practice requires specialized diagnostic, therapeutic, and office-type equipment and supplies. It is a pleasure to practice in a well-organized office with properly trained support staff, fully stocked with the right instruments and materials for treatment, with a well-established office infrastructure. Such a practice environment permits the best in patient care as well as the safest, most effective, and most satisfying practice for the clinician.

APPENDIX A

Samples of medical forms are from the authors' practices and are provided to assist other clinicians in developing their own forms. All materials are copyrighted protected. Always consult with your attorney for any legal form.

PATIENT INFORMATION FORMS

- General information about venous disease: educational video and brochures (Appendix B)
- Individualized practice brochure: professional help recommended
- Pre-and post-treatment instructions (Figure 1)

CHART FORMS

- Registration: demographics & insurance information: (Figure 2)
- Clinical history: general and vascular: (Figure 3)
- Physical exam, treatment and progress note: (Figure 4)
- Preoperative testing request: (Figure 5)
- Physiologic test results: Doppler mapping form: (Figure 6)
  - Digital PPG prints its own report.
- Duplex ultrasound mapping diagram: (Figure 7)
  - Written description would accompany this map.
- Treatment estimate/fee schedule consent: (Figure 8)
- General sclerotherapy information consent: (Figure 9)
- Consent form: (Figure 10)
- Alternative consent form: (Figure 11)

DRS. ROBERT AND MARGARET WEISS
AND DERMATOLOGY ASSOCIATES

OFFICES:

ASPEN MILL PROFESSIONAL CENTER
54 SCOTT ADAM ROAD, SUITE 301
HUNT VALLEY, MD 21030
(410) 666-3960
FAX (410) 666-3981

PERRY HALL PROFESSIONAL CENTER
9712 BELAIR ROAD, SUITE 200
BALTIMORE, MD 21236
(410) 529-0280
FAX (410) 529-0612

Sclerotherapy Instructions

- Leave cotton balls, tape, and stockings on until bedtime.

- If itching or burning develops, then remove the tape immediately.

- If you have redness or irritation in the areas of the tape, please call the office for a prescription cream.

- When returning for treatment, do not put any lotion or oil on your legs for 2 days *before* each treatment session.

- Do not shave your legs the morning of your treatment.

- If you prefer, you may bring a pair of shorts to wear during the treatment—some patients feel this is more comfortable.

- After you remove the tape, wear prescription or Delilah/Venosan support hose for two weeks, except to sleep.

- After treatments, there is no restriction on activity, but try not to bump the areas doing exercises, which can cause bruising. Weight lifting with the legs should be minimized for two weeks. We encourage walking.

- If something occurs (for example, illness or injury) that would interfere with normal walking, please postpone treatment.

- Please call us if you have any questions or problems.

Figure 1.   Pre- and post-treatment instructions

NEW PATIENT INFORMATION RECORD (PLEASE PRINT OR WRITE LEGIBLY)
PATIENT INFORMATION

PATIENT'S NAME (LAST, FIRST, MIDDLE)	SEX		MARITAL STATUS					DATE OF BIRTH	AGE	SOCIAL SECURITY NO.
	M	F	S	M	W	D	SEP			

STREET ADDRESS ☐ PERMANENT ☐ TEMPORARY	CITY AND STATE	ZIP CODE	HOME PHONE NO.
PATIENT'S EMPLOYER	OCCUPATION (INDICATE IF STUDENT)		BUSINESS PHONE NO.
EMPLOYER'S STREET ADDRESS	CITY AND STATE		ZIP CODE
DRUG ALLERGIES			
SPOUSE'S NAME			
SPOUSE'S EMPLOYER	OCCUPATION (INDICATE IF STUDENT)		
EMPLOYER'S STREET ADDRESS	CITY AND STATE		ZIP CODE
NEAREST RELATIVE	ADDRESS		HOME PHONE NO.

IF PATIENT IS A MINOR OR STUDENT

MOTHER'S NAME	STREET ADDRESS, CITY, STATE AND ZIP CODE	HOME PHONE NO.
MOTHER'S EMPLOYER	OCCUPATION	BUSINESS PHONE NO.
EMPLOYER'S STREET ADDRESS	CITY AND STATE	ZIP CODE
FATHER'S NAME	STREET ADDRESS, CITY, STATE AND ZIP CODE	HONE PHONE NO.
FATHER'S EMPLOYER	OCCUPATION	BUSINESS PHONE NO.
EMPLOYER'S STREET ADDRESS	CITY AND STATE	ZIP CODE

INSURANCE INFORMATION (PLEASE PRESENT INSURANCE CARDS TO RECEPTIONIST)

PERSON RESPONSIBLE FOR PAYMENT	SOCIAL SECURITY NO.		D.O.B.
☐ BLUE SHIELD (GIVE NAME OF POLICY HOLDER) OF MD	MEMBERSHIP NO.	GROUP NO. MAJOR MEDICAL	
☐ MEDICARE PRIMARY INSURANCE? YES NO	☐ MEDICAL ASSISTANCE EFFECTIVE DATES:		
☐ OTHER (WRITE IN NAME OF INSURANCE COMPANY)	POLICY NO./SOCIAL SECURITY NO. OF POLICY HOLDER-EMPLOYEE:		
OTHER INSURANCE COMPANY ADDRESS			
GROUP NO.:	POLICYHOLDER/EMPLOYEE NAME:		

MARYLAND ONLY

REFERRED BY
☐ PHYSICIAN _____ ☐ PATIENT _____ ☐ YELLOW PAGES
ADDRESS _____ ☐ OTHER _____

In order to control our costs of billing, we request that office visits be paid at the time the service is rendered.
We would rather control our billing costs than be forced to raise our fees.

AUTHORIZATION: I hereby authorize the physician indicated above to furnish information to insurance carriers concerning the illness/accident, and I hereby assign to the doctor all payments for medical services rendered. I understand that I am financially responsible for all charges whether or not covered by insurance.

_____ (Signature)

Figure 2. Registration, demographics, and insurance information

Name _____ Birthday _____ Occupation _____

Dermatologic History   **Referred By:** _____
1. Reason for visit _____
       How long has this been going on? _____
       What areas are affected? _____
       How has it been treated? _____
2. Other skin conditions _____
3. Topical (skin) medications _____
4. Other products applied to your skin _____
5. Family history of skin problems (what, in whom) _____

Office Use

Medical History (Includes system review)   Rx Plan   Y   N

Do you have or have you had any of the following?

	Yes	No		Yes	No		Yes	No
High Blood Pressure	[ ]	[ ]	Anemia	[ ]	[ ]	Stomach/Bowel Problem	[ ]	[ ]
Heart Disease	[ ]	[ ]	Glaucoma	[ ]	[ ]	Recent Weight Loss	[ ]	[ ]
Cardiac Pacemaker	[ ]	[ ]	Cancer	[ ]	[ ]	Tobacco Use	[ ]	[ ]
Rheumatic Fever	[ ]	[ ]	Arthritis	[ ]	[ ]	Keloids/excessive scar	[ ]	[ ]
Heart Murmur	[ ]	[ ]	Liver disease or hepatitis	[ ]	[ ]	Cold Sore/Fever Blister	[ ]	[ ]
Mitral Valve Prolapse	[ ]	[ ]	Hay Fever/Allergies	[ ]	[ ]	Radiation Therapy	[ ]	[ ]
Artificial Joints	[ ]	[ ]	Seizures	[ ]	[ ]	Ultraviolet light treatment	[ ]	[ ]
Stroke	[ ]	[ ]	Kidney/Bladder Problem	[ ]	[ ]	History of skin cancer	[ ]	[ ]
Diabetes	[ ]	[ ]	Asthma or Lung Problems	[ ]	[ ]			
HIV Infection	[ ]	[ ]						

Do you need antibiotics before surgical or dental procedures?   [ ]   [ ]

List any other medical problems or surgeries and explain any of above if needed

_____
_____
_____
_____

List any allergies (including medications)

_____

Please list all medications you are using (including non-prescription, aspirin, birth control pills, vitamins)

_____
_____
_____

Women Only: Are you . . .	Yes	No
Pregnant or think you may be?	[ ]	[ ]
Nursing (breast-feeding)?	[ ]	[ ]
Taking oral contraceptives?	[ ]	[ ]
Taking hormone replacements?	[ ]	[ ]

Information Request (check if you would like more information)

Wrinkle treatments	[ ]	Collagen	[ ]	Facial blood vessels	[ ]	Laser tattoo removal	[ ]
Chemical peels	[ ]	Leg veins	[ ]	Laser hair removal	[ ]	Dark spots (liver spots)	[ ]

_____   _____   _____   _____
Signature of patient (or parent if minor)   Date   Physician's initials   Date

Figure 3.   Clinical history: general and vascular

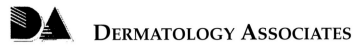

D▪ DERMATOLOGY ASSOCIATES

Patient Health History Form

Name: _____   Date: _____

Age: _____   Sex: M/F

Directions: Please answer the following questions, trying not to leave any blank spaces.

Past Medical History

1. Have you ever been in the hospital as a patient?   Yes   No
   If yes, for what reason _____

2. Have you ever had surgery?   Yes   No
   If yes, what type of surgery and when? _____

3. Have you ever had vein stripping surgery?   Yes   No
   If yes, when and which leg? _____
   _____
   _____

4. Have you ever had vein injections?   Yes   No
   If yes, when, where, and which leg? _____
   _____

5. Are you presently under the care of a physician?   Yes   No
   If yes, for what illness or purpose? _____
   _____

6. Do you have heart disease? . . . . .Yes   No
          lung disease . . . . .Yes   No
          high blood pressure . . . . .Yes   No
          hepatitis . . . . .Yes   No
          arthritis . . . . .Yes   No
          leg ulcer . . . . .Yes   No

7. Have you ever had a blood clot?   Yes   No
   If yes, which leg and when? _____

8. Have you ever had phlebitis?   Yes   No
   If yes, which leg and when? _____

Child Rearing History

1. Do you think you are presently pregnant?   Yes   No

2. How many times have you been pregnant?   _____

3. Do you intend to have any more children?   Yes   No

4. Are you presently breastfeeding?   Yes   No

Please *circle* the appropriate answer.

Figure 3.   Clinical history: general and vascular (*Continued*)

Family

Does anyone in your family have varicose veins, spider veins, leg ulcers, or swollen legs?

Father ....Yes   No
Mother ....Yes   No
Brother(s) ....Yes   No
Sister(s) ....Yes   No
Other _____

1. Do you experience any of the following?
   a. Aching/pain in your legs? ....   Yes   No
   b. Heaviness ....   Yes   No
   c. Tiredness/fatigue ....   Yes   No
   d. Itching/burning ....   Yes   No
   e. Swollen ankles ....   Yes   No
   f. Leg cramps ....   Yes   No
   g. Restless legs ....   Yes   No
   h. Throbbing ....   Yes   No
   i. Other_____

2. Have your veins gotten worse in recent months?   Yes   No

3. Do you elevate your legs to relieve discomfort?   Yes   No

4. Do you wear support hose prescribed by a doctor   Yes   No
   If yes, what type? _____

5. Do you wear light support hose (eg. sheer energy)?   Yes   No

6. Do they provide relief?   Yes   No

7. Do you have any problem walking?   Yes   No
   If yes, how does it affect you?_____

8. Do you stand much at work?   Yes   No
              at home?   Yes   No

9. How does this standing affect your legs?
   _____

10. Do you smoke?   Yes   No
    If yes, how many packs per day? _____

11. Have you ever had your veins evaluated before?   Yes   No
    If so, when and where? _____

12. Have you ever had any test(s) done on your veins?   Yes   No

Current Medical History

1. Do you have any allergies (medicines, food, pollen, etc.) Please list them and briefly
   describe your reaction (eg. rash, hives, shortness of breath, etc.)   Yes   No
   _____
   _____

2. Are you allergic to shrimp or shellfish (or any form of iodine, IVP dye)?   Yes   No

3. Are you presently taking any medication including prescription and/or non-prescription
   (over-the-counter) medicines (aspirin, vitamins)?   Yes   No
   If so, list them. _____
   _____

4. Do you take any blood-thinning medication?   Yes   No

5. Are you taking hormones or birth control pills?   Yes   No
   If yes, please list name(s). _____
   _____

Figure 3.   Clinical history: general and vascular (*Continued*)

DRS. ROBERT & MARGARET WEISS, M.D., P.A.
Dermatology and Dermatologic Surgery

<u>SCLEROTHERAPY RECORD</u>

Name _____   Date _____

_____

_____

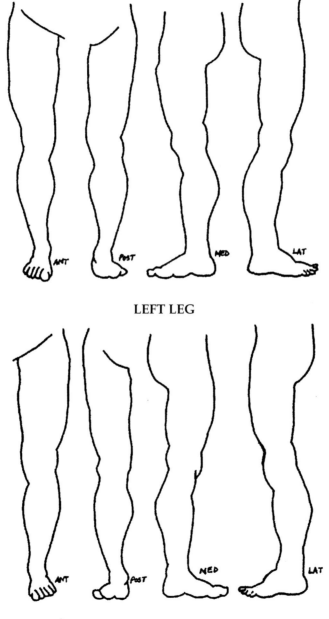

RIGHT LEG

LEFT LEG

Figure 4.   Physical exams, treatment, and progress note

Dermatology Associates
Pre-Operative Testing Request

Patient's Name _____   Date _____

Please check test(s) to be done. Keep in patient's chart.

1. _____ Doppler/PPG- bilateral study (1 hour)

2. _____ Doppler/PPG/Arterial- bilateral study (1 hour)

3. _____ Doppler/PPG/Duplex- bilateral study (2 hours)

4. _____ Doppler/PPG/Duplex- one leg (1 hour)

5. _____ Duplex- one leg or bilateral (1 hour)

6. _____ Duplex/PPG- one leg or bilateral (1 hour)

7. _____ No testing required

Any special requests _____

Please make sure that if the patient has an HMO, that they obtain a referral specifying what tests are to be done.

Figure 5.   Preoperative testing request

Dermatology Associates
DOPPLER EXAMINATION

PATIENT NAME (LAST, FIRST, MIDDLE INIT.)	DATE

RIGHT LEG

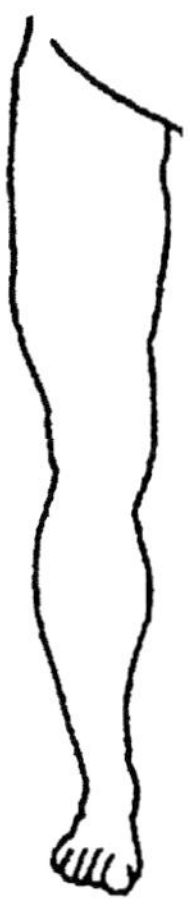

ANTERIOR 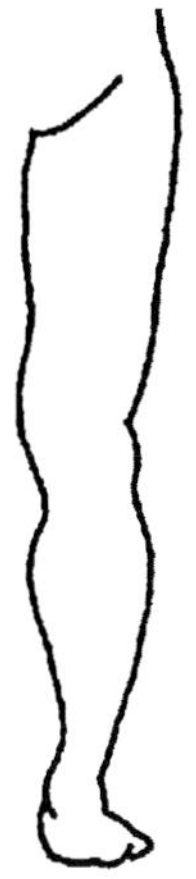   POSTERIOR

LEFT LEG

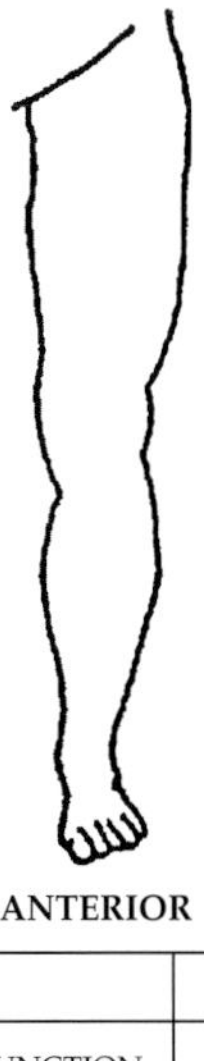

ANTERIOR 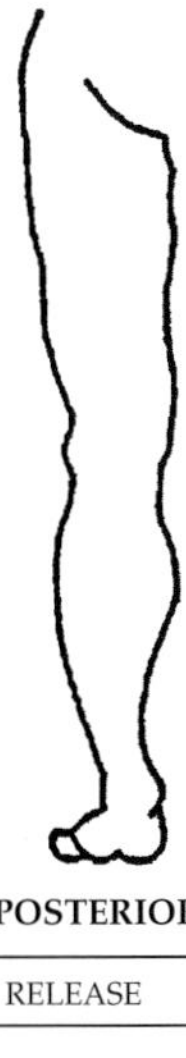   POSTERIOR

COMMENTS:

PERFORATOR LOCATIONS NOTED ON LEG DIAGRAM

	DISTAL COMPRESSION RELEASE	PROXIMAL COMPRESSION PHASE	VALSALVA MANEUVER
SAPHENOFEMORAL JUNCTION RIGHT			
SAPHENOFEMORAL JUNCTION LEFT			
SAPHENOPOPLITEAL JUNCTION RIGHT			
SAPHENOPOPLITEAL JUNCTION LEFT			

Figure 6. Physiologic test results: Doppler mapping form

**Dermatology
Associates**

NAME _____

DATE _____

PHYSICIAN _____

VENOUS REFLUX EXAMINATION

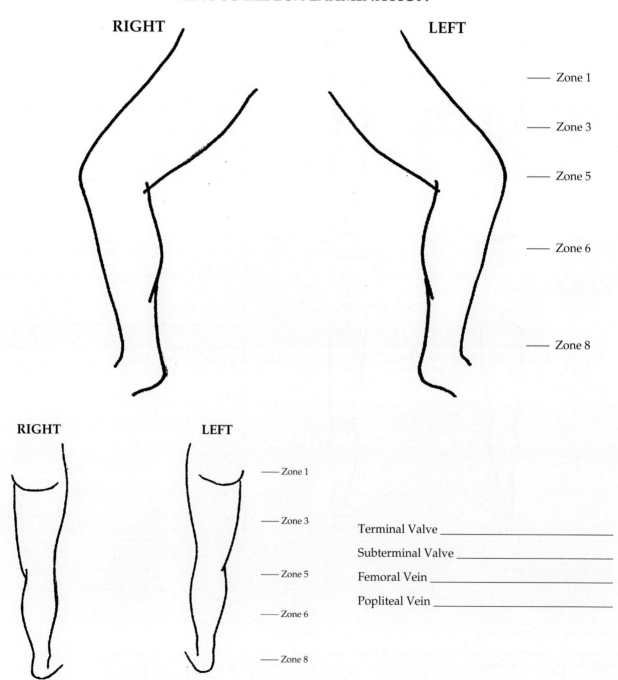

RIGHT   **LEFT**

—— Zone 1

—— Zone 3

—— Zone 5

—— Zone 6

—— Zone 8

RIGHT   **LEFT**

—— Zone 1

—— Zone 3

—— Zone 5

—— Zone 6

—— Zone 8

Terminal Valve _____

Subterminal Valve _____

Femoral Vein _____

Popliteal Vein _____

Figure 7.   Duplex ultrasound mapping diagram

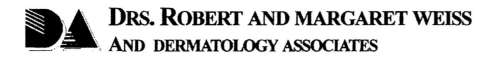

DRS. ROBERT AND MARGARET WEISS
AND DERMATOLOGY ASSOCIATES

SCLEROTHERAPY FEE SCHEDULE

Patient's name _____

Office Location _____

Date _____

Consultation with nurse _____

Pre-Operative Testing:

    Venous Doppler/PPG(93965) _____

    Venous Duplex Ultrasound (93970) _____

First Visit with Doctor-

    Office Visit _____

    Test Area (36470) _____

Subsequent Treatments (36471) _____

Duplex at time of treatment (93971) _____

Equipment Tray _____

Surgical Stockings_____

Delilah/Venosan_____

Samson Knee-highs (men)_____

Photography Fee (one time) _____

We make every effort to stay on schedule. Please call us if you will be delayed or cannot keep an appointment. There is a $50 charge for failure to cancel an appointment within 24 hours of its scheduled time.

Please remember that payment in full is due at the time of each treatment. We appreciate your cooperation with this policy.

An **average** session for many areas costs $250–350. Most patients need 2–4 sessions, spaced a month or so apart.

_____   _____

Patient   Witness

Figure 8. Treatment estimate/fee schedule

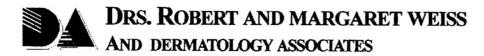

DRS. ROBERT AND MARGARET WEISS
AND DERMATOLOGY ASSOCIATES

SCLEROTHERAPY CONSENT AND FEE SCHEDULE

Name_____   Date _____

- Sclerotherapy is the method for eliminating superficial telangiectasias ("spider veins") and some varicosities by the injection of a solution, called a "sclerosing agent", into the veins. The vast majority of patients who have sclerotherapy will have significant clearing of the veins with at least good improvement. There can be no guarantee, however, that it will be effective in every case. Less than 10% of patients undergoing sclerotherapy will have poor results, in which the veins do not improve despite multiple injections. It is extremely rare for anyone's condition to worsen because of treatment.

- It is important to realize that sclerotherapy does not prevent development of new spider veins and varicosities over the years. Many people will require treatments from time to time to keep their legs clear. Standing occupations, pregnancy, and estrogen increase this tendency.

- It is difficult to predict the number of treatments needed to clear or improve the condition. Each vein may need to be injected one to five or more times, over a period of several months. Improvement is usually seen over a period of months, not weeks. In each treatment session, multiple areas can be treated, thus reducing the total number of sessions required. The total number of treatment sessions needed depends on the amount and severity of the veins (the average is three to five), with severe cases requiring as many as ten or more.

- Side effects of sclerotherapy are detailed in another handout which you will receive.

- Sclerotherapy is *not* usually covered by your insurance company, depending on the size of the veins and whether or not they cause symptoms. When the veins are small, the treatment is considered cosmetic and *not* covered. When the veins are large and "varicose", or cause pain or discomfort, then there is a *chance* that the sclerotherapy will be covered. Each patient has the responsibility for payment at the time of service, whether or not the treatments are successful, and whether or not the treatments are covered by insurance.

- All diagnostic testing and treatment must be paid for in full at the time the service is performed. At your request, we will send a detailed letter, photographs, and vascular test results to your insurance company. Each patient must submit their receipt to his/her insurance company for reimbursement.

FEE SCHEDULE

- ❖ Each treatment session lasts 10–15 minutes and will treat multiple areas and will cost $ _____.
- ❖ Each treatment session requires a "spider vein equipment tray" which cost $ _____.
- ❖ Some patients require prescription support hosiery, for which we charge $ _____. This is approximately half the charge made by pharmacies. Other patients require light support hosiery, for which we charge $ _____.
- ❖ Because of long waiting lines for appointments, we suggest scheduling several of your treatment sessions, a few weeks apart, at the same time. If your plans change, there is no charge for appointments canceled more than 24 hours in advance.
- ❖ IMPORTANT: There is a $50 charge for failure to cancel appointments within 24 hours of appointment time. I understand and agree to these items.

Patient _____   Witness _____

Figure 9.   General sclerotherapy information and consent to fee schedule

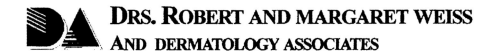

DRS. ROBERT AND MARGARET WEISS AND DERMATOLOGY ASSOCIATES

CONSENT FOR TREATMENT OF LEG VEINS

There have been many methods tried to remove unsightly "broken" or enlarged veins on the legs. Most do not work, and have been abandoned. The doctor uses a technique called sclerotherapy, which involves the following.

A tiny needle is threaded into the blood vessel and a small amount of a sclerosing agent is gently injected. This may sting for 20–30 seconds or cause a slight cramp. The injection "flushes" out the red blood cells temporarily, leading to an inflammatory reaction. This reaction causes "sclerosis", or the formation of fibrous tissue within the vessel, leading to the gradual disappearance of the vessel. This fading can take from a few weeks to a few months. Most areas will require between three to five treatments to fade.

A test area is injected first and observed for 4–6 weeks to see how well the procedure and particular solution achieves the desired result in that particular patient.

Some of the possible risks include:

1. The appearances of the veins may *not* improve. However, over 90% of patients see improvement.

2. Brown spots may appear that look like bruises or follow the path of the vein. These brown areas take several weeks to months to go away. It is rare for any discoloration to be permanent. Patients with naturally darker skin are more likely to experience this.

3. Blistering, redness, itching and irritation may develop as reaction to the adhesive tape used for compression.

4. Blistering, infection, ulceration, and scarring may develop if someone is exceptionally sensitive to the tiny amount of solution that may leak out during the injection. This occurs in less than 1% of patients. An allergic reaction to some of the solutions is also a rare possibility.

5. Tenderness, bruising, or a firmness (especially along the larger vessels) in the treated area may last for varying periods of time. This can be minimized by the use of support hose after the treatment.

6. Some people (less than 10%) may develop a "matt", or pink blush of the skin, which comes from a temporary enlargement of the tiny capillaries. This is rarely permanent, and can be treated.

7. Sometimes blood may accumulate in the larger veins treated by sclerotherapy. These accumulations may be treated by the physician to decrease any discomfort. Strict use of support hose minimizes this possibility.

8. Rarely, this accumulation of blood may form a clot. Although this is usually trapped in the treated vein, an extremely rare possibility is the extension of this clot into a deeper vessel causing phlebitis. The risk of this occurring is much less than 1%.

9. People with significant circulatory problems, uncontrolled diabetes or pregnant women should not undergo this procedure.

CONSENT

By signing this form, I attest that I have read and understand the procedure and its risks, and that it has been explained to my satisfaction.

Patient _____   Witness _____

Figure 10.   Sclerotherapy Informed Consent

I understand that I am being offered sclerotherapy as a treatment for venous insufficiency, and that the goal of treatment is to have better circulation and to look and feel better. I understand that my treatment plan will be adjusted as necessary to meet the needs of my particular problem. I understand that treatment may involve some or all of the following:

❑ **Medications**—Treatment will involve injection of sclerosant medications into the veins to be treated. There are many sclerosants that may be used. Three of the safest and most effective are:

    ❑ Sodium tetradecyl sulfate (FDA approved)

    ❑ Polidocanol (Most common drug used worldwide; not FDA approved)

    ❑ Hypertonic saline (FDA approved; "off-label usage")

❑ **Compression hose**—Prescription-strength compression stockings will enhance the results of treatment and reduce potential side effects.

❑ **Amount of clearing**—Treatment estimates are designed to give a typical patient about 80–90% clearing of all areas for which treatment is planned.

❑ **Appointment length**—Appointments are usually 30 minutes in length, including time for preparation and for placement of stockings.

❑ **Response visible only after second treatment**—Most patients do not notice any difference in treated veins until after the second treatment session. In many cases it seems as though the first treatment "sensitizes" the veins, and the next treatment closes them down in a noticeable way.

Side Effects:

I understand that any of the following side effects may occur:

❑ **Bruising/discoloration**—Like any other bruise, this will usually fade in a few days.

❑ **Inflammation and trapped blood**—Inflammation is a mild tenderness and/or slight swelling in treated veins that may last a few days. Most patients do not require any treatment for inflammation, but if you like, you may use Motrin®, Advil®, or any anti-inflammatory medication. Trapped blood is an uncommon problem that occurs when a little blood gets stuck in a closed section of the treated vein. Trapped blood feels like a firm, tender bump in the treated vein. Trapped blood resolves by itself in a few weeks or months, but sometimes we may use a tiny needle to remove trapped blood to speed up the healing.

❑ **Allergic reaction**—There is a very remote possibility of an allergic reaction to the medicine. Our medicines have an extremely low allergenicity in the general population. Temporary allergic reactions can include hives, tingling, flushing, or a brief feeling of shortness of breath. If you have a reaction we will treat you for the allergy and switch to a different medicine for your vein treatments.

❑ **Hyperpigmentation**—Often described as "staining," it is usually caused by iron from your own blood being deposited in the skin. It almost always fades away with time, but may take 6 months or more to fade away in patients with light skin, or even longer in patients with darker skin. In rare cases, staining may be permanent.

❑ **Telangiectatic matting**—This is a blush or flush that may occur in an area after treatment. Most matting (90%) fades away over 2 months. The more you wear your hose and stay active the faster it will resolve.

Figure 11.   Sclerotherapy Informed Consent—Alternative Form.

❑ **Ulcers**—An ulcer is a small sore caused by medicine irritating the skin. This is a rare problem, but it can occur with any injection. It will heal up completely, but may leave a small freckle scar. Generally, this will not be noticeable on normal skin.

❑ **Blood clots**—Surgical vein treatments cause a real risk of developing blood clots. Injection sclerotherapy may also cause a very small, theoretical (unproven) risk of getting blood clots. We reduce this possibility by having patients wear compression hose that are designed to prevent blood clots. We also keep patients active, thereby keeping blood flowing naturally and freely in the legs.

❑ **Recurrence of veins**—The veins that we treat completely will be gone forever, but most patients have a natural tendency to develop more abnormal veins, and new veins can always appear at a future time. About 25% of our patients like to come back in about 2–3 years for touch-up treatments on new problem veins.

The risks and benefits of treatment have been explained to me in a way that I can understand. Furthermore, I understand that medicine is not an exact science and that there are no guarantees of results in medicine. I also understand that there may be other treatment options, including the option to do nothing. With this in mind I am choosing to try compression sclerotherapy for treatment of my veins. I have read and understand this document, and my questions have been addressed and answered to my satisfaction. I understand and accept the terms of this agreement.

Patient: _____   **Date:** _____

Witness: _____   **Date:** _____

Figure 11.   Sclerotherapy Informed Consent—Alternative Form. (*Continued*)

Manufacturers

This is not meant to be an all-inclusive or comprehensive list of the many different manufacturers and distributors of quality medical supplies and equipment used in a phlebology practice. Technology, especially in the fields of photographic and vascular imaging, is evolving rapidly. Addresses, especially Internet, are subject to change. The authors have listed sources to serve as a starting point for the reader.

DIAGNOSTIC EQUIPMENT
Handheld Dopplers

Elcat GmbH
SchieBstattstraBe 29
D-82515 Wolfratshausen
Germany
Phone: 11-0049-08171-4214-0
Fax: 11-0049-08171-4214-47
Website: http://www.elcat.de
Email: info@elcat.de
Henry Schein, Inc.
135 Duryea Road
Melville, NY 11747
Phone: 800-472-4346
Fax: 1-631-843-5652
Website: http://www.henryschein.com
Email: webmaster@henryschein.com
Huntleigh Healthcare
40 Christopher Way
Eatontown, NJ 07724-3327
Phone: 732-446-2500
Fax: 732-446-1938
Website: http://www.huntleigh-healthcare.com
Imex Medical/Nicolet Vascular, Inc.
6355 Joyce Drive
Golden, CO 80403
Phone: 800-525-2519
Website: http://www.nicoletvascular.com
Email: info@NicoletVascular.com

Venous Function Measuring Devices
Digital PPG
Elcat GmbH
SchieBstattstraBe 29
D-82515 Wolfratshausen
Germany
Phone: 11-0049-08171-4214-0
Fax: 11-0049-08171-4214-47
Website: http://www.elcat.de
Email: info@elcat.de

Various Devices (PPG, Combinations):
Imex Medical/Nicolet Vascular, Inc.
6355 Joyce Drive
Golden, CO 80403
Phone: 800-525-2519
Website: http://www.nicoletvascular.com
Email: info@NicoletVascular.com

Duplex Ultrasound
Biosound Esaote, Inc.
8000 Castleway Drive
Indianapolis, IN 46250-0858
Phone: 317-849-1793
Fax: 317-841-8616
Website: http://www.biosound.com
Email: biosound@biomail.com
Agilent Technologies (formerly Hewlett-Packard)
MS390
3000 Minuteman Road
Andover, MA 01810
Phone: 1-800-934-7372
Fax: 978-689-9085
Website: http://www.agilent.com
Email: medsupplies_ecomm@agilent.com

PHOTOGRAPHY: DIGITAL AND 35-MM CAMERAS

Selection of an individual practitioner's medical imaging system depends on many factors. As of this writing, a website offering reviews of more than 40 digital cameras as well as selection criteria was http://www.imaging-resource.com

Canfield Clinical Systems
253 Passaic Avenue
Fairfield NJ 07004-2524
Phone: 973-276-0336/800-815-4330
Fax: 973-276-0339
Website: http://www.canfieldsci.com
Email: info@canfieldsci.com
Delasco/Dermatologic Lab & Supply Co., Inc.
608 13th Avenue
Council Bluffs, IA 51501-6401
Phone: 800-831-6273
Fax: 712-323-1156
Website: http://www.delasco.com
Email: questions@delasco.com
Lester A. Dine, Inc.
351 Hiatt Drive
Palm Beach Gardens, FL 33418
Phone: 800-624-9103
Fax: 561-624-9103
Website: http://www.dinecorp.com
Email: dinecorp@emi.net

NEEDLES
Acuderm, Inc.
5370 N.W. 35 Terrace, Suite 106
Fort Lauderdale, FL 33309
Phone: 954-733-6935/800-327-0015
Fax: 954-486-3602

Website: http://www.acuderm.com
Email: cust-service@acuderm.com
Distributes plastic and metal hub 30-gauge needles.
Air-Tite Products Co., Inc.
565 Central Drive
Virginia Beach, VA 23452
Phone: 800-231-7762
Fax: 757-340-2912
Website: http://www.air-tite.com
Email: atinfo@air-tite.com
Distributes German and Japanese 30-, 31-, and 32-gauge disposable needles.
Delasco/Dermatologic Lab & Supply Co., Inc.
608 13th Avenue
Council Bluffs, IA 51501-6401
Phone: 800-831-6273
Fax: 712-323-1156
Website: http://www.delasco.com
Email: questions@delasco.com
Distributes reusable 33-gauge and disposable 30-gauge needles, including Becton-Dickinson.
STD Pharmaceuticals
Fields Yard, Plough Lane
Hereford, HR4 OEL
England
Phone: 44-0-1432-353684
Fax: 44-0-1432-371314
Website: http://www.stdpharm.co.uk
Email: enquiries@stdpharm.co.uk
Distributes needles and other sclerotherapy supplies.

SYRINGES
Air-Tite Products Co., Inc.
565 Central Drive
Virginia Beach, VA 23452
Phone: 800-231-7762
Fax: 757-340-2912
Website: http://www.air-tite.com
Email: atinfo@air-tite.com
Distributes a variety of syringes, including Terumo.
Delasco/Dermatologic Lab & Supply Co., Inc.
608 13th Avenue
Council Bluffs, IA 51501
Phone: 800-831-6273
Fax: 712-323-1156
Website: http://www.delasco.com
Email: questions@delasco.com
Distributes variety of syringes, including Becton-Dickinson.

VACUTAINERS
Air-Tite Products Co., Inc.
565 Central Drive
Virginia Beach, VA 23452
Phone: 800-231-7762
Fax: 757-340-2912
Website: http://www.air-tite.com
Email: atinfo@air-tite.com

STERILE, EMPTY VIALS
Bayer Corporation
P.O. Box 3145
Spokane, WA 99220-3145
Phone: 800-992-1120
Website: www.hollister-stier.com

GLOVES
Nonsterile, disposable gloves with and without latex are very widely available through local as well as national medical suppliers. The authors encourage the readers to have their staff "shop around," as prices and quality may vary widely. Individual preference plays a great role in this choice.
Air-Tite Products Co., Inc.
565 Central Drive
Virginia Beach, VA 23452
Phone: 800-231-7762
Fax: 757-340-2912
Website: http://www.air-tite.com
Email: atinfo@air-tite.com
Delasco/Dermatologic Lab & Supply Co., Inc.
608 13th Avenue
Council Bluffs, IA 51501
Phone: 800-831-6273
Fax: 712-323-1156
Website: http://www.delasco.com
Email: questions@delasco.com
Henry Schein,Inc.
135 Duryea Road
Melville, NY 11747
Phone: 800-472-4346
Fax: 631-843-5652
Website: http://www.henryschein.com
Email: webmaster@henryschein.com

FOAM PADS (STD)
Delasco/Dermatologic Lab & Supply Co., Inc.
608 13th Avenue
Council Bluffs, IA 51501-6401
Phone: 800-831-6273
Fax: 712-323-1156
Website: http://www.delasco.com
Email: questions@delasco.com
STD Pharmaceuticals
Fields Yard, Plough Lane
Hereford, HR4 OEL
England
Phone: 44-0-1432-353684
Fax: 44-0-1432-371314
Website: http://www.stdpharm.co.uk
Email: enquiries@stdpharm.co.uk

COMPRESSION HOSE
Beirsdorf-Jobst, Inc.
5825 Carnegie Boulevard
Charlotte, NC 28209-4633
Phone: 704-554-9933
Fax: 704-551-8581

Website: http://www.jobst-usa.com
Email: jcustsrv@bdfusa.com
Carolon Company
601 Forum Parkway
Rural Hall, NC 27045
Phone: 800-334-0414
Fax: 336-969-6999
Website: http://www.carolon.com
Email: carolon@carolon.com
Note: All products are latex-free.
Gloria-Med America, Inc.
1417 N. Partin Drive Ste. 4
Niceville, FL 32578
Phone: 850-729-0717
Fax: 850-729-1696
"It Stays" (Adhesive)
Available through http://www.supportshop.com
Manufactured by Medi-USA, LP
JUZO
P.O. Box 1088
Cuyahoga Falls, OH 44223
Phone: 888-255-1300
Fax: 330-916-9165
Website: http://www.juzousa.com
Email: support@juzousa.com
MEDI USA, LP
76 W. Seegers Road
Arlington Heights, IL 60005
Phone: 800-396-2017
Fax: 800-633-4338
Website: http://www.mediusa.com
Sigvaris, Inc.
1119 Highway 14 South
Peachtree City, GA 30269
Phone: 770-631-1778
Fax: 770-631-4883
Website: http://www.sigvaris.com
Venosan North America
P.O. Box 1067
Asheboro, NC 27204-1067
Phone: 336-629-7181
Fax: 336-629-8006

MAGNIFIERS & VISUAL ENHANCERS

Delasco/Dermatologic Lab & Supply Co., Inc.
608 13th Avenue
Council Bluffs, IA 51501-6401
Phone: 800-831-6273
Fax: 712-323-1156
Website: http://www.delasco.com
Distributes variety of devices, ranging from simple binocular headbands to Heine loupes, including the Vein-Lite and Venoscope®.
Syris Scientific, LLC
P.O. Box 127
Gray, ME 04039
Phone: 800-714-1374
Fax: 207-657-7051
Website: http://www.syrisscientific.com

Email: info@syrisscientific.com
Formerly known as the Seymour Light, the headpieces (Syris v300 and v600) combine magnification with double-polarized light to enhance visualization of superficial veins.

PATIENT INFORMATION SOURCES

American Academy of Dermatology
930 N. Meacham Rd.
P.O. Box 4014
Schaumburg, IL 60168-4014
Phone: 847-330-0230
Fax: 847-330-0050
Website: http://www.aad.org
Distributes brochure on spider and varicose vein therapy.
American College of Phlebology
100 Webster Street Suite 101
Oakland, CA 94607-3724
Phone: 510-834-6500
Fax: 510-832-7300
Website: http://www.phlebology.org
Email: acp@amsinc.org
Distributes brochure on spider and varicose vein therapy.
American Society for Dermatologic Surgery
930 N. Meacham Road
Schaumburg, IL 60173-6016
Phone: 847-330-9830
Fax: 847-330-0050
Website: http://www.asds-net.org
Distributes brochure on spider and varicose vein therapy.
MJD Patient Communications
4641 Montgomery Avenue, Suite 350
Bethesda, MD 20814
Phone: 301-657-8010
Fax: 301-657-8023
Distributes brochure on spider and varicose vein therapy, as well as customized newsletters and practice brochures.
Venous Digest
2329 Barley Drive
Vista, CA 92083
Phone: 760-599-9456
Website: http://www.venousdigest.com
Distributes patient education video on spider and varicose vein therapy.

SCLEROSANTS

Delasco/Dermatologic Lab & Supply Co., Inc.
608 13th Avenue
Council Bluffs, IA 51501-6401
Phone: 800-831-6273
Fax: 712-323-1156
Website: http://www.delasco.com
Distributes 23.4% saline and sodium tetradecyl sulfate.
Kaye's Pharmacy
6913 Belair Road
Baltimore, MD 21206

Phone: 800-673-8277, 410-665-5192
Fax: 410-668-8533
Will prepare and ship mixture of dextrose and saline.
National Specialty Services, Inc.
556 Metroplex Boulevard
Nashville, TN 37211
Phone: 800-879-5569
Distributes Sotradecol™.
Chemische Fabrik
Kreussler and Co. GmbH
Rheingaustrasse 87-93
D-65203 Wiesbaden
Germany
Phone: 49-(0)-611-9271-0
Fax: 49-(0)-611-9271-111
Website: http://www.kreussler.de
Omega Laboratories, Ltd.
11,177 Hamon Street
Montreal, Quebec H3M 3E4
Canada
Phone: 514-335-0310 or 1-800-363-0584

Fax: 514-339-1407
Website: http://www.omegalaboratory.com
Distributes 23.4% saline, Sclerodex ™, sodium tetradecyl
sulfate, laureth-9 (polidocanol), Sclerodine ™, and Sali-
ject™, sodium salicylate.
STD Pharmaceuticals
Fields Yard, Plough Lane
Hereford, HR4 OEL
England
Phone: 44-0-1432-353684
Fax: 44-0-1432-371314
Website: http://www.stdpharm.co.uk
Distributes sodium tetradecyl sulfate, laureth-9 (polido-
canol), polyiodinated iodine, and chromated glycerin.
Wyeth-Ayerst Laboratories
P.O. Box 8299
Philadelphia, PA 19101
Phone: 610-902-2784
Fax: 610-964-3816
Website: http://www.ahp.com/wyeth_labs.htm
Distributes sodium tetradecyl sulfate.

Terminology for Billing and Encounter Forms

CPT-2000: CURRENT PROCEDURAL TERMINOLOGY CODES

36468: single or multiple injections of sclerosing solutions, spider veins (telangiectasia); limb or trunk.

36469: single or multiple injections of sclerosing solutions, spider veins, face

36470*: Injection of sclerosing solution, single vein, leg

36471*: Injection of sclerosing solution, multiple veins, same leg

36471-50*: Bilateral injection of sclerosing solution, multiple veins, two legs

37799: Unlisted procedure, vascular surgery

37720: Ligation and stripping of greater saphenous or lesser saphenous veins

37785: Ligation, and/or excision of recurrent or secondary varicose veins (clusters), one leg

93965: Non-invasive physiologic studies of extremity vein, complete bilateral study

93970: Duplex scan of extremity vein, complete bilateral study

93971: Duplex scan of extremity vein, unilateral or limited study

While the nuances of CPT coding are beyond the scope of this book, the asterisk* means that the surgical code listed above includes only the surgical procedure of sclerotherapy. This means that an appropriate evaluation and management code (e.g., level of service if "significant identifiable services" were actually provided in addition to the procedure), new or established patient, with the modifier '-25' may be theoretically added to the bill. However, this terminology has no bearing on whether or not an insurance company will actually pay for the added E&M visit charge. Many do not.

DIAGNOSIS CODES: ICD—9—CM

Telangiectasia	448.1
Varicosities	454.9
Varicosities with inflammation	454.1
Varicosities with ulceration	454.2
Varicosities with stasis dermatitis	454.1
Venous insufficiency	459.81
Venous ulcer	454.0
Venous leg pain	729.5

REFERENCES

Current Procedural Terminology, CPT-2000, American Medical Association, Chicago, 1999.

International Classification of Diagnoses-9, American Medical Association, Chicago, 1999.

Index

Page numbers in italics denote figures; those followed by "t" denote tables.

295